The Management of Infectious Diseases in Clinical Practice

ACADEMIC PRESS RAPID MANUSCRIPT REPRODUCTION

The Management of Infectious Diseases in Clinical Practice

WITHDRAWN

Edited by

PHILLIP K. PETERSON, M.D.
L. D. SABATH, M.D.
University of Minnesota School of Medicine
Minneapolis, Minnesota

ERNESTO CALDERÓN JAIMES, M.D.
Pediatric Unit General Hospital
Mexico City, Mexico

ALLAN R. RONALD, M.D.
University of Manitoba
Winnipeg, Canada

1982

ACADEMIC PRESS

A Subsidiary of Harcourt Brace Jovanovich, Publishers

New York   London
Paris   San Diego   San Francisco   São Paulo   Sydney   Tokyo   Toronto

ACADEMIC PRESS, INC.
111 Fifth Avenue, New York, New York 10003

United Kingdom Edition published by
ACADEMIC PRESS, INC. (LONDON) LTD.
24/28 Oval Road, London NW1 7DX

LIBRARY OF CONGRESS CATALOG CARD NUMBER: 81-20574

ISBN 0-12-788610-9

PRINTED IN THE UNITED STATES OF AMERICA

82 83 84 85   9 8 7 6 5 4 3 2 1

Contents

Contributors

Numbers in parentheses indicate the pages on which the authors' contributions begin.

David H. Ahrenholz, M.D. (93), Department of Surgery, University of Minnesota Hospitals, Minneapolis, Minnesota 55455

John E. Bennett, M.D. (331, 371), Clinical Mycology Section, National Institute of Allergy and Infectious Diseases, National Institutes of Health, Bethesda, Maryland 20205

Alberto Brown, M.D. (309), University of Panama Medical School, Complejo Hospitalario Metropolitano del Seguro Social and Hospital Santo Tomas, Panama City, Panama

Ernesto Calderón Jaimes, M.D. (135), Infectious Disease and Immunology Section, Pediatric Unit General Hospital, Health Department (S.S.A.), Mexico 13, D.F. Mexico

Robert E. Condon, M.D. (389, 419), Department of Surgery, The Medical College of Wisconsin, Milwaukee, Wisconsin 53226

William A. Craig, M.D. (409), Department of Medicine, University of Wisconsin, Veterans Administration Hospital, Madison, Wisconsin 53705

Michael Dan, M.D. (241), Division of Infectious Diseases, Department of Medicine, University of Alberta, Canada T6G 2G3

Enrique Diaz, M.D. (159), University of Panama Medical School, Complejo Hospitalario Metropolitano del Seguro Social and Hospital Santo Tomas, Panama City, Panama

Sam T. Donta, M.D. (61, 67), Infectious Disease Service, University of Iowa, Veterans Administration Medical Center, Iowa City, Iowa 52240

Randall Edson, M.D. (427), Division of Infectious Diseases, Mayo Clinic and Mayo Foundation, Rochester, Minnesota 55901

Robert Fekety, M.D. (103, 397), Division of Infectious Diseases, University of Michigan Medical School, Ann Arbor, Michigan 48104

Edgardo Fernández, M.D. (159), University of Panama Medical School, Complejo Hospitalario Metropolitano del Seguro Social and Hospital Santo Tomas, Panama City, Panama

Joseph E. Geraci, M.D. (171), Department of Infectious Diseases, Mayo Clinic, Rochester, Minnesota 55901

George Goldsand, M.D. (241), Division of Infectious Diseases, Department of Medicine, University of Alberta, Canada T6G 2G3

Jose J. Gutierrez-Nuñez, M.D. (181), University of Puerto Rico School of Medicine, San Juan, Puerto Rico 00936

Gonzalo Gutierrez T., M.D. (73), Jefatura de Enseñanza e Investigationes, Instituto Mexicano del Seguro Social, Mexico, DF

William E. Hauser, Jr., M.D. (341), Division of Infectious Diseases, Department of Medicine, Stanford University School of Medicine, Research Institute, Palo Alto Medical Foundation, Palo Alto, California 94301

Paul E. Hermans, M.D. (379, 427), Division of Infectious Diseases, Mayo Clinic and Mayo Foundation, Rochester, Minnesota 55901

Jesus Kumate R., M.D. (83), Immunochemistry Division, Biomedical Research Unit, National Medical Unit, Social Security, Mexico 12 D.F., Mexico

William J. Ledger, M.D. (15, 23), Department of Obstetrics-Gynecology, New York Hospital, Cornell Medical Center, New York, New York 10021

A. Martin Lerner, M.D. (263, 271), Department of Medicine, Wayne State University, School of Medicine, Hutzel Hospital, Detroit, Michigan 48201

Jacques E. Mokhbat, M.D. (33, 45), Department of Medicine, University of Minnesota Hospitals, Minneapolis, Minnesota 55455

Phillip K. Peterson, M.D. (125, 197), Department of Medicine, University of Minnesota Hospitals, Minneapolis, Minnesota 55455

Paul G. Quie, M.D. (359), Department of Pediatrics, University of Minnesota, Minneapolis, Minnesota 55455

Carlos H. Ramirez-Ronda, M.D. (181), University of Puerto Rico School of Medicine, San Juan, Puerto Rico 00936

Warren E. Regelmann, M.D. (359), Department of Pediatrics, University of Minnesota, Minneapolis, Minnesota 55455

Jack S. Remington, M.D. (319, 341), Division of Infectious Diseases, Department of Medicine, Stanford University School of Medicine, Research Institute, Palo Alto Medical Foundation, Palo Alto, California 94301

Allan R. Ronald, M.D. (3), Department of Microbiology, University of Manitoba, Winnipeg, Canada R3E 0W3

Carlos Russo, M.D. (309), University of Panama Medical School, Complejo Hospitalario Metropolitano del Seguro Social and Hospital Santo Tomas, Panama City, Panama

Corando Sáenz A., M.D. (145), Department of Internal Medicine, School of Medicine, University Hospital, Monterey, N.L., Mexico

L. D. Sabath, M.D. (33, 275), Department of Medicine, University of Minnesota, Minneapolis, Minnesota 55455

Rosa Maria Sanchez (135), Infectious Disease and Immunology Section, Pediatric Unit General Hospital, Health Department (S.S.A.), Mexico 13, D.F. Mexico

Jay P. Siegel, M.D. (319), Division of Infectious Diseases, Department of Medicine, Stanford University School of Medicine, Research Institute, Palo Alto Medical Foundation, Palo Alto, California 94301

Richard L. Simmons, M.D. (93, 211), Department of Surgery, University of Minnesota, Minneapolis, Minnesota 55455

Publio Toala, M.D. (159, 309), University of Panama Medical School, Complejo Hospitalario Metropolitano del Seguro Social and Hospital Santo Tomas, Panama City, Panama

Lewis W. Wannamaker, M.D. (231), Departments of Pediatrics and Microbiology, University of Minnesota, Minneapolis, Minnesota 55455

Walter R. Wilson, M.D. (171, 255), Department of Infectious Diseases, Mayo Clinic, Rochester, Minnesota 55901

Murray Wittner, M.D., Ph.D. (287, 299), Department of Pathology, Albert Einstein College of Medicine, Bronx, New York 10461

Isidro G. Zavala T., M.D. (115), Infectious Diseases Department, Angel Leaño Hospital, Guadalajara Autonomous University, Guadalajara, Jal., Mexico

Preface

Few areas of clinical practice have witnessed an accelerated growth of useful information during the past several years comparable to that seen in the field of infectious diseases. "New" etiologic agents and syndromes have been recognized, such as Legionnaires' disease, a variety of chlamydial infections, campylobacter enteritis, *Clostridium difficile* toxin-induced pseudomembranous colitis, and staphylococcal toxic shock syndrome. New guidelines for the management of "old" problems have been proposed—for example, shorter course treatment for tuberculosis and urinary tract infections. New insights have emerged into the mechanisms of host defense and of those infections that threaten the lives of our immunocompromised patients. In virology, important breakthroughs have occurred, and there has been a productive reawakening of interest in parasitology. Finally, new diagnostic methods have been introduced into practice, and there has been an almost explosive development of new antimicrobial agents.

Given the pace and complexity of many of these developments, it has become increasingly difficult for the clinical practitioner to keep abreast of those aspects that should have direct application to patient care. The main goal of this book is to facilitate this process. In this volume, an outstanding group of infectious disease specialists have summarized current approaches to the management of infections of greatest clinical importance. This book should be useful to virtually all primary care physicians—to the generalist, family practitioner, pediatrician, internist, and surgeon.

The book is organized into three subject areas: (1) infections of specific organ systems, (2) different types of pathogens, and (3) specific problem areas and general diagnostic and therapeutic considerations. The pathogenesis of each infectious disease is briefly reviewed; the main emphasis, however, is on a practical approach to diagnosis and treatment. For quick reference, there has been a liberal use of tables.

A "camera ready" form of manuscript preparation has been employed because it requires significantly shorter production time, and hence, facilitates the rapid availability and currency of the information covered.

The editors are deeply indebted to each of the authors of this book, to Jane Anderson for her assistance in its preparation, and to the staff of Academic Press for their encouragement and help in producing a timely publication.

PART I
GENITOURINARY TRACT INFECTIONS

URINARY TRACT INFECTIONS:
PRACTICAL APPROACHES TO DIAGNOSIS AND MANAGEMENT

Allan Ronald

Department of Medical Microbiology
University of Manitoba
Winnipeg, Manitoba

I. THE DISEASE ENTITY

Symptoms arising from infection of the urinary tract is a common problem in medical practice and experienced by most women at some time throughout life. Several studies have suggested that as many as 20% of women experience dysuria during the course of a year. One half of these women consult a physician about these symptoms for approximately 90 physician visits for dysuria per 1000 women per year (1). Urinary infection occurs frequently in female children (1-2 infections/year/100 schoolage girls) and in elderly men.

Table 1 summarizes definitions and presenting features useful as diagnostic entities in urinary infection. Unfortunately, no clinical presentation is uniquely associated with bacterial urinary infection and the diagnosis depends on careful microbiologic investigation of a clean voided urine with a quantitative culture.

Aerobic gram negative rods cause almost 90% of all urinary infections with Escherichia coli responsible for about 80% of community acquired infections. Coagulase negative Staphylococcus sp account for about 10% of infections. Infections acquired in hospital are more often due to P. aeruginosa, Proteus sp and Klebsiella sp.

The acute urethral syndrome is a diagnosis given to patients who have symptoms usually confined to the urethra

3

TABLE 1. Bacterial Urinary Infection Syndromes

Definitions and Presenting Features

Acute cystitis - Dysuria or painful urination with frequency, urgency, and a variable incidence of hematuria, malodorous urine, bladder spasms. Fever not more than 38°C. Pyuria and bacteriuria (usually more than 100,000 organisms per ml urine).

Acute urethral syndrome - Dysuria with variable bladder symptoms and "no growth" or low counts in urine cultures. Sometimes accompanied by vaginitis. May be due to bacteria or Chlamydia trachomatis.

Acute pyelonephritis - Fever and chills, flank pain, often accompanied by bladder and urethral symptoms. Bacteriuria with pyuria; sometimes with white cell casts. Usually inilateral. Bacteremia common.

Acute prostatitis - Severe perineal, rectal or penile pain with fever and chills. Bacteria in initial voided urine. Bacteremia common.

Chronic urinary infection - A diagnosis that defies a useful definition but implies recurrent bacterial urinary infection.

Chronic prostatitis - Recurrent usually low grade perineal discomfort, sometimes with intermittent episodes of bacterial cystitis or pyelonephritis. Etiology of non-bacterial prostatitis uncertain.

Chronic pyelonephritis - Roentenologic diagnosis based on pyelographic evidence of renal scarring and calyceal destruction with loss of fine details of calyceal structure. May be accompanied by recurrent renal symptoms, bacteriuria, and pyuria. Renal impairment may be present often with an inability to concentrate urine normally after fluid deprivation.

Asymptomatic bacteriuria - Bacteriuria sometimes accompanied by pyuria. May be confined to the bladder or involve in addition one or both upper tracts. Of uncertain significance in most populations. Should be treated if present during pregnancy or if complicated by intermittent symptoms or evidence of destructive changes in the upper tracts.

(continued Table 1)

Reinfecting recurrent urinary infections – New organism from
  outside the urinary tract ascending the urethra and
  establishing infection at a variable interval after
  eradication of a prior infection.

Relapsing recurrent urinary infection – Persistence of the
  organism within the urinary tract (usually in a focus in
  the prostate or kidney) with emergence (regrowth) after
  therapy.

without a positive urine culture (< 100,000 organisms/ml).
Recent studies have shown that these patients can be categorized
by the presence of inflammatory cells. Patients with pyuria
usually have either "low count" bacteriuria or Chlamydia trachomatis urethritis. A ten day course of doxycycline has been
found effective for most patients (2). Patients without pyuria
do not respond to antimicrobial agents and the etiology of their
symptoms remains uncertain.

Most urinary pathogens gain access to the bladder and kidneys
by ascending against the urinary stream. Only S. aureus and
Candida albicans reach the kidney in most instances via the
hematogenous route. In women, the propensity to frequent reinfections appears to be due to a biologic defect that permits
heavy prolonged colonization of the perineum with gram negative
rods. Probably this is due to increased adherence of E. coli
to uroepithelial cells. In a recent study, we have shown that
sexual intercourse is an important antecedent event in women
with recurrent infection. About 80% of infections in sexually
active young women occur on a postintercourse day. Voiding
patterns and residual urine are presumably also important factors in urinary infection pathogenesis.

Bacteria can readily ascend to the kidneys if vesicoureteral
reflux is present. However, only 20% of patients with acute
bacterial cystitis and 40% of patients with asymptomatic bacteriuria, have organisms in the upper tracts. The presence of renal
calculi or of unilateral renal disease, permit organisms to persist in the upper tract despite antimicrobial therapy.

The antimicrobial coated bacteria test has been used to
localize the site of infection in patients who are either asymptomatic or have symptoms confined to their lower urinary tract.
Organisms eminating from the kidneys are coated with antibody
to the osomatic antigen. This antibody is produced within renal
tissue in response to invasive infection. Bacteria that originate from the bladder are not coated with antibody. Unfortunately, this test as presently carried out, is only useful for epidemiologic and therapeutic investigation and is not reliable for
the treatment of the individual patient.

II. ITS NATURAL HISTORY

In the absence of treatment, the natural history of various
urinary infection syndromes is uncertain. Patients with acute
cystitis and occasionally even patients with acute pyelonephritis experience symptomatic improvement despite continuing
bacteriuria. In one series, asymptomatic women with bacteriuria
were followed for one year. One third spontaneously resolved
during the year, one third became symptomatic and one third continued to have asymptomatic bacteriuria (3).

TABLE 2: Prognostic Factors in Urinary Infection

	Usually More Simple to Treat	Usually More Difficult to Treat and Prone to Recur
Source of infection	Community acquired	Institutionally acquired
Presenting symptoms	Acute cystitis	Acute pyelonephritis Acute prostatitis Asymptomatic infection
Etiology	Susceptible organisms, such as E. coli	Resistant organisms, such as P. aeruginosa
Site of infection (localization by ACB or single dose therapy)	Infection confined to the bladder	Asymptomatic or recurrent infection localized to the kidney or prostate
Underlying disease	None	Infection complicated by obstruction, calculi, congenital anomalies, neurologic disease
Pattern of recurrence	Reinfections after previous curative regimens	Relapse after previous courses of treatment
Renal function	Normal	Impaired
Sex	Females	Males

III. MANAGEMENT OF EPISODIC INFECTION

The response to therapy is variable but can be predicted by
several prognostic factors. Several of these are outlined in
table 2.
Single dose treatment has been popularized during the past
five years through at least eight studies, each of which have
shown that a single dose of an antimicrobial agent can cure more
than 90% of women and girls with acute cystitis or asymptomatic
infection localized to the bladder (4,5). Single dose therapy
is inexpensive, rarely associated with side effects, and does
not predispose to the acquisition of resistant pathogens.
Those patients who have failed single dose therapy have not
recurred with symptoms or signs of renal infection within the
initial weeks of follow-up. However, all patients treated with
single dose therapy must have a follow-up to identify those
patients who will recur.
The identification of patients with renal infection who require more prolonged intensive therapy and additional investigation, is the most important advantage of single dose therapy.
Studies with single dose therapy that have used localization
techniques, have determined that failure of single dose therapy
in females is an excellent indicator of renal infection
(specificity of over 90%) and failure of single dose therapy
will detect all patients who have urologic or anatomic abnormalities in their urinary tract.
No single dose studies have yet been reported in males.
Many males with symptoms confined to their lower urinary tract
also have concomitant prostate infection. Two weeks or more of
therapy is required, usually with an agent such as trimethoprim/
sulfamethoxazole, that enters prostatic tissue (6).
Patients with upper tract symptoms are usually ill with
symptoms and signs of acute pyelonephritis. They should be
treated with wide spectrum parenteral antimicrobial therapy
until a clinical response occurs and the susceptibility of the
infecting organisms is known. An aminoglycoside such as gentamicin or tobramycin together with ampicillin is appropriate
initial therapy. Some patients with renal infection are not
acutely ill and can be treated without hospital admission with
an oral well absorbed wide spectrum antimicrobial agent such as
cephalexin or trimethoprim/sulfamethoxazole. The prevelance of
ampicillin resistant organisms in most community acquired
urinary infection studies, makes ampicillin or amoxicillin a
less effective choice for the initial treatment of acute upper
tract infection prior to susceptibility testing.
Patients with hospital acquired infection particularly
associated with catheterization who develop invasive renal

infection, require parenteral antimicrobial therapy. Drugs
should be selected with knowledge of the susceptibility pattern
of nosocomial urinary pathogens. An aminoglycoside such as
amikacin and an antipseudomonas penicillin such as carbenicillin
or ticarcillin may be necessary for initial therapy. All
patients with acute pyelonephritis who do not respond to parenteral therapy within 48 hours, should be investigated radio-
graphically to exclude urinary obstruction or suppurative complications such as a cortical or perinephric abscess.

Patients started on parenteral therapy for renal infection
can be discharged on appropriate oral therapy as soon as they
have become afebrile and susceptibility results are known. Oral
therapy should be continued in females for at least two weeks
and in men for at least six weeks in order to cure the majority
of patients with renal infection. All patients with presumed
renal infection require follow-up urine cultures to identify
individuals with a continuing focus of persisting infection
within the urinary tract.

IV. MANAGEMENT OF RECURRENT URINARY INFECTIONS

Recurrent urinary infections are to be anticipated in
patients with urinary infection. One half of women will experience a second attack of cystitis within 12 months of the initial
episode. Recurrences should be categorized into bacteriologic
reinfection, relapse or persistence of the infecting organism.
Table 3 outlines features that characterize each of these
recurrence patterns. Reinfections occur from re-entry of organisms from the perineal fecal reservoir and account for the vast
majority of recurrences in females. Reinfections can be prevented by prolonged continuous low-dose prophylaxis with
trimethoprim/sulfamethoxazole every other day (40 mg of trimethoprim and 200 mg of sulfamethoxazole) (7). Resistance rarely
develops. Nitrofurantoin 50 mg daily can also prevent most
recurrences. Infections can also be prevented by postintercourse
chemotherapy with either one of these two agents. Intermittent
self administration of single dose therapy for lower tract
symptoms may be a suitable alternative to chemoprophylaxis in
selected women.

Patients can also recur due to persistence with continuing
positive cultures throughout therapy due to inadequate activity
in the urine or bacterial resistance (table 4). It should be
noted that bacteriologic eradication often does not correlate
very exactly with clinical response. A variety of alternate
explanations should be considered if a patient fails to improve
after initiation of therapy (table 4).

Patients who recur with the same organisms (relapse) after
initially negative urine cultures need careful radiographic and

TABLE 3: Characteristics of reinfecting, relapsing and persistent urinary infection recurrences.

	Relapse	Reinfection	Persistence
Organism	Identical species and serotype to that present before treatment	Often different organism from previous infection	Same organism as that present before treatment
Culture on therapy	No growth	No growth	Positive
Mode of presentation	Variable Often asymptomatic or renal	Bladder most common	Continuing symptoms on therapy
Underlying disease	Often none May be calculi, chronic pyelonephritis, diabetes mellitus	Usually none May be increased residual urine	Often renal impairment
Precipitating events	Usually none	Often related to inter-course, vaginitis, catheterization	Often failure to take antimicrobial agents
Relation to previous therapy	Recurrence usually within one week of stopping therapy	Recurrence at an un-predictable interval after therapy	None
Response to single-dose therapy	Relapse again	Usually cured	Failure

TABLE 4:   Reasons For Bacteriologic or Clinical Failure During
            Treatment

A.   Bacteriologic persistence (Urine culture remains positive)

     1.   Inadequate antibacterial activity in urine
               Patient noncompliance
               Inadequate dosage or frequency of dosing
               Drug malabsorption
                    Primary G.I. pathology
                    Interaction with food or other drugs
               Renal insufficiency

     2.   Bacterial resistance
               Wrong initial drug choice
                    i.e., not susceptible in vitro
               Development of resistance
               Mixed urinary infection with selection of resistant
                    strain
               Superinfection with new exogenous resistant strain
               "Specious" infection due to contamination with
                    perineal resistant strain

B.   Lack of clinical response

     1.   Error in diagnosis - not a bacterial infection

     2.   Obstruction within the urinary tract

     3.   Undrained pus, e.g., renal or perinephric abscess

     4.   Foreign body or renal calculi

     5.   Unrealistic expectation of rapid response

     6.   Complications of therapy

     7.   Immune defects

     8.   Bacteriologic persistence

sometimes urologic investigation to exclude a calculus or other anomaly to account for persistence of organisms in renal or prostatic tissue. Women with normal urinary tract should be treated for six weeks; men for 12 weeks. Trimethoprim/sulfamethoxazole is effective for many men with presumed prostatic foci of relapsing infection. Patients with renal or prostatic calculi non amenable to surgical extrapolation can be maintained on long term suppressive antibacterial therapy for years and remain free of infection on suppression.

It is important to emphasize the difference between suppression and prophylaxis. Prophylaxis prevents new organisms from entering the urinary tract from the fecal perineal reservoir. Suppression keeps patients asymptomatic by suppressing but not curing bacterial growth within the urinary tract.

Routine radiography is not indicated in all patients even with recurrent urinary infection (8). It should be reserved for females of any age with relapsing infection and all males. Repeated examinations are seldom warranted in either sex at any age; in the absence of obstruction, renal scarring and radiographic changes of "chronic pyelonephritis" are unlikely to develop in adults despite frequent infection recurrences.

Excessive urologic manipulation and unproven surgical procedures may befall patients with recurrent infection. The literature is replete with a variety of surgical techniques which, after a short period of popularity, are recognized as without benefit to the patient's illness. These procedures include bladder neck operations in women such as YV plasty, urethral surgery or urethral stenosis, ureteral reimplantation for minimal vesicoureteral reflux, and ileal conduits for pyelonephritis. Careful prospective studies are necessary before these procedures are given widespread acceptance by the medical community. However, judicious use of surgery is of unequivocal value in patients with obstructing lesions within the urinary tract if they can be relieved without major anatomical alterations of the drainage system.

Patients with an indwelling urethral catheter become infected within 2 to 4 days of catheter installation unless a closed drainage system is used to prevent infections. All patients catheterized for a month or longer routinely become infected. Superinfection with very resistant organisms can be avoided by limiting the use of antimicrobial therapy for acute symptoms in these patients. Long term suppression with systemic or local antibacterial agents is of no proven value in patients with indwelling catheters.

VI.   PROBLEMS FOR THE FUTURE

With increased understanding of the pathogenesis of urinary infection particularly as it relates to bacterial adherence, therapeutic intervention to forestall attachment of organisms to uroepithelial cells may be developed. Perhaps a specific vaccine directed against fimbriae (pili), the organ of adherence, will replace long-term continuous prophylactic regimens. We also require antimicrobial agents that can gain access more readily to "priviledged" areas such as prostatic tissue and kill organisms even in the presence of calculi.

REFERENCES

1.   Waters, W.E. (1969). Br J Prev Soc Med 23, 263.
2.   Stamm, W.E., et al.(1981). N Engl J Med 304, 956.
3.   Asscher A.W., et al. (1973). In "Urinary Tract Infection –
          Proceedings of the Second National Symposium, chap 7,
          p. 51. Oxford University Press.
4.   Rubin, R.H., et al. (1980). JAMA 244, 651.
5.   Ludwig, P., et al. (1980). Curr Chemother Proc 11th Int
          Cong Chemother 2, 1297.
6.   Smith, J.W., et al. (1979). Ann Intern Med 91, 544.
7.   Harding, G.K.M., et al. (1979). 242, 1975.
8.   Fowler, J.E. Jr., et al. (1981). N Engl J Med 304, 462.

VAGINITIS
Practical Approach to Diagnosis and Therapy

William J. Ledger

Department of Obstetrics and Gynecology
The New York Hospital
Cornell Medical Center
New York, New York

INTRODUCTION

Vaginitis is an important clinical problem for the physician caring for women. It is not life threatening, but the patient with an excessive, uncomfortable, vaginal discharge has a number of serious problems that need to be addressed in a comprehensive way by the physician. Some are immediate. The discomfort may preclude normal sexual function, and the odor or irritation of the discharge may make it difficult for the patient to contemplate participation in any social function. "I feel like a leper" was the way one patient described the social impact of the symptomatology. Other problems may be deeper and even more debilitating. The fear of a "serious" venereal disease is often present, and must be investigated by the physician. After appropriate microbiologic studies, these patients need reassurance that their sexual partners will not re-infect them and that they will not be a source of future infection to their male partners. All of these concerns must be acknowledged by the physicians.

GENERAL APPROACH

The goal of any physician evaluating the patient with an excessive, uncomfortable vaginal discharge is to make an accurate diagnosis. This requires a thorough history and physical examination of the patient, so that specific causes of vaginitis will be discovered. Symptomatic treatment without this evaluation is too often associated with a delay in more appropriate therapy. A number of important entities must be ruled out in patients with this complaint. In sexually active women, there is a significantly higher incidence of positive cultures for *Neisseria gonorrhea* among patients presenting with an abnormal vaginal discharge (1). A culture for *Neisseria gonorrhea* should be obtained in these women. The retention of a foreign object within the vagina can be associated with an excessive, malodorous discharge. This may be the cause of a vaginitis in a pre-menarchal girl who has pushed a small toy into her vagina. It also can be present in an adult woman who has forgotten to remove a tampon or a diaphragm. Symptomatic treatment of these patients without an examination is poor therapy. Finally, an excessive vaginal discharge or vulvar irritation may be a sign of a genital tract malignancy. Careful examination should include a Pap smear, as well as specific biopsies if there is an abnormal gross appearance at the time of examination of genital tract tissue.

SPECIFIC CAUSES OF VULVO-VAGINITIS

Candida albicans vaginitis

Vaginitis, due to the yeast *Candida albicans*, is the most common form of this clinical infection seen by doctors. A number of alterations from normal seem to increase the incidence and sometimes the severity of this infection as well. Recent exposure to broad spectrum antibiotics, particularly ampicillin and the tetracyclines, eliminates much of the normal bacterial flora of the vagina and permits overgrowth of *Candida albicans* and the subsequent development of symptomatology. Pregnancy also seems to predispose women to an increased incidence of this yeast vaginitis. The reasons for this more common occurrence in pregnancy are not known, although it may be related to the higher rate of glycosuria associated with pregnancy. There are conflicting views on

the impact of oral contraceptives on Candida vaginitis. Although
most clinicians believe more frequent infections are seen with
women using this form of contraception, at least one study could
not demonstrate this relationship (2). Finally, there is an
increased frequency of this infection in diabetic women who are
in poor metabolic control. Evaluation of blood sugars should be
done in those women with persistent Candida infections. All
of these altered states will increase the frequency of this form
of vaginitis and should be considered as possible factors in
the patients with a diagnosed Candida vaginitis. All of these
conditions help to contribute to the frequency with which this
infection is seen.

The diagnosis of *Candida albicans* vaginitis should be obvious
when an appropriate workup has been performed. There are
suggestions from the history of an irritating discharge, particularly when the patient has had perineal itching. The index
of suspicion will be particularly high when the patient is
pregnant or has had recent therapy with broad spectrum antibiotics. On examination, there often is a whitish, curd-like
discharge, and often these women have an inflamed, reddened
perineum. Some patients will not have any of these typical
expected findings. Because of this, the definitive diagnosis
depends upon microscopic examination and culture of the
vaginal secretions. A drop of vaginal secretions is placed in
a drop of warm saline, covered with a coverslip and examined
under the microscope. This is a good screening examination and
the presence of mycelia or hyphae is strongly suggestive of the
diagnosis. A most helpful diagnostic aid is to place another
sample of vaginal secretion onto a drop of 10% potassium hydroxide solution. This will lyse the other cellular elements and
permit an easier identification of the yeast-like forms. These
microscopic examinations will provide the diagnosis in the
majority of cases, but the definitive diagnosis requires a
culture and this should be employed in every patient with these
symptoms in whom the diagnosis is not obvious on microscopic
examination. If these steps are followed in every patient,
the diagnosis should be made in every patient with this infection.

The treatment of a patient with *Candida albicans* vaginitis
is usually restricted to the area of infection. For years,
preparations made with mycostatin were used locally in the form
of vaginal tablets for two weeks or more. The recent introduction of miconazole, a more potent antifungal agent, has
resulted in treatment success with shorter therapy durations of
three to seven days. Preparations with this agent added include
a vaginal cream and vaginal suppositories. There are other
techniques that seem to help in the care of these women.
Restrictive undergarments made of synthetic fibers will increase
the chances for continued perineal irritation. Although the
male is usually not a factor in the woman maintaining an
infection or having a reinfection, occasionally an uncircumcised

male will need local therapy. Although the gastrointestinal
tract will house these yeast forms, no definitive studies have
shown that oral mycostatin therapy will lower the frequency of
re-infection in normal women, by reducing gastrointestinal
yeast colonization. The patient with a persistant Candida
vaginal infection should be evaluated for the possibility of
abnormal glucose tolerance. Although one recent report showed
diminished cellular immune response in women with chronic
Candida vaginitis (3), this has not been translated into a
treatment regimen.

Trichomonas vaginalis vaginitis

Vaginitis, caused by the protozoa, *Trichomonas vaginalis,*
is a common office problem that requires care of both the male
and female sexual partners. The awareness of the two patients
is involved in the successful treatment of these uncomfortable
women, for most males who are carriers of this organism are not
symptomatic.

The diagnosis of Trichomonas vaginitis is straightforward.
These women usually complain of an excessive, malodorous
discharge, and frequently have discomfort or burning with intercourse. On examination, the vaginal discharge often has a
"bubbly" appearance and small punctate hemorrhagic areas may be
visible on the cervix or vagina. Many women with a symptomatic
vaginal infection will show no typical gross signs of the disease.
Because of this, the cornerstone of diagnosis is an examination
of these vaginal secretions in warm saline. The motile trichomonads are easily identified. Culture techniques are available,
but these are usually reserved for the patients who fail to
respond to therapy.

The treatment of Trichomonas vaginitis is systemic rather
than local. In the past, local medications would eliminate
trichomonads from the vaginal surface, but recurrences were
frequent because these organisms often resided in sites as
Skene's and Bartholin's glands, where the vaginal creams would
not penetrate and the trichomonads repopulate the vagina after
local therapy was completed. The introduction of an effective
systemic anti-protozoal agent, metronidazole, revolutionized
the care of these women. One gram of metronidazole daily in
four divided doses for three to seven days would eliminate
the disease in females. When it became apparent that
asymptomatic male carriers could reinfect these women, concomitant
treatment of the male resulted in a higher percentage of permanent
cures. Despite this improved therapeutic picture, there are a
number of increasingly difficult issues in the treatment of these
women. The widespread availability of non-barrier methods of
contraception, such as the pill and the intrauterine contraceptive
device, plus changes in social standards, have increased the pool

of adult men and women who have more than one sexual partner.
In this context, one asymptomatic male may start a chain of
infection that results in many men and women requiring treatment
and the successful treatment of an infected couple may not be
permanent if any member becomes infected again outside of that
relationship. In addition to these problems, the view of
metronidazole is undergoing alteration. A major concern is
the report in experimental animals that it causes cancer (4).
Although carcinogenesis has not been confirmed in the human to
date (5), this does give the prescribing physician some pause.
The gastrointestinal disturbance with metronidazole and the need
to abstain from alcohol during therapy have led to interest
in a one large (i.e. two gram) dosage regimen (6). This is an
acceptable alternative to the longer treatment course. A more
disturbing recent development is the report of the appearance
of *Trichomonads* which are resistant to metronidazole (7).
This resistance is obvious in the laboratory, and is not related
to poor absorption of the drug by the patient. To date, an
alternative form of systemic therapy has not been successful
and local therapy has been ineffective in eliminating the
carriage of this organism.

Non-specific vaginitis

Non-specific vaginitis is a term applied to a group of women
with a recognized clinical entity. These are women in the
child-bearing age range, with a gray, homogenous, odorous
vaginal discharge that on examination yields no presence of mo
trichomonads. This is a frequent clinical problem easily
recognized by clinicians.

There is controversy about the microbiologic etiology of
specific vaginitis. Herman Gardner feels that a specific gra
negative bacillus, known variously as *Hemophilus vaginalis,*
Corynebacterium vaginalis, and *Gardnerella vaginalis*, is the
cause of this vaginal infection (8). He bases this on the
finding of this organism in women with this symptomatology,
elimination of symptomatology with eradication of the organi
and the ability to reproduce symptomatology when this bacter
species is introduced into the vagina of normal healthy wom
There is not uniform acceptance of this microbiologic theor
because of these observations. This organism has been reco
from the vagina of asymptomatic women who are allegedly not
sexually active (9), from asymptomatic women (10), and from
in whom antimicrobial therapy has eliminated symptomatolog
My own impression is that the overgrowth of this organism
vagina occurs concomitantly with an overgrowth of anaerobi
bacteria and produces the symptomatology in these women.
ation of the anaerobic bacteria that produce these foul sm
amines will result in a clinical cure.

There is controversy about the diagnosis of non-specific vaginitis. In the evaluation of women with typical symptoms, a number of ancillary tests must be done. A wet mount in warm saline of vaginal secretions should be done to eliminate the possibility of Trichomonas infection. Gardner has stressed the importance of "clue" cells on a vaginal smear, but some investigators have found clue cells present in asymptomatic women (10). The most specific test is the presence of a "fishy" odor when vaginal secretions are placed in 10% KOH.

The treatment of non-specific vaginitis is currently undergoing change. Although the standard therapy in the past has been the use of local sulfa creams, these have largely been abandoned. Oral ampicillin was popular therapy for many years, but a recent report indicates metronidazole 500 mg twice daily for seven days has a much higher rate of success (12). Most authors believe the male should be treated concomitantly.

OTHER CAUSES OF VAGINITIS

A number of women may present to the doctor with an excessive vaginal discharge, or an irritated vagina or perineum, with no evidence of Candida, Trichomonas, or non-specific vaginitis. There are a number of other possibilities. Vaginitis due to estrogen lack can be seen in post-menopausal women. If other more common causes of vaginitis are eliminated, this is a possible diagnosis. If there is concern about the accuracy of this diagnosis in a woman who has had a hysterectomy performed, for this eliminated amenorrhea as a symptom, a serum FSH can be measured. Elevated levels are compatible with estrogen lack and appropriate replacement therapy with oral unconjugated estrogens, with daily doses of 0.375 mg to 2.5 mg should be utilized. The lowest dose needed to eliminate symptomatology should be employed. The woman with estrogen lack vaginitis and a uterus in place probably is at some increased risk for the development of endometrial carcinoma (13). She should be warned of this possibility before this therapy is begun and endometrial biopsies should be done at six month intervals to detect any early changes. Genital herpes usually causes much discomfort and there usually is no question of the diagnosis. In some women, the recurrence may be mild and not recognized as such. Careful physician examination is important and a viral culture should be employed if there is any clinical suspicion of this disease. A patient with a cervicitis due to Chlamydia may have an excessive vaginal discharge. If a patient grossly has a marked cervicitis, a Chlamydia culture should be obtained if available, and therapy with either tetracycline or erythromycin can be employed. Finally, there are a small group of women in whom no microbiologic etiology can be assigned. Some of these women may have psycho-

somatic vulvovaginitis. This can be a possibility if a history
is elicited of the onset of symptomatology with a traumatic
emotional event, particularly when a careful physical examination
and microbiologic workup has revealed no known etiology of the
vaginitis (14). I am quite concerned about the premature use
of this term by physicians when the workup has not been thorough
and complete. In my own referral practice of vaginitis, a number
of women had psychologic problems with the unresolved symptoms
of their vaginitis, which disappeared when the vaginitis was
correctly diagnosed and treated.

REFERENCES

1. Cunan, J.W., Redtorff, R.C., Chandler, R.W., et al. (1975).
    Relationship of female gonorrhea to abnormal uterine bleeding,
    urinary tract symptoms, and cervicitis. *Obstet. Gynecol.*
    45, 195.
2. Spellacy, W.M., Zaias, N., Buhi, W.C., et al. (1971). Vaginal
    yeast growth and contraceptive practices. *Obstet. Gynecol.*
    38, 343.
3. Syverson, R.E., Buckley, H., Gibian, J., et al. (1979).
    Cellular and humoral immune status in women with chronic
    Candida vaginitis. *Amer. J. Obstet. Gynecol. 134,* 624.
4. Rustia, M., and Shuhib, P. (1972). Induction of lung tumors -
    malignant lymphomas in mice by metronidazole. *J.N.C.I. 48,* 721.
5. Friedman, G.D. (1980). Cancer after metronidazole. *N. Engl.*
    J. Med. 302, 519.
6. Csonka, G.W. (1971). Trichomonal vaginitis treated with one
    dose of metronidazole. *Brit. J. Ven. Dis. 47,* 456.
7. Muller, M., Meingassner, J.G., Miller, W.A., et al.
    Three metronidazole resistant strains of *Trichomonas vaginalis*
    from the U.S.A. *Amer. J. Obstet. Gynecol.*
8. Gardner, H.L., and Dukes, C.D. (1955). *Hemophilus vaginalis*
    vaginitis. *Amer. J. Obstet. Gynecol. 69,* 962.
9. McCormick, W.M., Hayes, C.H., Rosner, B., et al. (1977).
    Vaginal colonization with *Corynebacterium vaginale (Haemo-*
    philus vaginalis). J. Infect. Dis. 136, 740.
10. Levison, M.F., Trestman, I., Quach, R., et al. (1979).
    Quantitative bacteriology of the vaginal flora in vaginitis.
    Amer. J. Obstet. Gynecol. 133, 139.
11. Eschenbach, D. Personal communication.
12. Pheifer, T.A., Forsyth, P.S., Durfee, M.A., et al. (1978).
    Nonspecific vaginitis. *N. Engl. J. Med. 298,* 1429.
13. Ziel, H.K., and Finkle, W.D. (1975). Increased risk of endo-
    metrial carcinoma among users of conjugated estrogens.
    N. Engl. J. Med. 293, 1167.
14. Dodson, M.G., and Friedrich, E.G. Jr. (1978). Psychosomatic
    vulvovaginitis. *Obstet. Gynecol. 51,* 235.

INTRAPELVIC INFECTIONS

William J. Ledger

Department of Obstetrics and Gynecology
The New York Hospital
Cornell Medical Center
New York, New York

INTRODUCTION

The Obstetrician-Gynecologist caring for a woman with a pelvic infection uses different criteria to measure the clinical response to therapy than do other infectious disease experts in medicine and surgery. Most of the women seen with pelvic infections are less than 50 years of age and few have any serious underlying disease or are receiving immunosuppressive therapy that could influence host response to infection. As a result, death from sepsis, with the pelvis as the primary site of infection, is a rare event. Evaluation of treatment success or failure, of necessity, must use parameters other than mortality. There is a narrow focus of treatment efficacy. The patient response to initial antibiotic therapy is evaluated by the requirement to use additional antibiotics for cure. The need for operative intervention for cure, in the form of drainage or removal of an abscess, must be noted. More important, the impact of the infection and treatment upon future pelvic function has to be measured. For example, in the case of salpingitis there must be some note of the ability of the treated women to become pregnant in future years.

There has been a remarkable change in the microbiologic understanding of pelvic infection in women. In the past, the emphasis was upon a single pathogen, such as *Neisseria gonorrhea, Escherichiae coli,* or the Group A beta hemolytic streptococcus as the cause of disease. A number of recent studies (1,2) have demonstrated the polymicrobial nature of pelvic infections with many different bacteria isolated. Anaerobes seem to have special significance in pelvic infections for they are isolated from the majority of infection sites in the pelvis (1,2), from the blood stream in 25% or more of women with associated bacteremia (3), and are the predominant isolates from patients with a pelvic abscess requiring operative care (4). All of these observations indicate that antibiotic strategy for the woman with a pelvic infection should include consideration of anaerobes.

There are many parallels in the human to the animal model of infection developed by Bartlett and his co-investigators (5,6). In the animal, there was a biphasic response to fecal bacterial contamination of the peritoneal cavity, with early onset sepsis due to gram negative aerobic bacteria and late onset abscess formation in which anaerobic bacteria predominate. In the human, the early onset sepsis can be related to gram positive aerobic bacteria as well as all anaerobic bacteria, but the importance of anaerobes in abscesses seems the same.

There is a marked difference in the prognosis to therapy in the human, depending upon the timing of antibiotic treatment. In patients seen early in the course of infection, with symptomatology of five days or less and no pelvic masses, the therapeutic response is usually favorable. Of 403 patients treated with a variety of antibiotics effective against anaerobes, 337 (83.6%) were cured with the initial regimen and only 26 (6.4%) required some form of operative intervention (7). The therapeutic response in the patient with a well established infection is not nearly as good. In 98 patients with a well established infection, a cure with systemic antibiotics was achieved in 47 (48%) and operative care was necessary in 50 (51%). These different prognoses must be acknowledged in the antibiotic strategy for patients with a pelvic infection.

Because of the vast differences in outcomes, a classification of pelvic infection needs a focus upon early onset and well established infections. Within these two major divisions, a number of sub-categories will be noted.

EARLY ONSET INFECTION

Endomyometritis following vaginal delivery, is a pelvic
infection with an excellent prognosis. The number of women
who develop an infection after a vaginal delivery is much
lower than those who become infected after cesarean section (8).
Of equal predictive importance is the observation that serious
infections following vaginal delivery occur infrequently (9).
At least one factor in this low risk infection population
is the infrequent number of difficult vaginal deliveries done
in the 1980's. The complicated vaginal delivery of an infant
presenting as a breech or the difficult mid-forceps delivery
with associated soft tissue trauma is rarely performed.
Because of the infrequent serious infection, these early onset
infections can be treated with single antibiotic regimens.
Ampicillin, cefoxitin (10), cefamandole (11), and metronidazole (12) have all been successfully used in these women.
Although some women are treatment failures requiring other
antibiotics for cure, the patient requiring operative
drainage of an abscess is a rare event.
Endomyometritis following cesarean section is a much more
serious problem for the physician: infection is a more frequent
event (8) and the severity of infection is much greater (9).
The most serious hospital acquired infections in obstetric-
gynecologic patients follow cesarean section on the patient
in labor. These women can develop difficult to treat abdominal
wound infections or a pelvic abscess that may require extir-
pation of the pelvic organs for cure. Because of this, there
has been a great interest in a number of antibacterial
regimens that will avoid these serious complications. Some of
the more standard antibiotic regimens have had a consistent
rate of treatment failures in which serious problems were seen.
The frequently used combination of penicillin and an aminoglycoside (13) or a first generation cephalosporin and an
aminoglycoside (14) have had a small percentage (less than
5%) of women who have had serious infectious complications.
A somewhat higher number of patients requiring operative
intervention for cure was seen when penicillin and tetracycline were used (15). Utilizing the excellent results achieved
in animal experiments with clindamycin and gentamicin as the
basis for the experiment, the clindamycin regimen was compared
to the then more standard penicillin and aminoglycoside
combination (16). The clinical results were impressive and
are noted in Table 1. Clearly this combination avoided the
serious problems seen in the past. The major question still
to be resolved is the propriety of using, in every patient,

Table I. Comparison of the Two Regimens

	Clindamycin-gentamicin	Penicillin-gentamicin	Significance
No. of patients	100	100	N.S.
Therapy completed, no problems	86	64	p< 0.001
Poor clinical results:			
No response—third antibiotic	5	29	p< 0.001
Abdominal wound infection	8	16	N.S.
Operative drainage only	6	4	N.S.
Prolonged febrile course after drainage	2	12	p< 0.02 (Fisher's exact test)
Serious problems:			
Pelvic abscess, total abdominal hysterectomy, bilateral salpingo-oophorectomy	0	4	p< 0.06
Wound evisceration	0	1	
Heparin	0	2	
Reaction during antibiotics:	4	3	N.S.
Rash	2*	2	
Hematuria	0	1+	
Diarrhea	2	0	
Indirect measures of morbidity:			
Hospital days	7.4	8.7	p< 0.01 (Mann-Whitney U test)

Table 1.   Comparison of the Two Regimens (continued)

	Clindamycin- gentamicin	Penicillin- gentamicin	Significance
(Indirect measures of morbidity - cont.)			
Fever index in degree hours			
Median	77.3	91.3	p< 0.02
Mean	81.2	110.7	
+ SD	+40.6	+89.6	
+ SE	+ 4.06	+ 9.0	

N.S. = Not significant

* Drug continued, rash disappeared, one patient.

+ Drug continued, hematuria stopped.

this antibiotic combination with its toxic potential in order
to avoid serious problems in less than 5%. Because of these
concerns, prospective studies with the newer cephalosporins
have been done. Cefamandole given intravenously at a dose 12-
16 grams per day, had a high incidence of successful response,
but a few patients still developed abscesses (11,17).
Cefoxitin used in this situation has had a high rate of success
without abscess formation (10). Moxalactam was less effective
in the 3.0 gram per day range, than when 6 grams were used (18).
Prospective comparative studies of cefoxitin, cefamandole, or
moxalactam against clindamycin-gentamicin need to be done to
establish the efficacy of these single antibiotic regimens.

Medical thinking on the infected abortion has dramatically
changed in the past decade. In the 1960's, septic shock in
the patient with an infected abortion was a feared complication. The more widespread availability to women of all social
classes of both better contraceptive techniques and pregnancy
termination for the patient with an unwanted pregnancy have had
a marked impact on this type of infection. The number of
women with an infected abortion has diminished and the frequency of life threatening infections has decreased as well (9).
These patients have the most favorable prognosis for a response to treatment of all of the women with a soft tissue
pelvic infection. Evaluations of the treatment of a patient
with an infected abortion indicate that the curettage is the
single most important aspect of therapy (19), but there are
differences in the therapeutic response when different antibiotics are employed. Antibiotics with activity against
anaerobes and gram-negative aerobes provide a better clinical
response than does clindamycin used alone (19). In this
setting, antibiotic coverage with a cephalosporin alone seems
to provide adequate treatment for women with an infected
abortion.

The patient with salpingo-oophoritis seen early in the
course of infection presents a therapeutic dilemma to the
physician. There are so many unanswered questions. It has
not been established whether or not outpatient treatment is
adequate for these women although both of the standard
treatment regimens with either a penicillin or a tetracycline
alone have unacceptably high failure rates (20). Of even more
importance is the lack of information about the effect of
various antibiotic regimens upon future fertility of these
women. A percentage of women with salpingitis will have tubal
blockage and subsequent infertility (21). A critical issue
is the pelvic response to the various antibiotics that can
be employed in such women when they first seek treatment.
Until this information is provided by prospective study,
definitive recommendations cannot be given. Based upon the

initial response to therapy, the newer tetracyclines, particularly doxycycline, seem very effective in women with salpingitis. This may be due to the recovery of chlamydia from tubal biopsies of 30% of patients with acute salpingitis (22). The newer cephalosporins, particularly cefoxitin and cefamandole, have also been clinically effective in this situation even though they are ineffective against chlamydia. These agents have particular appeal because of their in vitro effectiveness against the penicillin resistant strains of *Neisseria gonorrhea*. This organism may have a great deal of significance for the physician who is treating pelvic infections in future years.

WELL ESTABLISHED INFECTIONS

Patients with a well established salpingitis, i.e., a history of symptomatology for five days or more, or a pelvic mass, have a markedly different prognosis. The major concern in these women should be the presence of a pelvic abscess and the antibiotic strategy should include antibiotics effective against anaerobes and gram negative aerobic organisms. Despite this broad spectrum antibacterial coverage, some patients will remain febrile and require operative drainage or removal for a cure. This operative intervention is usually not required because of the presence of bacteria resistant to the antibiotics employed pre-operatively. In one evaluation of women receiving three antibiotics, only two women of forty requiring operations had bacteria isolated from the abscess that were resistant in the laboratory to the antibiotics employed pre-operatively (23). Since the failure rate of antibiotics is so high in this clinical situation, it is important to use the most effective antibiotics primarily. Since the anaerobic spectrum of clindamycin, chloramphenicol, and metronidazole is superior to the newer cephalosporins, these should be the drugs of choice in this situation. This theoretical concern seems verified by the poor results with cefoxitin and cefamandole in the treatment of well established infections. One clinical study demonstrated no clinical differences when either clindamycin or chloramphenicol were employed (23). To date, a comparative study of metronidazole has not been done.

Well established infections can be seen in post-operative and post partum infections. The clinical histories of these women follow a similar pattern. These women have been discharged from the hospital, evidently free of infection, and subsequently are readmitted febrile with a pelvic mass. Again, the major therapeutic concern should be a pelvic abscess in which anaerobes and gram negative aerobes are the predominant organisms. The antibiotic selection should reflect this concern and the combination of clindamycin and gentamicin has been popular in this situation. In those patients who show no evidence of a clinical response after three or more days of therapy, operative intervention for drainage or removal of an abscess is indicated.

REFERENCES

1. Thadepalli, H., Gorbach, S., and Keith, L. (1973). Anaerobic infections of the female genital tract: Bacteriologic and therapeutic aspects. *Amer. J. Obstet. Gynecol. 117,*1034.
2. Swenson, R.M., Michaelson, T.C., Daly, M.J., et al. (1973). Anaerobic bacterial infections of the female genital tract. *Obstet. Gynecol. 42,* 538.
3. Ledger, W.J., Norman, M., Gee, C., et al. (1975). Bacteremia on an Obstetric-Gynecologic service. *Amer. J. Obstet. Gynecol. 121,* 205.
4. Ledger, W.J. (1975). Anaerobic infections. *Amer. J. Obstet. Gynecol. 123,* 111.
5. Weinstein, W.W., Onderdonk, A.B., Bartlett, J.G., et al. (1974). Experimental intra-abdominal abscesses in rats: Development of an experimental model. *Infect. Immun. 10,*1250.
6. Onderdonk, A.B., Kasper, P.L., Mansheim, B.J., et al. (1979). Experimental animal models for anaerobic infections. *Rev. Inf. Dis. 1,* 291.
7. Ledger, W.J. Unpublished observation.
8. Gassner, C.B., and Ledger, W.J. (1976). The relationship of hospital acquired maternal infections to invasive intrapartum monitoring techniques. *Amer. J. Obstet. Gynecol. 126,* 33.
9. Ledger, W.J., Kriewall, T.J., and Gee, C. (1975). The fever index - a technique for evaluating the clinical response to bacteremia. *Obstet. Gynecol. 45,* 603.
10. Sweet, W.J., and Ledger, W.J. (1979). Cefoxitin: Single agent treatment of mixed aerobic-anaerobic pelvic infection. *Obstet. Gynecol. 54,* 193.
11. Cunningham, F.G., Gilstrap, L.G. III, and Kappus, S.S. (1974). Treatment of obstetric and gynecologic infections with cefamandole. *Amer. J. Obstet. Gynecol. 133,* 602.
12. Platt, L.D., Yonekura, K.L., and Ledger, W.J. (1979). The role of anaerobic bacteria in postpartum endomyometritis. *Amer. J. Obstet. Gynecol. 135,* 814.

13. Gibbs, R.S., Jones, P.M., and Wilde, C.J. (1978). Antibiotic therapy of endometritis following cesarean section. Treatment of successes and failures. *Obstet. Gynecol. 52,* 31.

14. Sen, P., Apuzzio, J., Reyelt, C., et al. (1980). Prospective evaluation of combination of antimicrobial against for endometritis after cesarean section. *S.G.O. 151,* 89.

15. Cunningham, F.G., Hauth, J.C., Strong, J.D., et al. (1978). Infectious morbidity following cesarean section. *Obstet. Gynecol. 52,* 656.

16. Di Zerga, G., Yonekura, L., Roy, S., et al. (1980). A comparison of clindamycin-gentamicin and penicillin-gentamicin in the treatment of post cesarean section endomyometritis. *Amer. J. Obstet. Gynecol. 137,* 914.

17. Gall, S.A., and Hill, G.B. (1980). High dose cefamandole therapy in obstetric and gynecologic infections. *Amer. J. Obstet. Gynecol. 137,* 914.

18. Cunningham, F.G., Hemsell, D.L., DePalura, R.T. et al.(1981). Moxalactam for obstetric and gynecologic infections. *Amer. J. Obstet. Gynecol. 139,* 915.

19. Chow, A.W., Marshall, J.R., and Guze, L.B. (1977). A double blind comparison of clindamycin with penicillin plus chloramphenicol in treatment of septic abortion. *J. Inf. Dis. 135,* 535.

20. Cunningham, F.G., Hauth, J.C., Strong, J.D., et al. (1977). Evaluation of tetracycline or penicillin-ampicillin for treatment of acute pelvic inflammatory disease. *N. Engl. J. Med. 296,* 1380.

21. Westrom, L. (1980). Incidence, prevalence and trends of acute pelvic inflammatory disease and its consequences in industrialized countries. *Amer. J. Obstet. Gynecol. 138,* 880.

22. Mårdh, P.A., Ripa, K.T., Svensson, L., et al. (1977). *Chlamydia trachomatis* infections in patients with acute salpingitis. *N. Engl. J. Med. 296,* 1377.

23. Ledger, W.J., Gee, C., Lewis, W.P., et al. (1977). Comparison of clindamycin and chloramphenicol in the treatment of serious infections of the female genital tract. *J. Inf. Dis. 135,* 530.

SEXUALLY TRANSMITTED DISEASES

L.D. Sabath
Jacques E. Mokhbat

University of Minnesota
Minneapolis, Minnesota

GENERAL COMMENTS

It is a remarkable fact that several of the most important venereal diseases are treatable with a safe, inexpensive antibiotic, benzylpenicillin (Penicillin G). Therefore one would expect that these diseases would have diminished markedly or possibly even have disappeared. Nothing could be further from the facts. One of these diseases, gonorrhea, has increased manyfold over the last several decades and syphilis is currently increasing in numbers of cases. It has been suggested that several radical changes in social behavior have led to increased inter-human contact in which infection with these agents is more likely to occur. These changes in attitude towards sex, the liberalization and increasing safety of abortion, the widespread use of a variety of birth control devices and medications, especially "the pill", are all thought to have contributed to the increase in venereal diseases. The fact that the term "venereal diseases" is being replaced by the term "sexually transmitted diseases" also reflects a change in attitude toward these diseases.

Whereas twenty years ago it was considered that "the venereal diseases" comprised 5 specific diseases (syphilis, gonorrhea, chancroid, lymphogranuloma venereum and granuloma inguinale), it is now widely recognized that there is a very large spectrum of sexually transmitted disease; most remarkably the most common STD in the United States and Britain (and probably other countries as well) is not even among the traditional five (this new disease is chlamydial infection, due to the organism *Chlamydia trachomatis*).

NEW ASPECTS OF STD

The field of sexually transmitted diseases has encompassed
enormous changes in basic observations, epidemiology, concepts
and practice of therapeutic modalities, and pathogenesis of
these diseases, but it is only possible here to give a brief
mention of some of the most important developments.

A. *Antibiotic Resistance to Neisseria gonorrhoeae, the Organism
    Causing Gonococcal Disease*

Whereas *N. gonorrhoeae* was frequently inhibited by 0.002 µg/ml
penicillin G at the outset of the penicillin era, this is no
longer the case and the dosage (detailed below) required to
cure such an infection has increased considerably. This is
primarily due to emergence of relatively resistant organisms
that require higher concentrations of penicillin G for inhibition,
but do not inactivate the antibiotic with β-lactamases. A second
type of penicillin resistance which has caused considerable concern is that due to penicillin inactivation by β-lactamases.
Basic studies suggest the plasmid bearing the penicillinase gene
in *Neisseria gonorrhoeae* had its origin in *Escherichia coli*.
Fortunately these organisms are relatively uncommon and account
for only a small proportion of the penicillin resistance and
treatment failure in patients with this disease.
    In addition to gonococcal resistance to penicillin G there
is also a problem of gonococcal resistance to other antibiotics.
Most troublesome is the emergence of spectinomycin resistant
gonococci. These were first reported from Denmark in 1973 and
since then an additional case from Denmark, one from Holland
and one from the United States before the recent (May, 1981)
isolate of a spectinomycin resistant isolate of *Neisseria
gonorrhoeae* that was also a penicillinase producing organism.
    In addition to the common occurrence of penicillin resistant
gonococci and the much rarer existance of spectinomycin resistant
gonococci, there is also variable degrees of resistance of
gonococci to the tetracyclines and to erythromycin.

B. *New Antibiotics for Use in Treatment of Gonococcal Infections*

In addition to the antibiotics mentioned above, some of the
newer β-lactam antibiotics have been and are being tested for
efficacy in treating gonococcal infections. Among those that
appear most promising are cefoxitin, piperacillin, cefonicid
and cefuroxime.

C. *Increased Number of Etiologic Agents of Sexually Transmitted Diseases*

Table 1 indicates the broadened spectrum of sexually transmitted diseases classified by the type of microorganism and Table 2 lists some non-classical sexually transmitted organisms. Of considerable importance in Table 2 is that *Chlamydia trachomatis* is listed; infections due to *Chlamydia trachomatis* are more common than those due to any of these other agents. These agents listed in Tables 1 and 2 are often responsible for one or more syndromes and the correlation of etiologic agents and presenting syndromes are organized in Table 3.

TABLE 1. Sexually Transmitted Diseases

Organism group	Disease
Bacteria	Gonorrhoea
	Chancroid
	Lymphogranuloma venereum
	Granuloma inguinale
Viruses	Herpes simplex
	Genital warts
	Molluscum contagiosum
Spirochaetes	Syphilis
	Balanitis
Protozoa	Trichomoniasis
Fungi	Candidosis
	Tinea cruris
Parasites	Scabies
	Pediculosis pubis
Uncertain	Non-specific genital infection

TABLE 2. Some Non-Classical Sexually Transmissible Organisms

Group	Organism
Bacteria	Chlamydia trachomatis
	Ureaplasma urealyticum
	Mycoplasma hominis
	Herellea vaginicola
	Listeria monocytogenes
	Mima polymorph
	Haemophilus spp.
	Corynebacteria
	Group B streptococci
	Shigella
Viruses	Hepatitis B virus
	Cytomegalovirus
	Epstein-Barr virus
	Marburg virus
Protozoa	Entamoeba histolytica
	Giardia lamblia

D. New Information on the Biology of Neisseria gonorrhoeae

There are recent observations that men may harbor the organism in the urethra without symptoms, and thus be asymptomatic carriers. Another newer observation is that women with genital infections may, on close questioning, admit to a variety of pelvic symptoms. There is increasing and abundant evidence that gonococci that cause disseminated gonococcal infection (DGI) tend to be very sensitive to penicillin G whereas those that are predominantly genital in location include among their numbers the more resistant strains. An association has been noted between patients with deficiencies of C6, C7 and C8 (the later elements in the complement cascade) and bacteremia due to *Neisseria gonorrhoeae* or *Neisseria meningitidis*. This information has led to the conclusion that the serum bactericidal activity rather than opsonic activity is the more important feature of host defense against dissemination of gonococcal infection. In addition, there is some recent evidence that IgA proteases are produced by some gonococcal strains causing disseminated infection. Thus a specific parasite virulence factors and defects in host defense factors are being clarified as important in dissemination of gonococcal infection.

TABLE 3. *Selected Syndromes and Complications with Corresponding Sexually Transmitted Etiologic Agents[a]*

PRESENTATION	ETIOLOGIC AGENT
Male urethritis	N. gonorrhoeae, C. trachomatis, herpes simplex virus, ?U. urealyticum
Lower genitourinary infection in women	Vulvitis: C. albicans, herpes simplex virus
	Vaginitis: T. vaginalis, C. albicans, H. vaginalis
	Cervicitis: N. gonorrhoeae, C. trachomatis, herpes simplex virus
	Female urethritis: N. gonorrhoeae, C. trachomatis
Genital ulceration	Herpes simplex virus, Treponema pallidum, H. ducreyi, Cal. granulomatis, C. trachomatis (LGV)
Pelvic inflammatory disease	N. gonorrhoeae, C. trachomatis
Proctitis	N. gonorrhoeae, herpes simplex virus, ?C. trachomatis
Acute arthritis with genital infection	N. gonorrhoeae, ?C. trachomatis
Neonate and infant:	
"TORCHES" syndrome	Cytomegalovirus, herpes simplex virus, T. pallidum
Other infant and childhood mortality	Conjunctivitis: C. trachomatis, N. gonorrhoeae
	Pneumonia: C. trachomatis
	Otitis media: C. trachomatis
	Sepsis, death: Group B streptococcus
	Cognitive impairment: Cytomegalovirus, herpes simplex virus, T. pallidum
Infertility:	
Postsalpingitis, postobstetric, postabortion	N. gonorrhoeae, C. trachomatis, M. hominis
Spontaneous abortion	Herpes simplex virus, ?N. gonorrhoeae, ?C. trachomatis, fetal wastage

[a]*For each of the above syndromes and complications, a variable proportion cannot yet be ascribed to any cause and must currently be considered idiopathic.*

E.   STD in Homosexual Men

There has been special attention paid to the phenomenon of a variety of the sexually transmitted diseases occurring much more frequently and often with much greater severity in homosexual males. For example, homosexual males are especially important reservoirs of syphilis, cytomegalovirus (CMV) disease, hepatitis B, as well as many of the other sexually transmitted diseases listed in Tables 1 and 2. It should be noted that Kaposi's sarcoma and pneumocystis pneumonia have been diagnosed with remarkable frequency in homosexual men. During the 30 months preceding July 3, 1981, Kaposi's sarcoma was diagnosed in 26 homosexual men (20 in New York City, 6 in California). Six of the Kaposi's sarcoma patients also had pneumonia (four biopsy confirmed as due to *Pneumocystis carinii*). Since September, 1979, 15 cases of pneumocystis have been reported in homosexual men in California.

The question is frequently asked what impact does homosexual preference have in sexually transmitted diseases in females. The massive problems seen in homosexual males are not seen in homosexual women. The explanation generally accepted is that homosexual women are usually monogamous and that they have far less sexual contact than do homosexual men. These behavioral factors would explain the great disparity in STD between the two sexes of homosexuals.

GONOCOCCAL INFECTIONS

A much wider range of gonococcal infection is now recognized than a generation ago. The major gonococcal infection syndromes are: 1) uncomplicated gonococcal infection in men and women, 2) anorectal infection in men, 3) pharyngeal infection, 4) ocular gonococcal infection, 5) gonococcal arthritis, 6) acute pelvic inflammatory disease, 7) acute epididymitis, 8) disseminated gonococcal infection.

The diagnosis of acute urethral gonococcal infection in men still remains the gram stain showing numerous polymorphonuclear leukocytes with intracellular gram negative diplococci. Cultures are rarely indicated in patients with discharge. In contrast, culture is a major means of diagnosing female genital gonococcal infection although some interest in the possible use of the gram stain is being explored currently. Gonococcal pelvic inflammatory disease is frequently not diagnosed bacteriologically directly unless there is surgery of the fallopian tubes. Gonococcal infection of the epididymis is diagnosed by culture and gram stain of aspirated material. Gonococcal arthritis may have negative cultures and gram stain; when these are positive the diagnosis is clear. Disseminated gonococcal infection has

negative blood cultures in a surprising proportion of cases; the
clinical manifestations, especially if cutaneous, are pustular
lesions seen around the fingers and wrists and occasionally
ankles. It has been suggested that more than a dozen cutaneous
lesions is inconsistent with disseminated gonococcal infection.

The treatment of these various gonococcal infections is
detailed in Table 4.

For penicillinase producing gonococci treatment should be
given as either tetracycline (as recommended in the table),
spectinomycin, 2 gm I.M., or cefoxitin, 2 gm I.M. Spectinomycin
has been ineffective in treating gonococcal pharyngitis and the
CDC has recommended trimethoprim-sulfamethoxazole tablets (400 mg
sulfamethoxazole/80 mg trimethoprim tablets), 9 tablets daily
for 5 days for the infection when penicillin is inappropriate.

In the first 4½ months of May, 1981, 99 infections due to
penicillinase producing gonococci were reported in Florida alone,
accounting for over half of those reported in the United States
during that period of time. With the possible exception of
Florida or other areas where penicillinase producing strains of
gonococci are especially prevalent, the recommended therapy
would nonetheless be as indicated in the table.

VAGINITIS SYNDROMES

The often troublesome problem of the various vaginitis syndromes has received increasing attention recently. The
diagnostic features and current suggested therapy of these are
summarized in Table V.

CHLAMYDIA TRACHOMATIS INFECTIONS

Although the organism *Chlamydia trachomatis* was first
recognized as a pathogen causing the ocular disease trachoma,
it is now recognized to cause a very wide range of human infections. The most commonly occurring infection due to this
organism in the United States is urethritis (infections of this
nature are occasionally called nongonococcal urethritis [NGU]
or nonspecific urethritis [NSU]). Other important infections
caused by *Chlamydia trachomatis* are neonatal ophthalmitis, pneumonia in infants during the first four months of life (the latter
two infections being acquired during the birth process), epididymitis, pelvic inflammatory disease, pneumonia in the immunocompromised adult, possibly pneumonia in other adults, perihepa-
titis, Reiter's syndrome, cervicitis, meningitis (one case
report). Possible other disease entities due to this organism
are diarrheal disease, arthritis, and conjunctivitis of the

TABLE 4.   *Recommended Treatment for Gonococcal Infection*

Diagnosis		Treatment of Choice
Uncomplicated gonococcal infection in men and women		Aqueous procaine penicillin G (APPG), 4.8 million units injected intramuscularly, at two sites with 1.0 g probenecid by mouth
	OR	tetracycline 0.5 g by mouth four times a day for 5 days (total dosage 10.0 g)
	OR	ampicillin 3.5 g (or amoxicillin 3.0 g) single oral dose, given with 1.0 g probenecid by mouth
Anorectal infection in men		APPG, 4.8 million units, with 1.0 g probenecid
Pharyngeal infection, either sex		APPG, 4.8 million units, with 1.0 g probenecid
Treatment failures		Spectinomycin, 2.0 g intramuscularly
Penicillinase-producing N. gonorrhoeae		Spectinomycin, 2.0 g intramuscularly
Gonorrhea in pregnancy		APPG, 4.8 million units intramuscularly with 1.0 g probenecid by mouth (if pregnant patient is allergic to penicillin, spectinomycin 2.0 g intramuscularly is recommended)
Acute PID, outpatient		Tetracycline 0.5 g orally four times a day for 10 days
	OR	APPG 4.8 million units intramuscularly plus 1.0 g probenecid orally, followed by ampicillin 0.5 g orally four times a day for 10 days
Acute PID, hospitalized		Aqueous crystalline penicillin G, 20 million units intravenously each day until improvement occurs, followed by ampicillin 0.5 g orally four times a day to complete 10 days of therapy. Since optimal therapy for hospitalized patients has not been established, alternative regimens, such as gentamicin plus clinda-

TABLE 4 CONTINUED NEXT PAGE

TABLE 4.   *Recommended Treatment for Gonococcal Infection – continued*

Diagnosis	Treatment of Choice
(Acute PID, hospitalized – cont.)	mycin, or chloramphenicol, are often used for severe PID in hospitalized patients.
Acute epididymitis	Tetracycline 0.5 g orally four times a day for 10 days
Disseminated gonococcal infection	Aqueous crystalline penillin G, 10 million units intravenously per day until improvement occurs, followed by ampicillin 0.5 g four times daily to complete 7 days of therapy
	OR ampicillin 3.5 g orally with probenecid 1.0 g, followed by ampicillin 0.5 g orally four times a day for 7 days
	PENICILLIN ALLERGY: Tetracycline 0.5 g orally four times daily for 7 days.
Pediatric gonococcal infection	See "Gonorrhea–CDC recommended treatment schedules"

TABLE 5. *Vaginitis Syndromes with Diagnosis and Therapy*

Etiology	Diagnostic features	Therapy
Trichomonas vaginalis	Motile trichomonads pH = 5.5-6.0 Amine odor volatilized by adding 10% KOH	Metronidazole 2.0 g single oral dose Metronidazole 250 mg three times daily for 10 days
Candida albicans	Yeast, pseudomycelia pH < 4.5 No odor with 10% KOH Isolation of C. albicans	Nystatin vaginal tablet twice daily for 7 days Imidazole (clotrimazole or miconazole) intravaginally once daily for 7 days
Hemophilus vaginalis	Clue cells pH > 4.5 Amine odor with 10% KOH Isolation of H. vaginalis	Ampicillin 500 mg four times daily for 7 days Metronidazole 500 mg twice daily for 7 days
Uninfected	Normal vaginal secretions pH < 4.5 No odor with 10% KOH	No medications

adult. There is increasing data that *Chlamydia trachomatis* may be one of the causes of the urethral syndrome, usually seen in young women. It should be emphasized that although *Chlamydia trachomatis* is the most common cause of NGU in the United States it is by no means the only cause of each. Making the diagnosis of *Chlamydia trachomatis* infection may be by direct demonstration of inclusion bodies in the pus from an infection (as in conjunctivitis or trachoma) but this is far less sensitive than growing the organism (in tissue culture). There are serologic tests but their current use is controversial. Laboratory kits for growing the organism are now readily available. Few laboratories perform the serologic tests for chlamydial infection.

The major therapeutic agents used in treating chlamydial infection are tetracyclines and erythromycin. In vitro, rifampin is the most active agent against Chlamydia, but its status in therapy remains to be determined. One frequent regimen of infection is tetracycline, 0.5 gm p.o. q6h for 7-10 days, but this therapy has not as yet been officially approved by the Food and Drug Administration of the United States. Other tetracyclines have been used successfully in treating chlamydial infections. In the newborn and infant, where tetracyclines are contraindicated, erythromycin is the usual agent used.

GENITAL HERPES INFECTION

An extraordinarily painful, annoying, basically unsolved problem in sexually transmitted diseases is that of genital herpes infection. These infections are usually caused by Herpes simplex type II, but may be caused by Herpes Type I. The problem of survival of the virus in nerve tissue and recrudescence is the basis of these troublesome infections. Like Herpes simplex infections elsewhere in the body, the precise factors that make one patient subject to painful recrudescence and others subject possibly to only one infection without recurrence are unknown. The occurrence of these lesions also enters into the differential diagnosis of penile and cervical-vaginal ulcerative lesions (Table 6). In addition to the problems of pain, recurrence and transmission of disease to the sexual partner, the major problem with genital herpes is that of transmission of disease from a pregnant mother to her offspring. Estimates are that the risk of neonatal infection is 10% if the genital herpes infection occurs before the 32nd week of gestation, whereas if the infection is present at the time of delivery, 40-80% of the offspring are affected.

If intrauterine infection occurs, the usual outcome is fetal death, whereas if the virus is present at the time of delivery, it is recommended that cesarean section be performed prior to the rupture of fetal membranes to avoid the high risk of herpes neonatorum.

The manifestations of herpes virus infection in the newborn occur 2-12 days after delivery. The infected newborn may have one or more of the following manifestations of infection: conjunctivitis, keratitis, rash (vesicular), jaundice, cyanosis, GI bleeding, CNS manifestations (including seizures) and other additional organ involvement. Two-thirds of the infants with disseminated infection survive. A high proportion of survivors have significant morbidity.

TABLE 6. *Penile Ulcers, Differential Diagnosis*

Disease (cause)	Identifying Characteristics
Chancroid	painful; small gram-negative rods
Genital herpes	painful, recurrent, multiple lesions, positive Tzanck smear
Syphilis	painless, positive dark field
Trauma	milder pain
Lymphogranuloma venereum	systemic symptoms, isolation of C. trachomatis

SYPHILIS

Syphilis will be considered in a separate chapter of this book.

REFERENCES

Young, Alex W. (1972). Herpes genitalis. *Med. Clin. N. Amer.* *56,* 1175-1192.

Willcox, R.R. (1972). A world look at the venereal diseases. *Med. Clin. N. Amer. 56,* 1057-1071.

Holmes, K.K. (1980). Gonococcal infections. *In* Harrison's Principles of Internal Medicine, 9th Ed. (K.T. Isselbacher, R.D. Adams, E. Braunwald, R.G. Petersdorf, and J.D. Wilson, eds.), p. 624-629. McGraw-Hill Book Company, New York.

Holmes, K.K., and Ronald, A.R. Chancroid. *Ibid.* p. 657-658.

Holmes, K.K. Sexually transmitted diseases. *Ibid.* p. 589-594.

Tack, K.J., *et al.* (1980). Isolation of *Chlamydia trachomatis* from the lower respiratory tract of adults. *Lancet i,* 117-120.

Schneider, N.J., Rarick, H.R., Frazier, D.E., Wroten, J., and Gunn, R.A. (1981). Infections due to penicillinase-producing *Neisseria gonorrhoeae* - Florida. *MMWR 30,* 245-247.

Friedman-Kien, A., Laubenstein, L., Marmor, M., *et al.* (1981). Kaposi's sarcoma and *Pneumocystis pneumonia* among homosexual men - New York City and California. *MMWR 30,*305-308.

Adams, H., Ashford, W., Potts, D.W., *et al.* (1981). Spectinomycin resistant penicillinase-producing *Neisseria gonorrhoeae* - California. *MMWR 30,* 221-222.

Lerner, A.M. (1981). Infections with Herpes simplex virus. *In* Harrison's Principles of Internal Medicine, 9th Ed. (K.T. Isselbacher, R.D. Adams, E. Braunwald, R.G. Petersdorf, and J.D. Wilson, eds.), p. 847-852. McGraw-Hill Book Company, New York.

SYPHILIS

Jacques E. Mokhbat

Department of Medicine
University of Minnesota
Minneapolis, Minnesota

EPIDEMIOLOGY

Syphilis is the third most frequently reported communicable disease in the United States. In a survey of STD clinics, syphilis ranked seventh in all recognized sexually transmitted diseases, accounting for an average of 1.5 cases per 100 visits to the clinics. The trend of reported primary and secondary syphilis has changed several times during the past 40 years. After a dramatic decrease in the late 1940's, the average reported case rate in the U.S. is 10 to 15 per year per 100,000 population, while the rates of latent and late syphilis average 30 cases per year per 100,000 population. In 1980, 27515 cases of primary and secondary syphilis were reported, representing an increase of about 10% over 1979. The number of unreported cases has been estimated to be two or three times greater.

The reported incidence of syphilis appears higher in non-whites than in whites and in urban than in rural areas. These differences partly reflect the fact that indigent urban racial groups are treated in public clinics where case reporting is complete.

Syphilis is most common in the sexually active years peaking between 20 and 24 years of age, with a range of most new cases occurring between 15 and 40 years of age. The male-female ratio of early cases is about 2 to 1 in the U.S.

Interviews of patients with early syphilis disclose an average of 2.8 contacts at risk per patient and about 50% of these contacts will become infected. This leads to the discovery of a cluster which is especially common in homosexuals. Since a number of these contacts will be incubating the disease, "epidemiologic"

treatment of all recently exposed persons regardless of their
symptomatology has been strongly recommended. Other important
data for the epidemiologist have been the serologic testing
of pregnant women, hospital admissions, military recruits and
pre-marital screening.

A relatively new aspect is the increased incidence in homosexual men. A recent report from the CDC (Henderson 1977)
indicates that nearly half the male patients with primary,
secondary or early latent syphilis claim homosexual or bisexual
contact. This increased risk is related to the anonymity and
large number of patients. Another factor is the difficulty in
diagnosing early syphilis in gays because of the common location
of chancres in the anorectal area, because of the atypical
presentation such as a painful superinfected chancre and because
of the failure to suspect syphilis in the evaluation of an anal
lesion in men. Female homosexuals have a lower prevalence of
STD because of the absence of male urethra, the virtual absence
of anonymity in lesbian sexual intercourse and the much lower
number of partners.

The overwhelming majority of cases are acquired by sexual
contact with highly infectious lesions such as the chancre, the
mucous patches or the condylomata lata. Other modes of transmission are much rarer; they include transfusions of blood or
blood products which is very rare because of the serologic
screening of blood donors and of the non-survival of *Treponema
pallidum* for more than 24-48 hours in stored blood. Syphilis can
also be transmitted through accidental direct inoculation by
needle or infected clinical material. Congenital infection
occurs most frequently by transplacental transmission almost
exclusively in the last five months of pregnancy. There are few
reported cases of infection of the neonate while passing through
the birth canal.

CLINICAL MANIFESTATIONS

Syphilis has always been described as the "great imitator"
of infectious diseases and dermatological ailments.

Primary Syphilis

The classical primary chancre begins at the site of inoculation as a painless papule, within 3 to 90 days of the infection,
most commonly within three weeks. It quickly erodes, becomes
indurated with a cartilaginous consistency and is typically
painless, unique, without discharge. Chancres can occasionally
be multiple or painful with discharge when superinfected. The
most common site is the external genitalia but has been des-

cribed in the cervix, anal canal, oral mucosa and in almost any
mucocutaneous site. An inguinal lymphadenopathy appears within
one week of the lesion, is bilateral, painless, nonsuppurative.

The chancre heals within 3-4 weeks (range 2-12 weeks) and
leaves no or a minimal scar. The lymphadenopathy usually persists
for months.

The differential diagnosis is with genital herpes, chancroid
and traumatic supra-infected genital lesions, all with which
syphilis can coexist. Other diseases are early condyloma acumin-
ata, LGV, granuloma inguinale, cutaneous tuberculosis and other
mycobacterial infections, tularemia, rat-bite fever, squamous
cell carcinoma, cutaneous amoebiasis.

Secondary Syphilis

Secondary syphilis usually follows the onset of the chancre
by 9 to 90 days (average 21 days). In 24% of the cases, this
secondary stage relapses during the following 5 years with 85% of
relapses occurring during the first two years. Condyloma lata
are particularly common during these relapses.

TABLE 1.   *Secondary Syphilis*

<u>*Early constitutional symptoms*</u>   *70%*
    Headache
    Fever (even FUO)
    Arthralgias
    Sore throat
    Nasal discharge, lacrimation
    Pruritus (rare)

<u>*Lymphadenopathy*</u>   *85%*
    Diffuse, rubbery, symmetrical, painless, small
    Areas (by frequency):   inguinal
                           cervical and occipital
                           axillary
                           epitrochlear (most characteristic)

TABLE 1 continued on following page

TABLE 1. *Secondary Syphilis (cont.)*
Skin and mucous membranes   90%

Lesion	Description	Distribution
macular rash (roseola)	rosy red macules fades in 2 weeks	trunk, shoulders, inner thighs
maculopapular	coppery red	face, chest, back, abdomen, flexor surfaces of forearms, palms and soles
mucous patches	grayish white erosion with an erythematous raised border	lips, tongue, gums, buccal mucosa, palate, pharynx, glans, foreskin, labia
papular	large brownish red papules or follicular, sometimes papulosquamous or annular	same distribution as maculopapular + moth eaten nonscarring alopecia of scalp, beard, eyebrows
condylomata lata	hypertrophic, purplish, flat-topped, moist, coalesced papules	moist areas (mucocutaneous junctions and intertriginous)
pustular	necrotic papules	generalized, periungeal, palms and soles

CNS
   Asymptomatic
   Symptomatic: Meningismus
                 "Aseptic meningitis"
                 Cranial nerve involvement (II-VIII)
      Eyes: Anterior uveitis   5-10%
Other
   Immune complex glomerulonephritis and nephrotic syndrome
   Hepatitis
   Intestinal ulcerations and infiltrations
   Arthritis, periostitis

Latent Syphilis

    The diagnosis of latent syphilis is made by the discovery of
a positive treponemal serologic test in the absence of any other
manifestation of syphilis. It is divided into early (2-4 years)
during which relapses of secondary lesions can occur.   The
patient is usually infectious. Late latent syphilis is usually
characterized by relative resistance to infection and absence

of relapses. The patient is usually non-infectious, although
rare instances of transmission transplacentally or via blood
transfusions have been reported.

Late (or Tertiary) Syphilis

If left untreated, up to 28% of patients will develop
symptomatic tertiary syphilis. This includes three major syndromes, which can coexist: neurosyphilis, in 6.5%; cardiovascular
syphilis, in 10%; benign tertiary syphilis or gummas in 16%.

TABLE II. Presentation of Late (or Tertiary) Syphilis

Neurosyphilis
    Asymptomatic: 20-30% of untreated patients
            CSF: high protein level
                  pleiocytosis
                  positive serology
    Symptomatic: 6.5% of untreated patients
        -Meningovascular   5-10 years after onset
            Seizures: focal
                        generalized
            Stroke
            Transverse myelitis
        -Parenchymatous
            General paresis   15-20 years
                changes in personality, megalomania,
                    delusions; illusions
                hyperreactive reflexes
                Argyll-Robertson pupils
                optic atrophy
            Tabes dorsalis   25-30 years
                ataxia, Romberg
                paresthesia (lightening pains)
                impotence
                bladder disturbances
                areflexia
                loss of pain and temperature sensation
                Charcot joints, mal perforans (rare)
                cranial nerves (II)
Cardiovascular   10.4% of untreated patients
    Aortic insufficiency
    Aortic ectasias (particularly ascending thoracic aorta)
    Coronary artery stenosis
     (now very rare)

TABLE II continued on following page

TABLE II.   Presentation of Late (or Tertiary) Syphilis
            (continued)

Gummas
    Skin: painless nodule, ulceration, arciform scar, mucosae
    Bone: pain, pathologic fractures, joint destruction
    Upper respiratory tract: nasal septal perforation
                              palatal perforation
    Gummatous hepatitis: FUO, cirrhosis

Congenital Syphilis

    See Table III.

TABLE III.   Manifestations of Congenital Syphilis

Abortion
Stillborn
Latent infection
Neonatal disease:
    434 cases reported in 1978 (6.4% decrease since 1977)
    - Mucocutaneous: rhinitis (snuffles)
                      bullae, vesicles
                      diffuse papulosquamous desquamative rash
                      mucous patches, condylomata lata
    - Skeletal: osteochondritis
                 periostitis (progressive)
                 saddle nose, saber shin
    - Hepatosplenomegaly, jaundice
    - Thrombocytopenia, leucocytosis
    - Anemia and paroxysmal cold hemoglobinuria
    - Immune complex glomerulonephritis and nephrotic syndrome
Later manifestations (after 6-12 months)
    - Interstitial keratitis with deep vascularization of
        cornea (age 5-25)
    - Deafness
    - Recurrent arthropathies (Clutton's joints)
    - Hutchinson's teeth, Moon's molar
    - Frontal bossa, poor maxillary development
    - Rhagades
    - Neurosyphilis
    - Gummas

LABORATORY DIAGNOSIS

Darkfield Examination

Darkfield examination of fresh lesions in primary, secondary
or early congenital syphilis is the most important tool in confirming the diagnosis. Syphilis should not be ruled out until
three examinations have been negative on three successive days.
Some suggest to repeat this examination weekly until the diagnosis is made. The application of antiseptic solution on the
lesion will immobilize the treponema and falsify the diagnosis.

Serology

The value of serology is unquestionable. Forty-three million
tests for syphilis were performed in the U.S. in 1977, 1.5
million of which were positive.

TABLE IV. Untreated Syphilis

	Primary	Secondary	Late latent	Late (tertiary)
VDRL	76%	100%	70%	70%
FTA-ABS	86%	100%	96%	97%
TPI	53%	98%	89%	93%

Non-treponemal. These are based on the detection of antibodies (reagin) directed against purified cardiolipin combined
with lecithin. The most commonly used are the flocculation
tests, namely the VDRL, RPR (rapid plasma reagin) and the ART
(automated reagin test). Initially nonreactive in early syphilis,
they convert 4-8 weeks after the infection. They are almost always positive in secondary and early latent syphilis, with a
considerable decrease in their sensitivity in the late and late
latent phases.
Quantitative nontreponemal tests are useful in assessing
activity of disease and response to treatment. A rising titer
may indicate a recently acquired infection, a reinfection or a
relapse in serofast individuals. A patient with early latent
syphilis will respond to treatment by decreasing his titers to
seronegativity in two to four years while a patient in late
latent phase may become very slowly seronegative in 44% of
patients within 5 years with 56% remaining persistently positive.

Quantitative testing is helpful in differentiating congenital syphilis from passive transplacental transfer of reagins. A non-infected infant will see his titer rapidly decline to sero-negativity within three months; it may also mean that the mother and the infant are responding favorably to a treatment given to the mother during pregnancy. A large number of infected neo-nates can be non-reactive at birth and start to show positive serology at 4-12 weeks of age. In treated congenital syphilis, the titers may fluctuate without any relationship to disease activity.

In seronegative primary syphilis, treatment can prevent sero-conversion, although some may show a transient reaginemia. In seropositive primary syphilis or in secondary phase, the non-treponemal tests usually revert to seronegativity within one and two years, respectively, after treatment. In late latent and late syphilis, although the titers bear minimal relation-ship to disease activity, a fourfold increase in titer should prompt retreatment.

A prozone reaction is found in 1-2% of secondary syphilitics and leads to false negative tests. This is alleviated by serial dilutions of the serum. False positive reactions are reported in 3 to 40% of positive tests.

TABLE V. Acute False Positive Serology (<6 months duration)

Infections due to:	*Bacteria: pneumococcal, chancroid, scarlet fever, rat bite fever*
	Protozoa
	Viruses: measles, chickenpox, infectious mononucleosis, hepatitis
	Chlamydia: LGV
	Mycoplasma
	Rickettsiae
	Spirochetal: leptospirosis, relapsing fever
Immunizations (smallpox)	
Pregnancy	

TABLE VI.   Chronic False Positive Serology (>6 months)

Leprosy
Tuberculosis
Malaria
Infective endocarditis
Trypanosomiasis
Drug addiction
Blood transfusions
"Old age"
Autoimmune disorders :   Lupus
Rheumatoid arthritis
MCTD
Hasimoto's thyroiditis
Various diseases with hypergammaglobulinemia

Treponemal Tests. These are useful in confirming the diagnosis in a patient with unclear history and positive VDRL, in detecting false positive VDRL and in patients who have a negative VDRL but in whom syphilis is strongly suspected such as in later stages. *Treponema pallidum* immobilization test (TPI) is the most specific but also the most difficult, dangerous and requires high technicity and a live source of treponemas. The most commonly used is the FTA-ABS using lyophilized Treponema as antigen for an immunofluorescence test. The serum is first treated with extract of cultivable Reiter's treponemes containing group antigens to prevent cross reactions with group antibodies.

This test is not quantified but is evaluated on the intensity of fluorescence and therefore is relatively subjective.

FTA can be negative in 18% of early syphilis and 5% in the latent or late stages.

The TPHA (Treponema pallidum hemagglutination test) is less expensive, easier to perform and more specific, but less sensitive. False positive reactions are reported in pregnancy, leprosy, connective tissue diseases, infectious mononucleosis. Although seroconversion occurs later than with the FTA, it is as sensitive in the later stages of the disease.

It is important to note that the non-venereal treponematoses (yaws, pinta, endemic syphilis) give true-positive treponemal and non-treponemal serology.

TABLE VII. *False Positive FTA-ABS (rare)*

Beaded fluorescence:
  Malignancy
  SLE
  Rheumatoid arthritis
  Scleroderma
  MCTD

Borderline homogenous fluorescence:
  Discoid, systemic and drug induced lupus
  Rheumatoid arthritis
  Lymphosarcoma
  Autoimmune hemolytic anemia
  Alcoholic cirrhosis
  Pregnancy
  Herpes
  Vaccination
  Normal individuals

The FTA-ABS IgM test was developed for diagnosis of congenital syphilis but has been so far disappointing.

The CSF examination can be abnormal in the secondary stage and returns invariably to normal after standard penicillin therapy. Therefore the only indication for CSF examination is in late latent syphilis or in suspected neurosyphilis. Three tests are performed: VDRL, protein content, cell count. A reactive VDRL is almost always an indication of neurosyphilis but doesn't distinguish between active, inactive or treated disease. Disease activity can be more reliably evaluated by a high protein of more than 40 mg/dl or a cell count of more than 4 mononuclear cells per mm^3. Following treatment the cell count drops to normal within 6 months while protein count remains elevated up to two years. The CSF VDRL declines slowly and can remain reactive for years. Three to 5% of patients with neurosyphilis can have normal values in their CSF and in one series, CSF VDRL was positive in only 56.7% of 176 patients with neurosyphilis. False positive reactions seldom occur. A syphilitic with a meningitis from other etiology can have a reactive VDRL by crossing of antibodies through the choroid plexuses. Patients with tuberculous meningitis, cerebral neoplasms or medullary tumors may have reactive serology in the CSF. A CSF contaminated by blood in a traumatic lumbar puncture can also give a reactive VDRL.

TREATMENT

These are the latest recommendations of the CDC (Venereal Disease Control Advisory Committee) in 1976 (see Table VIII).

In pregnancy, the treatment is the same as for non-pregnant patients; however, if the patient is allergic to penicillin, erythromycin (stearate, ethylsuccinate or base), not tetracycline, should be used.

All patients should have a follow-up quantitative serology 3, 6 and 12 months after treatment. Patients with syphilis of more than 1 year's duration should also have a serologic testing at 24 months. Retreatment is considered when:

1) Clinical signs of symptoms of syphilis persist or recur.
2) Sustained fourfold increase in the titer.
3) An initially high titer fails to show a fourfold decrease within a year.

The Jarisch-Herscheimer reaction occurs mostly in secondary stage but also in primary or early latent disease and is thought to be due to release of endotoxin by lysis of the treponemes.

With neurosyphilis, (asymptomatic or symptomatic), some authors suggest an intravenous treatment with aqueous crystalline penicillin G 2 to 4 million units IV every 4 hours for 10 days, or the addition of probenicid to the Procaine penicillin protocol.

CONCLUSION

One interesting aspect is that it is possible that a large number of cases of syphilis are aborted by the early penicillin treatment of gonorrhea, frequently coexisting and therefore preceding syphilis. It is possible that with the increasing numbers of resistant gonococci requiring non-penicillin treatment such as spectinomycin, we start seeing an increase in the cases of early syphilis.

TABLE VIII. Treatment Schedules for Syphilis

	1st choice	Penicillin allergy
Early Syphilis (Primary, Secondary or latent less than 1 year's duration)	*Benzathine penicillin G 2.4 million U IM (one dose)* OR *Aqueous procaine penicillin G 600000 U IM daily for 8 days* OR *Procaine penicillin G in oil with 2% aluminum monostearate 2.4 million U followed by 1.2 million U for 2 subsequent visits 3 days apart*	*Tetracycline 500 mg 4 times per day for 15 days* OR *Erythromycin 500 mg 4 times per day for 15 days*
Late latent, cardiovascular, late benign, neurosyphilis	*Benzathine penicillin G 2.4 million U IM weekly for 3 successive weeks* OR *Aqueous procaine penicillin G 600000 U IM daily for 15 days*	*Tetracycline 500 mg 4 times a day for 30 days* OR *Erythromycin 500 mg 4 times a day for 30 days*
Congenital Syphilis Abnormal CSF	*Aqueous crystalline penicillin G 50000 U/Kg IM or IV in two divided doses daily for at least 10 days* OR *Aqueous Procaine penicillin G 50000 U/Kg IM daily for at least 10 days*	
Normal CSF	*Benzathine penicillin G 50000 U/Kg IM one dose*	

REFERENCES

Center for Disease Control. (1976). Syphilis: Recommended treat-
    ment schedules. *Ann. Int. Med. 85,* 94-96.
Chapel, T.A. (1978). The signs and symptoms of secondary syphilis.
    Sex. Transm. Dis. 5, 68-70.
Clark, E.G., Danbolt, N. (1964). The Oslo study of the natural
    course of untreated syphilis. *Med. Clin. N. Am. 48,*
    613-623.
Dunlop, E.M.C., Al-Egaily, S.S., Houang, E.T. (1979). Penicillin
    levels in blood and CSF achieved by treatment of syphilis.
    JAMA 241, 2538-2540.
Felman, Y.M., Nikitas, J.A. (1980). Syphilis serology today.
    Arch. Dermatol. 116, 84-89.
Fiumara, N.J., Giunta, J.L., Collins, P.S. (1978). Nasolabial
    condylomata lata: Report of a case. *Sex. Transm. Dis. 5,*
    112-114.
Fiumara, N.J. (1979). Serologic responses to treatment of 128
    patients with late latent syphilis. *Sex. Transm. Dis. 6,*
    243-246.
Fiumara, N.J. (1980). Treatment of primary and secondary syphi-
    lis: serological response. *JAMA 243,* 2500-2502.
MMWR *28*:61-63, 1979; *28*:433-434, 1979; *29*:632, 1981.
Owen, W.F. (1980). Sexually transmitted diseases and traumatic
    problems in homosexual men. *Ann. Int. Med. 92,*
    805-808.
U.S. Department of Health, Education and Welfare. (1968).
    Syphilis, a synopsis. Public Health Service No. 1660.

PART II
GASTROINTESTINAL AND INTRAABDOMINAL INFECTIONS

DIARRHEA IN THE NON-TRAVELER
WORK-UP AND TREATMENT

Sam T. Donta

Department of Medicine
University of Iowa and Iowa City
Veterans Administration Medical Center
Iowa City, Iowa

I. EPIDEMIOLOGIC FACTORS

A. *Age, Seasonal, and Geographic Variations*

Diarrhea in the indigenous population may be caused by factors and etiologic agents similar to those experienced by travelers. Depending on the geographic area, there will be differences in the incidence of diarrhea due to a particular agent. Diarrhea associated with *Yersinia enterocolitica*, for example, is more prevalent in the Scandinavian and Canadian countries than it is in the United States and Central America. Certain viruses (e.g., Norwalk agent) may be more prevalent in some areas, while unrelated viruses prevail in other areas. Whereas toxigenic *E. coli* appears to be a common cause of diarrhea in Central American countries, its importance in the United States is essentially restricted to the Southwest.

Infants appear to have a high incidence of rotavirus-associated diarrhea. These viruses have been reported to cause diarrhea in older children and adults, although other viruses are probably of greater importance in these older age groups. The susceptibility of neonates and infants to diarrheal disease of any etiology appears to be generally greater than older age groups. Diarrhea associated with *Clostridium difficile* appears to have a greater prevalence among older patients (mean age of 55 yrs), even though this organism and its toxin can be found in asymptomatic infants.

Different seasons are sometimes associated with higher inci-
dences of particular etiologic agent-induced diarrheal disease.
Cholera, for example, follows the rainy seasons, and entero-
viruses are more prevalent in the summertime in the United States.
In general, sporadic diarrheal disease is more prevalent during
the warmer months.

B. Food Poisoning

Epidemic diarrhea is most frequently associated with an
infected, common-source, food. Throughout the world, the three
major etiologic agents appear to be *Staphylococcus aureus*,
Clostridium perfringens, and *Salmonella sp.* Food poisoning due
to *S. aureus* is a result of contamination of food by the handler,
with subsequent multiplication of the organism and enterotoxin
production if the food is not properly refrigerated. The enterotoxin is acid-stable and is absorbed in the proximal gut, and
evokes a central nervous system-induced vagal response, resulting
in a clinical syndrome characterized by prominent vomiting, as
well as diarrhea.

Food poisoning associated with *C. perfringens* and *Salmonella sp.* is the result of residual contamination and subsequent
growth of the organisms in improperly stored foods. With *C.
perfringens*, it is impossible to rid the meat of spores, which
can germinate under room-temperature conditions. Similar problems with spores occur with *Bacillus cereus*, an important cause
of grain-associated food poisoning.

There are numerous other microbial and chemical causes of
food poisoning. Table I lists only the major etiologic agents
along with their usual implicated food sources.

TABLE I. Etiologic Agents of Food Poisoning

Organism	Usual Food Source
S. aureus	Salads, Custards, Creams
C. perfringens	Roasts, Gravy
Salmonella sp.	Poultry
V. parahemolyticus	Shellfish
B. cereus	Grains, Cereals
C. botulinum	Canned Vegetables, Smoked Fish

II.   PATHOPHYSIOLOGY OF THE DISEASE

A.   *Establishment of Infection*

Ingested organisms and toxic materials must survive the host's defenses, as discussed in the chapter on traveler's diarrhea. With the exception of staphylococcal enterotoxin and botulinum toxin, the other toxins are susceptible to inactivation by gastric acid. It may be, however, that some ingested toxin is able to escape inactivation because of the presence of food and other buffering agents.

Organisms differ both in their intrinsic virulence and in their host range. Thus, *Shigella dysenteriae* is more virulent than *Salmonella sp.*, which is more virulent than either *E. coli* or *V. cholerae*. Cholera and shigellosis appear to affect only higher primates, and even *E. coli* has a restricted host range. In contrast, salmonellosis is a disease of most vertebrates, although considerable host-specificity often exists.

Some of the restrictions in host-range and tissue tropism may be related to the presence or absence of specific receptors for the attachment of microorganisms. *E. coli* bearing K88 fimbrial antigens will only attach to porcine intestine, whereas those bearing K99 antigens attach only to bovine epithelium. Although the mechanisms underlying specific tissue tropism remain to be identified, there appear to be preferential sites of colonization for different organisms (e.g., duodenum-giardia, strongyloides; jejunum and ileum-*E. coli*, *V. cholerae*; colon-shigella, ameba).

Once colonization is established, the pathogen may secrete a toxin or invade tissues, and the associated clinical syndrome is often related to the particular virulence mechanism.

B.   *Secretory vs. Inflammatory Diarrhea*

The possible mechanisms mediating a secretory or inflammatory diarrhea are discussed in the chapter on traveler's diarrhea. In Table II are listed the usual causative agents of infectious diarrhea and their associated virulence mechanisms.

TABLE II.   Infectious Agents of Diarrhea

Organism	Secretory	Inflammatory
S. aureus	+	-
C. perfringens	+	-
Salmonella sp.	?	+
V. parahemolyticus	+	-
B. cereus	+	-
V. cholerae	+	-
E. coli	+	(rarely)
Shigella sp.	(rarely)	+
Yersinia enterocolitica	+	(sometimes)
Campylobacter fetus	+	+
Giardia lamblia	+	-
Ent. histolytica	-	+
Viruses	(sometimes)	+

III.   CLINICAL FEATURES

As previously discussed, organisms associated with secretory diarrheas will be more likely to be associated with clinical syndromes of watery diarrhea in the absence of fever and inflamed bowel mucosa.   In most cases, these disorders are self-limited and non-debilitating, and patients have generally recovered in 3-5 days.   It is with the inflammatory disorders that the etiologic agent needs to be identified, as antibiotic therapy may be needed to abort the clinical syndrome.

IV.   DIAGNOSTIC CONSIDERATIONS

In patients with suspected inflammatory diarrhea, fresh fecal material should be examined for the presence of WBCs and trophozoite forms.   Stool cultures should be ordered, and special procedures instituted for the detection of campylobacter, vibrios, and yersinia.   Stool cultures will not be helpful in the diagnosis of food poisoning due to S. aureus or C. perfringens, nor in the detection of enteropathogenic E. coli (both toxigenic and invasive); special tissue culture and other assays will be needed to detect the virulence products of these agents.   Examination of duodenal aspirates may be helpful in finding the giardia.   Radiographic procedures may be helpful in the diagnosis of colitis, but care should be exercized in the performance of Barium enema examinations, and these procedures should be done only after adequate examination of the stools and colonic mucosa with sigmoidoscopy.

V. TREATMENT

A. *Supportive Measures*

The mainstay of therapy is fluid replacement. Fluids containing salts and glucose should help restore the body's losses.
In infants and elderly, debilitated, individuals, intravenous
fluid replacement may be needed to avert hypovolemic shock and
renal failure. Glucose or sucrose in oral fluids is especially
useful, as its absorption is unimpaired by the action of enterotoxins and its absorption carries with it obligatory water
transport.

The use of antimotility agents carries with it the risk of
increasing the severity or prolongation of the enteric disease,
by allowing the organisms and toxic products to be retained for
longer periods of time. Antimotility agents are probably less
harmful in the secretory, non-inflammatory diarrheal states.

Adsorptive agents such as kaolin-pectin mixtures may help
reduce stooling, but their use is probably better restricted to
the secretory diarrheas.

Restoration of the normal flora is a highly desirable goal,
but this objective is not easily achieved by exogenous therapy.
The use of lactobacillus preparations, even that utilizing the
human strains (*L. acidophilus*) has not proven to be very
effective.

Specific antimicrobial therapy may be indicated for some of
the inflammatory disorders. Although great controversy still
exists about the use of any such agents in salmonellosis, these
agents may need to be used for more severe cases of salmonella
gastroenteritis, and in disorders associated with persistent or
extensive disease. In Table III are listed some suggested
regimens.

TABLE III. Antimicrobial Therapy of Diarrhea

Etiologic Agent	Antimicrobial Regimen (Adults)
Shigella sp.	Ampicillin 2 gm daily x10-14 days or Trimethoprim/Sulfamethoxazole 2 tabs daily x10-14 days
Campylobacter fetus	Erythromycin 2 gm daily x10-14 days
Salmonella sp.	Ampicillin 2 gm daily x14 days or Trimeth/Sulfa 2 tabs daily x14 days
Giardia lamblii	Metronidazole 750 mg daily x10 days
Ent. histolytica	Metronidazole 750 mg daily x10-14 days (may need repeat treatment, or additional agents)

DIARRHEA IN TRAVELERS
CAUSES, PREVENTION, AND THERAPY

Sam T. Donta

Department of Medicine
University of Iowa and Iowa City
Veterans Administration Medical Center
Iowa City, Iowa

I. GENERAL CONSIDERATIONS

A. *Epidemiology of Disease*

Diarrhea in travelers may be the result of either exogenous or endogenous factors. While greater emphasis has been placed on disease caused by the ingestion of foreign substances or organisms, it is apparent that this means of disease acquisition is not solely responsible for traveler's diarrhea. The stress of travel, the exposure to new diets and climates, and a variety of other factors associated with travel probably induce changes in the composition of the intestinal microflora, and perhaps in intestinal function, that somehow is translated into diarrhea. It should not be surprising, therefore, that in only 25%-45% of cases can an etiologic agent be readily identified.

Depending on the geographic area, the traveler may be exposed to particular potential pathogens. Exposure to *Vibrio cholerae*, for example, is more likely to occur in certain areas of the Near East and Africa than it is in the Mediterranian and the Americas. Exposure to non-cholera vibrios (e.g., non 0-1 *V. cholerae*, *V. parahemolyticus*) is also more likely to occur in certain coastal areas than in inland regions. In general, travel to tropical areas is associated with higher rates of traveler's diarrhea than is travel to more temperate and cooler climates.

The pathogens responsible for traveler's diarrhea are likely similar to those responsible for enteric disease in the indigenous population. Thus, in Central America, enterotoxigenic *E. coli* are the leading cause of severe diarrhea in a pediatric population, as well as being the most prominent pathogen associated with travel to this área (1, 2). The mechanisms of spread and reservoirs of *E. coli* need better definition. Food and water-borne transmission appear to be important, although the high carriage rate among humans in indigenous areas makes it likely that human-to-human transmission also takes place.

B. *Determinants of Organism Virulence*

In general, pathogens are thought to cause enteric disease because of their ability to produce a toxin or to be invasive. The ability to invade may be linked to certain toxins as well. In fact, the organisms must first have the ability to adhere to specific mucosal sites and to be present in sufficient numbers to successfully colonize a particular section of the intestinal tract.

The term enterotoxin has been used to describe substances elaborated by enteric pathogens that induce an intestinal secretory response. Experimentally, this is measured in ligated intestinal loop model systems. There appear, however, to be several types of toxins, some of which (e.g., cholera, *E. coli*) induce a true secretory response with little or no histopathologic changes, while others (e.g., *Shigella dysenteriae*) cause a more necrotizing response.

C. *Host-defense Factors*

In order for pathogens to cause disease, they must be able to escape the various host-defense systems. For enteric pathogens, they must be able to survive passage through gastric acid and pancreatic enzymes, and withstand the inhibitory effects of the existing microflora. Humoral immune mechanisms, both IgA and IgG, are important in prevention of attachment and in antitoxicity, and cellular immune mechanisms are important in limiting the invasive potential of the organism. Finally, the normal shedding of intestinal epithelial cells and intestinal motility help provide an exodus for the pathogens.

II. ETIOLOGIC AGENTS

The major defineable etiologic agent of traveler's diarrhea appears to be *Escherichia coli*, which is responsible for 20%-40% of cases. Many other organisms are also potential pathogens. In Table I are listed the various etiologic agents, along with their associated virulence mechanisms.

TABLE I. Etiologic Agents of Traveler's Diarrhea

Organism	Toxin	Invasive
Esch. coli	LT, ST	sometimes
Salmonella sp	?	yes
Shigella sp	cytotoxin	yes
V. cholerae	LT	no
non 0-1 *V. cholerae*	cytotoxin, LT (rarely)	no
V. parahemolyticus	?	?
Yersinia enterocolitica	ST	yes
Aeromonas sp	cytotoxin	?
Giardia lamblia	?	no
Ent. histolytica	cytotoxin	yes
Viruses	no	yes
? Campylobacter fetus	?	?

III. CLINICAL MANIFESTATIONS AND EVALUATION

A. *Pathophysiologic Correlations*

Organisms that evoke a secretory response will be associated with clinical syndromes consisting primarily of watery diarrhea for 3-4 days in the absence of other systemic symptoms or signs. In contrast, organisms which are invasive or produce cytotoxins that cause cell necrosis are likely to be associated with clinical symptoms and signs of inflammation, i.e., abdominal cramping, fever, and diarrhea that is less watery, but containing mucus or blood.

The mechanisms responsible for the secretory response appear to have been well-formulated for only toxigenic *E. coli* and *V. cholerae*. These organisms produce a heat-labile toxin (LT) that activates the adenylate cyclase system of intestinal epithelial cells, with concomitant production of cyclic AMP. The effect of cyclic AMP on intestinal cells promotes chloride excretion and inhibits sodium absorption, with associated loss of water. Some strains of *E. coli* and *Yersinia enterocolitica* produce a heat-stable toxin (ST), which activates granylate cyclase to generate cyclic GMP. Through similar effects on absorption and secretion, losses of water and electrolytes ensue.

Invasive organisms may be able to evoke a secretory response through cyclic AMP, by first causing a submucosal inflammatory response, with subsequent generation of prostaglandins and secondary activation of adenylate cyclase by these products of inflammation.

B. *Diagnostic Aids*

The clinical history should help in the classification of the diarrhea as secretory or inflammatory. Most patients with secretory diarrhea will experience a transient 3-4 day illness; hence, the physician is more likely to see patients with inflammatory illnesses that have not resolved in a few days.

For patients with diarrhea persisting for more than a few days, examination of the stool for WBCs, using Giemsa stain or methylene blue, may help further classify the diarrhea. Smears should also be done, looking for trophozoites. Stool cultures will be helpful in identifying patients with Salmonella or Shigella, but will not be useful in the diagnosis of toxigenic *E. coli* disease. Even for organisms such as vibrios, aeromonads, *Yersinia sp.*, and campylobacter, the laboratory will often need to use special procedures for their identification. Until better immunologic assay systems are developed, tissue culture assays in specialized settings will need to be used to confirm the diagnosis of toxigenic diarrhea.

IV.   THERAPEUTIC APPROACHES

A. *Prophylaxis of Infection*

It should be theoretically possible to prevent diarrhea caused by exogenous agents through proper immunization or other means of augmenting host-defenses. Because of the wide variety of agents responsible for the disease, this goal will not be totally achieved. Should common pili that are responsible for attachment of organisms be identified, it might be possible to design an effective vaccine directed at the attachment process. Otherwise, vaccines directed against whole organisms are of limited value in prevention of traveler's diarrhea. The development of antitoxic immunity may be an important means of prevention, and this area is under active study.

Short of major changes in sanitation systems and alterations in farming practices, it will not be possible to reduce the risk of exposure to large numbers of human pathogens during travel to underdeveloped nations. Attempts, therefore, to restrict dietary habits to certain foods and beverages, and to certain eating establishments will probably be of only limited value in avoiding exposure to the organisms. Nonetheless, it seems prudent to avoid drinking or using water that has not been specially processed, and to avoid eating fresh garden vegetables that are uncooked. The use of antacids and frequent meals may impair the effectiveness of gastric acid.

Adsorbents such as bismuth subsalicylate (Pepto-Bismol) and kaolin-pectin mixtures may help adsorb organisms and toxins, but their use seems rather impractical as prophylactic agents. They do appear to reduce by 50% the diarrheal attack rate.

Most of the recent publicity surrounds the use of anti-microbial agents for the prevention of traveler's diarrhea. Doxycycline (100 mg. daily) has been shown to be effective in reducing traveler's diarrhea to Africa, but its effectiveness in travelers to Central American nations still needs to be proven. Doxycycline's effectiveness may not be a direct result of its action on enterotoxigenic *E. coli*, but may represent a stabilizing effect on the intestinal microflora. In one of the African studies, there appeared to be a rebound increase in diarrhea following discontinuation of the antibiotic. And the only serious case of diarrhea developed in an individual taking doxycycline who required hospitalization for treatment of shigellosis. This problem may be magnified in parts of the world where tetracycline resistance is common. Trimethoprim/sulfamethoxazole in combination may afford broader protection, but its effectiveness needs further documentation.

B. *Therapy of Acute Illness*

Most traveler's diarrhea is self-limiting, and requires only supportive measures of fluids and rest, as indicated. Oral rehydration programs are effective for all forms of diarrhea, and the inclusion of glucose or sucrose in the fluids will help reverse water losses, as the absorption of glucose is unimpaired. The normal shedding of intestinal epithelial cells and the development of immunity help limit most cases of infectious diarrhea to 5-7 days and to make the use of antimicrobial agents unnecessary. Specific therapy for patients with shigellosis, amebiasis, giardiasis, and severe cases of salmonellosis is, however, often indicated.

REFERENCES

1. Donta, S.T., Wallace, R.B., Whipp, S.C., and Olarte, J. (1977). Enterotoxigenic *Escherichia coli* and Diarrheal Disease in Mexican Children. *J. Infect. Dis.* *135*, 482-485.
2. Merson, M.H., Morris, G.K., Sack, D.A., Wells, J.G., Feeley, J.C., Sack, R.B., Creech, W.B., Kapikian, A.Z., and Gangarosa, E.F. (1976). Travelers' Diarrhea in Mexico. A Prospective Study of Physicians and Family Members Attending a Congress. *New Engl. J. Med.* *294*, 1299-1305.

GASTROENTERITIS IN CHILDREN

Gonzalo Gutiérrez

Jefatura de Enseñanza e Investigación
Instituto Mexicano del Seguro Social
México, D.F.

Gastroenteritis or infectious diarrhea is one of the main causes of disease and death throughout the world. In the rich media with satisfactory sanitary levels, it is a frequent complaint at consultation; but oppositely to what occurs in the less affluent and ill-sanitized media, in the former, infectious diarrhea is very rarely the cause of death, whereas in the latter it constitutes the main cause of fatalities and is also one of the basic components of infantile malnutrition. This situation, and the fact that in the last decade important advances have been achieved in the knowledge of the etiopathogenesis and the treatment of this infectious syndrome, makes it necessary to review, even though briefly, certain concepts related with this entity.

I. THE DISEASE ENTITY

A. Pathogenesis

The advances in the knowledge of the etiopathogenesis of diarrheal disease and the development of new techniques for their study in the present decade have changed the concepts related with the frequency and distribution of the infectious agents that cause this syndrome, and presently we know that the microorganisms most frequently identified are the following (1,2,3):

Virus	Toxigenic bacteria	Invasive bacteria
Rotavirus	V. cholerae	E. coli
Norwalk agent	E. coli	Shigella
Coronavirus	Cl. difficile	Salmonella
Astrovirus	S. aureus	C. yeyuni
Minireovirus		Y. enterocolitica
Others		

Other bacteria	Parasites
Enteropathogenic E. coli	E. histolytica
V. parahemolyticus	G. lamblia

The frequency of these etiologic agents varies according to age, time of year and sanitary conditions fundamentally. In table No. 1 the most frequently identified etiologic agents in children in Mexico City are presented, from a study performed in 1976 and 1977 (4).

TABLE 1
INFECTIOUS DIARRHEA
PATHOGENIC AGENTS ISOLATED IN
CHILDREN IN MEXICO CITY (1976-77)

Pathogenic agent	No.	%
Rotavirus	58	17.1
Adenovirus	3	0.9
Shigella species	46	13.6
Salmonella species	41	12.1
Toxigenic E. coli	24	7.1
Toxigenic Proteus	12	3.5
Invasive E. coli	2	0.6
Toxigenic Aeromonas	0	-
G. lamblia	6	1.8
E. histolytica	7	2.1
Not identified	135	39.7

Recently, it has also been found that in children in Mexico City Campylobacter fetus is responsible for approximately 14% of cases, and it is known that Yersinia enterocolitica is responsible only in isolated cases.

In infectious diarrheas caused by bacteria, three different pathogenic mechanisms have been identified, each one corresponding to a different anatomopathologic lesion:
- Multiplication in the intestine, without invasion of the mucosa or production of enterotoxins.
- Invasion of the intestinal mucosa.
- Invasion of the submucosal tissues.

In the first category, different strains of E. coli predominate which are capable of producing at least two types of enterotoxins denominated one as thermolabile and the other as heatstable. The first has a mechanism of action similar to that of Vibrio cholerae, which exerts its pathogenic effect by stimulating adenyl-cyclase of the epithelial cell of the small intestine, causing an increase in the intracellular concentration of cyclic AMP and as a final effect it inhibits the absorption of sodium and increases the secretion of chlorides, bicarbonate, potassium, and water towards the lumen of the intestine. Such a mechanism of action of the thermostable toxin is unknown. The information to synthetize these enterotoxins is found in different plasmids or episomes that may be acquired or lost with relative ease, as well as be transferred to other bacteria by sexual conjugation, in such a way that certain strains of Klebsiella, Pseudomonas, and Proteus are known to be capable of producing diarrhea by this mechanism. More recently, another factor of pathogenicity has been discovered in different strains of E. coli, known as the colonization factor, which allows bacteria to adhere to intestinal mucosa and multiply besides, a step which is considered presently as indispensable, or at least a coadjuvant in the enteropathogenicity of bacteria of this group. This factor is also regulated by a plasmid which determines the formation of structures on the surface of bacteria known as "pili" or "fimbria".

The bacteria which are capable of invading the intestinal mucosa are various strains of the Shigella gender and certain strains of Escherichia coli which do not produce enterotoxins. The lesions are located initially in the small intestine and later in the colon, where they produce ulceration and inflammation of the mucosal epithelium; Shigella dysenteriae produces also a cytotoxic enterotoxin to the cells of the capillary endothelium; certain strains of E. coli are also capable of producing a similar toxin.

The different species of Salmonella gender penetrate the intestinal epithelium and reach the lamina propia, where they give rise to an inflammatory response of the submucous tissues of the polynuclear type, which stimulates the production of prostaglandins and in turn increases the activity of adenyl-cyclase and triggers the previously described process, which leads to the production of diarrhea.

Viruses capable of causing diarrhea, mainly rotavirus, do so fundamentally in children, by invasion and replication in the mucous epithelium of the duodenum and the upper part of the jejunum, where shortening of the villi can be observed with mononuclear infiltration of the lamina propria and cuboidal transformation of the epithelial cells. In a high proportion of these cases, there is a diminished production of saccharase, lactase, and maltase with the consequent development of intolerance to the corresponding sugars, usually during the acute phase of the disease.

Giardia lamblia produces prolonged diarrhea generally, by adhering to the duodenal mucous epithelium and E. histolytica invades the tissues of the intestinal wall in different degrees.

B. Clinical Features

The clinical findings that are observed in gastroenteritis may be grouped conventionally in four basic syndromes: diarrheal syndrome, dysenteric syndrome, infectious syndrome (5) and complications. The diarrheal syndrome is manifested as a sudden increase in the number of stools and in their liquid content; there may be blood and mucus, or they may consist fundamentally of liquid fecal matter; there may also be colics. The dysenteric syndrome is characterized by mucus and blood, with scarce fecal matter and almost always accompanied by colics, straining and tenesmus. The infectious syndrome is characterized by fever, anorexia, vomiting, and deterioration of the patient.

TABLE 2

MAIN CLINICAL CHARACTERISTICS ACCORDING TO THE ETIOLOGIC AGENT

ETIOLOGIC AGENT	INFECTIOUS SYNDROME		DIARRHEAL SYNDROME		DYSENTERIC SYNDROME	DURATION IN DAYS
	FEVER	VOMITING	BLOODY STOOLS	WITHOUT BLOODY STOOLS		
VIRUS						
ROTAVIRUS	+	+ +	−	+ +	−	5- 7
NORWALK AGENT	+	+	−	+	−	1- 2
TOXIGENIC BACTERIA						
V. CHOLERAE	−	+	−	+ + +	−	2- 7
E. COLI	−	+ +	−	+ +	−	5- 10
CL. DIFFICILE	+ +	+ +	+	+ +	−	VARIABLE*
S. AUREUS	−	+ + +	−	+	−	1 - 3
INVASIVE BACTERIA						
E. COLI	+ +	+	+	−	+ +	5- 10
SHIGELLA	+ +	+	+ +	−	+ +	2 - 14
SALMONELLA	+	+	+ +	+	−	3 - 10
C. YEYUNI	+ +	+	+ +	−	+	1 - 2
Y ENTEROCOLITICA	+	+	+	+ +	−	3 - 14
OTHER BACTERIA						
ENTEROPATHOGENIC E. COLI	+	+	+	+	−	5- 10
V. PARAHEMOLYTICUS	+	+	−	+ +	+	2 - 5
PARASITES						
E. HISTOLYTICA	+	+	+	−	+ +	5- 14
G. LAMBLIA	−	+ +	−	+ +	−	15

* SYMPTOMS GENERALLY DIAPPEAR AFTER DISCONTINUING THE ANTIBIOTIC.

These syndromes may be present simultaneously or successively in the same patient, or else the clinical picture may correspond to only one; however, in order to make the diagnosis, it is necessary to have at least the presence of diarrhea or dysentery. The frequency and intensity of the symptoms and the type of syndrome vary with the pathogenic agent, which permits the clinician a reasonable etiologic orientation; however, the margin for error is high and hence, the laboratory tests are indispensable when an etiologic diagnosis is to be established. In table No. 2 a qualitative and semiquantitative relation is presented between the clinical manifestations and the main etiologic agents.

The most frequently observed complication is dehydration and in a smaller proportion of patients septicemia may develop, as well as renal insufficiency, paralytic ileus, pneumatosis intestinalis, infarction or perforation of the intestine, the description of which is beyond the scope of this paper.

Transitory intolerance to lactose is another relatively frequent complication which may be observed in up to 60% of cases produced by rotavirus. In gastroenteritis produced by other etiologic agents, it is observed much less frequently (4).

C. Morbidity and Mortality

According to reports of the World Health Organization (6,7), gastroenteritis constitutes the main cause of death in the developing countries, representing in general terms between 20 and 30% of the mortality in those countries. In Latinamerica, the mortality rates due to enteritis and other diarrheal diseases vary between 10 and 280 per 100,000 inhabitants, which reveals the great diversity of socioeconomic levels of this region, which sometimes is considered a uniform area.

In Mexico, gastroenteritis is one of the main reasons for seeking medical attention and for hospitalization and presently occupies second place among the causes of death in the Mexican Republic. In 1974, 50,842 deaths were recorded for this cause. It is more frequent in badly sanitized areas and where malnutrition is prevalent; it predominates in infants, mainly during the first months of life, and the frequency diminishes gradually until the final stage of pre-school age; in later ages, the incidence is similar. In general terms, gastroenteritis is present in endemic form with epidemic rises.

The severity of the clinical picture and hence the mortality of this disease is related more directly with the conditions of the host than with the etiologic agent and is higher in children aged less, particularly in newborns and in young infants, as well as in malnourished children. In our country, according to different series that have been published, the lethality of gastroenteritis in hospitalized patients varies between 10 and 20% in these type of patients and in these groups of age (5).

II. DIAGNOSIS

A. Key Diagnostic Tests

The diagnosis of gastroenteritis is relatively easy to establish; the presence of acute diarrhea almost always indicates the existance of intestinal infection, especially if it is accompanied by the other clinical manifestations already mentioned. However, it must be remembered that though it is rare in our country, acute diarrhea may be of a non-infectious nature. The confirmation of an infectious enteropathogenic agent can only be made by laboratory tests. The enormous number of cases of gastroenteritis and the fact that the majority follow a benign course, curing spontaneously within a few days, make it impossible or unnecessary to practice these studies in all cases. They are only indicated in the following circumstances:

- In newborns, in children with advanced malnutrition, or in patients with immunodepressive diseases.
- When the diarrhea is very abundant and is accompanied by clinical deterioration of the patient.
- In the presence of blood and mucus in the stools.
- In the presence of severe complications.

The tests that are available to any clinical laboratory are direct microscopic examination of fecal mucus to investigate leukocytes, parasites or mycelia, and a stool culture. The first allows to distinguish the cases produced by invasive bacteria, by parasites, and the rare cases with fungi; the culture will identify enteropathogenic bacteria in approximately one third of individuals studied (8).

The technique to investigate toxigenic bacteria in the intestine of the rabbit, or of newborn rat, or by the morphologic alterations of tissue cultures; the study of the invasive capacity by inoculation in the conjunctiva of a guinea-pig (Sereny test) or in tissue cultures; the determination of serum antibodies to thermolabile toxin or to rotavirus; the identification of these by electronic microscopy, or by other procedures, are part of the new technology that has permitted a better knowledge of the infectious diarrheal diseases, but for the time being they are only reserved to specialized laboratories; it is certain that in the immediate future simple methods will be available within reach of the clinical laboratories (9).

It is important to mention that serotypification of E. coli with commercial sera that are presently available, is not clinically useful, since many of the serotypes traditionally considered as enteropathogenic have lost this characteristic, while others not considered as such have acquired it. This is due to the fact that these characteristics are determined by plasmids which may be lost or acquired.

B. Differential Diagnosis

In general terms it is not difficult to make the differential diagnosis between acute infectious diarrhea and diarrhea of another etiology: the sudden onset of the clinical picture, the characteristics of the stools and frequent presence of the infectious syndrome allow to establish the diagnosis of gastroenteritis of an infectious etiology without much difficulty in the majority of cases.

III. PREVENTION AND THERAPY

Even though at present various groups are working on the development of vaccines against the different infectious agents that are capable of causing gastroenteritis, up to this moment total success has not been achieved in this field of investigation and for that reason their prevention must be sought by environmental sanitation. In relation to this disease, there are three fundamental chapters: an adequate supply of drinking water, hygienic food and a correct elimination and handling of excreta and garbage, all this linked to campaigns of nutrition and hygiene education.

Presently it is considered that treatment of gastroenteritis must have two fundamental objectives (10):

1. The prevention and correction of dehydration, by means of the
    administration of water and electrolytes.

2. The prevention and correction of malnutrition.

The discovery that intestinal absorption of glucose and sodium are united and that the first accelerates the absorption of
water and solutes is a medical advance of great importance (11),
which has permitted the prevention and treatment of dehydration
due to accute diarrhea, by means of oral administration of glucose
solution with electrolytes. The most accepted solution is the one
recommended by the World Health Organization with the following
composition:

Sodium chloride	3.5 g.	
Potassium chloride	1.5 g.	
Sodium bicarbonate	2.5 g.	
Glucose	20.0 g.	
Water	1	liter

A number of studies have demonstrated that the oral administration of this solution in amounts varying between 25 and 100
ml/Kg at intervals of 4 to 24 hours, depending on the age and severity of the disease, may prevent dehydration or achieve rehydration in approximately 90% of cases, as long as it is not used
on patients in a state of shock or with other complications which
may contraindicate this therapeutic procedure (12,13). In infants,
it is recommendable to administer the electrolyte solution alter-
nately with plain water, breast milk, or milk formula diluted 50%,
to avoid the risk of hypernatremia.

There is no evidence to suggest that total fasting may be useful for the treatment of infectious diarrheas, whereas different
studies have demonstrated that despite the diarrhea, nutrients can
be absorbed efficiently. Therefore, the prescription of a fast
during an episode of diarrhea is an erroneous practice; it is an
important cause of malnutrition, a situation which by itself originates an increase in the frequency and severity of gastroenteritis. The correction of dehydration is usually followed by the re-
cuperation of an appetite. If the child is receiving breast milk,
he should be kept on it. If he is fed milk formula, it is convenient to dilute it 50% during periods no longer than 24 to 48
hours and then resume normal dilution. Only in cases with clinical and biochemical evidences of intolerance to lactose, should
milk be withdrawn while this complication exists. Solid food must
be given normally at all times according to the child's age, once
vomiting has ceased, when present.

Antimicrobial treatment is not indicated in a large majority
of cases (10) since they are not effective and because an important proportion of patients course spontaneously to a cure within
a few days. Their indication, efficacy and dose are expressed in
tables 3 and 4.

TABLE 3

ACUTE GASTROENTERITIS

ANTIMICROBIALS OF CHOICE BY ETIOLOGIC AGENT

MICROORGANISM	ANTIMICROBIAL	EFFICACY	INDICATIONS	DOSE
VIRUS				
ROTAVIRUS	NONE	—	—	—
NORWALK AGENT	NONE	—	—	—
TOXIGENIC BACTERIA				
V. CHOLERAE	TETRACYCLINE	LIMITED	SEVERE CASES	USUAL, DURING 5 DAYS
E. COLI	NONE	—	—	—
CL. DIFFICILE	VANCOMYCIN	PROVEN	SEVERE CASES	USUAL, UNTIL DISAPPEARANCE OF SYMTOMS.
S. AUREUS	NONE	—	—	—
INVASIVE BACTERIA				
E. COLI AND SHIGELLA	TRIMETHOPRIM-SULPHAMETHOXAZOLE / AMPICILLIN	VARIABLE	SEVERE CASES	USUAL, DURING 5 DAYS
SALMONELLA	NONE	—	—	USUAL, DURING 5 DAYS
Y. ENTEROCOLITICA	TETRACYCLINE / TRIMETHOPRIM-SULPHAMETHOXAZOLE	DOUBTFUL	SEVERE CASES	USUAL, DURING 5 TO 10 DAYS
OTHER BACTERIA				
ENTEROPATHOGENIC				
E. COLI	AMINOGLUCOSIDES / COLIMYCIN	DOUBTFUL	SEVERE CASES	USUAL, DURING 5 DAYS
V. PARAHEMOLYTICUS	FURAZOLIDONE / TETRACYCLINE	DOUBTFUL	SEVERE DYSENTERIC FORMS	USUAL, DURING 5 DAYS
PARASITES				
E. HISTOLYTICA	METRONIDAZOLE / EMETINE	PROVEN	ALL CASES	USUAL, DURING 5 TO 10 DAYS
	DIIODOHYDROXY-QUINOLINE / QUINACRINE	VARIABLE	CARRIERS	USUAL, DURING 10 DAYS
G. LAMBLIA	METRONIDAZOLE / FURAZOLIDONE	PROVEN	PROLONGED DIARRHEA	USUAL, DURING 5 DAYS

NOTE: ANTIMICROBIAL RESISTANCE IN BACTERIA, ESPECIALLY IN ENTEROBACTERIA IS VARIABLE AND IN GENERAL IT IS INCREASING.

TABLE 4
INFECTIOUS DIARRHEA
SELECTION OF ANTIMICROBIALS

CLINICAL PICTURE	CLINICAL AND LABO-RATORY DATA	MOST FREQUENT ETIOLOGY	CHOICE OF ANTIMICROBIALS
DIARRHEA WITHOUT BLOOD	— SELF-LIMITED (LESS THAN ONE WEEK). — ABSENCE OF LEOUKOCYTES IN FECAL MUCUS. — IDENTIFICATION OF PATHOGEN	ROTAVIRUS TOXIGENIC E.COLI	NONE
	— PROLONGED (MORE THAN TWO WEEKS). — IDENTIFICATION OF GIARDIA IN DUODENAL FLUID OR STOOLS.	G. LAMBLIA	QUINACRINE METRONIDAZOLE FURAZOLIDONE
	— PROLONGED, EXPLOSIVE WITH METEORISM AND GLUTEAL ERYTHEMA. — POSITIVE TESTS TO SUGAR INTOLERANCE.	DEFFICIENCY OF DISACCHARIDASES	NONE
DYSENTERY DIARRHEA WITH BLOOD	— FEVER INITIALLY, FOLLOWED BY DIARRHEA. — POLYMORPHONUCLEAR CELLS IN FECAL MUCUS — SHIGELLA IN CULTURE	SHIGELLA OR OTHER INVASIVE BACTERIA	TRIMETHOPRIMSULPHAMETHOXAZOLE AMPICILLIN
	— ABSENCE OF POLYMORPHONUCLEAR CELLS IN FECAL MUCUS. — TROPHOZOITES OF E. HISTOLYTICA.	E. HISTOLYTICA	EMETINE METRONIDAZOLE

The use of the so called "antidiarrheal drugs" like diphenoxylate and loperamide is not only unjustified, they should be proscribed, since they are inefficient and their effect of retaining water in the intestinal lumen in an apparent therapeutic effect to decrease the stools, is noxious, plus the knowledge of the frequent intoxications it produces fundamentally in children (14).

IV. PERSPECTIVES ON NEW AND FUTURE DEVELOPMENTS

Various groups of investigators in different countries are working intensely on the development of vaccines and of new diagnostic techniques within the reach of clinical laboratories which will allow the prevention and an opportune etiologic diagnosis of the gastroenteritic diseases.

Regarding the vaccines, work is proceeding in the development of immunizing agents against rotavirus, mainly toxigenic E. coli, Salmonella, Shigella, and E. histolytica (9,15,16).

Despite that prevention should be led fundamentally through sanitation, in certain countries this will be achieved only after many years, while on the other hand, even in highly sanitized countries, the frequency and severity of some cases is still high, as occurs with gastroenteritis of viral origin. Hence the potencial importance that vaccines have against the causal agents of infectious diarrhea.

REFERENCES

1. Giannella, R.A. (1981) Pathogenesis of acute bacterial diarrheal disorders. Ann. Rev. Med. 32, 341.
2. Blacklow, N.R. (1981) Viral gastroenteritis. N. Engl. J. Med. 304, 397.
3. Gutiérrez, G. (1981) Características principales de la amibiasis invasora en niños. Arch. Inv. Med. (Méx.) 11 (Supl.1) 281.
4. Muñoz, O., Coello-Ramírez, P., Serafín, F. et.al. (1979) Gastroenteritis infecciosa aguda. Etiología y su correlación con las manifestaciones clínicas y el moco fecal. Arch. Inv. Med. (Méx.) 10,135.
5. Gutiérrez, G. (1980) Gastroenteritis infecciosa. Manual de Infectología (7a.Ed.) Ediciones Médicas del Hospital Infantil de México. Mexico. p. 34.
6. Anonymous (1974) Las condiciones de salud en las Américas. Organización Panamericana de la Salud. O.M.S. Washington, D. C.
7. Puffer, R.R. and Serrano, C.V. (1975) Patterns of Mortality in Childhood. W.H.O. Washington, D.C.
8. DuPont, H.L. and Horwick, R.B. (1973) Clinical approach to infectious diarrhoeas. Medicine. 52, 265.
9. Scientific working group reports (1980) Programme for control of diarrhoeal disorders. W.H.O. Geneve. CCD/80.1.
10. Scientific working group reports (1980) A manual for the treatment of acute diarrhoea. W.H.O. Geneve. CCD/80.2.
11. Anonymous (1975) Oral glucose/electrolyte therapy for acute diarrhoea. Editorial. Lancet. 1,79.
12. Pierce, N.F. and Hirschhorn, N. (1972) Oral fluid. A simple weapon against dehydration in diarrhoea. W.H.O. Chronicle. 31, 87.
13. Palacios-Treviño, J., Jaimes-Malacara, A., Bonilla-Suárez, J. and Dumois-Muñoz, R. (1981) Rehidratación por vía bucal en niños hospitalizados de la Ciudad de México. Rev. Med. I.M.S.S. (Méx.)19, 417.
14. Montoya-Cabrera, M.A., Furuya, M.E., Palacios-Treviño, J. and Hernández-Zamora, A. (1980) Intoxicación por loperamida en niños. Gac. Med. Mex. 116, 31.
15. Levine, M.N. and Edelman, R. (1979) Acute diarrhoeal infections in infants. Epidemiology, treatment, and prospects for immunoprophylaxis. Hosp. Pract. 15, 89.
16. Sepúlveda, B. (1980) Inducción de inmunidad antimibiásica en primates subhumanos con antígeno lisosomal de Entamoeba histolytica I. Introducción. Arch. Inv. Med. (Méx.) 11 (Supl. 1) 245.

IMPORTANT PARASITIC DISEASES
OF THE GASTROINTESTINAL TRACT

Jesus Kumate

I. AMEBIASIS

Intestinal amebiasis results from the invasion of large intestine by trophozoites of Entamoeba histolytica which produce an inflammatory reaction with ulcers accompanied by diarrhea with blood and mucus in the stools.

Pathogenesis

The Trophozoites in contact with the cecal or colonic epithelium produce dissappearance of microvilli, marked alterations of cytoplasm, separation of the adjoining cells and final extrusion of the epithelial cells into the lumen with penetration of the amebae to the lamina propria. (1)

The extensive ulceration in cecum, colon and rectum is accompanied by severe inflammatory reaction which may reach deeper layers and occasionally it may occur an intestinal perforation.

There is evidence that some isoenzymes (zymodemes) of E. histolytica are significantly associated with symptomatic intestinal amebiasis whereas others are found in subclinical conditions. (2,3)

Other factors associated with pathogenicity are under study and are not completely elucidated. Some of them are: the association of intestinal microbial flora, the high-carbohydrate, low-protein diet or the high serum cholesterol levels.

Clinical Features

The most frequent clinical conditions is diarrhea with blood and mucus, accompanied by tenesmus, abdominal cramps and moderate fever. It corresponds to the recto-colonic location without - complications. In many cases the symptoms decrease in severity within 7-10 days.

In pre-school children and infants the conditions may be indistinguishable from shigella or salmonella gastroenteritis with nausea, vomiting, high degree fever and profuse diarrhea with severe dehydration.   In 1/5 children with amebiasis an additional enteropathogen coexists. (4)

The clinical spectrum of intestinal amebiasis which encompasses amebic dysentery or amebic colitis, appendicitis, ameboma and colonic perforation is presented in Table I including adults and children. (5,6)

TABLE I. Clinical spectrum of Intestinal Amebiasis

Clinical condition	Adults (3,000 cases)	Children (439 cases)
Amebic Colitis	2,805 - 94.5%	403 - 91.8%
Appendicitis	20 - 0.7%	10 - 2.3%
Ameboma	60 - 2.0%	3 - 0.7%
Intestinal Perforations	115 - 3.8%	23 - 5.2%

In other series with 450 cases, (4) 1.7% presented intestinal intussuception involving large and terminal small intestine.

In pre-school children and infants with severe proteincalorie malnutrition cutaneous and gastrointestinal hemorrhages are more frequent then in well-nourished children of the same age.

In amebic appendicitis common findings are an edematous cecum, appendix perforation, spastic colon and clinical and laboratory signs of hepatic dysfunction or hepatic abscess. In ameboma there coexists an episode of amegic colitis with an abdominal mass shich mimics an intraabdominal neoplasia. It is more frequent in adults and the usual localizations are the cecal and sigmoidal regions.

In colonic perforations, the ulcer with submucosal involvement evolves through stages which comprise necrosis of myenteric plexuses with marked colonic dilatation, paralytic ileus and septic shock. This condition previous to perforation is called "toxic colon".

The colonic perforation corresponds to acute peritonitis with abdominal tenderness, cutaneous abdominal hyperesthesia, marked dilatation of colon and small intestine, dissappearance of hepatic dullness and signs corresponding to septic shock. In one third of the cases there is hepatic amebiasis with multiple abscesses.

Morbidity and Mortality

Information on attack rates are non-existent or unreliable due to under- and overdiagnosis of clinical intestinal amebiasis. Microbiologic examination of stools from children with diarrhea in Mexico results in less than 5% with trophozoites of E. histolytica.

In autopsies practiced in Latin America, amebiasis appears as the primary cause of death in 1.2% Costa Rica, El Salvador 1.4%, Colombia 3.5%, Mexico 5% and Venezuela 1.9-6.2%. (7)

Diagnosis

The diagnosis rests on the demonstration of hematophagous trophozoites, size larger than 12 μ and frequently between 30-40 μ. There is clear separation of ecto- and endoplasm and the locomotion is active and directed with several pseudopodia.

Indirect immunofluorescence and coagglutination may identify amebic antigens in recently emitted stools and are very promising as rapid, sensitive and specific tests which circumvents the morphologic pitfalls in the microscopic examination of feces.

Differential Diagnosis

From the clinical standpoint amebic dysentery may be differentiated from bacterial gastroenteritis because fever is not very elevated, nausea and vomiting are less intense and dehydration is not as marked as in salmonellosis or shigellosis. The blood and mucus in amebic stools are more abundant than in bacterial diarrheas but there is much overlapping in the proportions in both conditions.

The microscopic examination of stools must be performed with a calibrated ocular micrometer to differentiate E. histolytica and E. hartmanii which are very similar. E. hartmanii never exceeds 12 μ and E. histolytica is consistently larger. Macrophages or even polymorphonuclear leukocytes may cause confusion and it is recommended to perform periodical audits with fixed preparation which will be stained with ferric hematoxylin.

Prevention and Therapy

Prevention is possible by avoiding fecal contamination of food, water and beverages all along the way from the sources of production to transport, distribution and consumption. Personal uses in fecal toilet and hand washing are contributory factors. There are no vaccines available.

Nitroimidazoles, i.e.: Metronidazole and others, are the drugs of choice for intestinal and extraintestinal amebiasis. In children, 30 mg/kg/day x 7, by oral route divided in three doses. In adults 800 mg t.d. x 7-10 days. Other regimes use a single dose of 2.4 g during 5 days. All series are consistent in report more than 90% of successful results.

It is a common practice to associate an anti-amebic drug with activity limited to the intestinal lumen. The more active agents in this group are dichloroacetamides, i.e.: Clefamide, Diloxanide furoate and Etofamide. The recommended doses are 7,10 and 20 mg/kg/day x 7-10 for Clefamide, Diloxanide and Etofamide respectively.

In cases of colonic perforation, amebic appendicitis and ameboma, it is possible to administer Metronidazole by intravenous route. A dose of 200 mg in isotonic glucose should be administered during a 3 hour period and up to a total daily dose of 1.6 g. The addition of 2-dehydroemetine, 1.5 mg/kg/day by intramuscular route is useful to reinforce the amebicidal activity. The total daily dose must not surpase 90 mg during a maximum period of 10 days.

II   GIARDIASIS

The infection by Giardia lamblia is mainly an asymptomatic one. In acute cases it is a self-limited disease with propensity to develop malabsorption syndromes and prolonged course in immunodeficient individuals.

Pathogenesis

The infecting cysts present in water or in some foods, are usually destroyed by the gastritic acidity. However, if the inoculum is very large or there is achlorydria or marked hypochlorhydria, some may reach the duodenum where the minimum inoculum is very small: 10 viable cysts.

Multiplication of trophozoites is essential for epithelium damage through a combination of irritation of the microvilli, toxigenicity and limited invasive capacity. If the number of trophozoites is very large, they may cover an important area duodenal and jejunal segments.

As a consequence of damaged microvilli there is abnormal function of disaccharidases, peptidases and subnormal absorption of vitamins A and B_{12}.

The malabsorption mechanisms are not completely known. Some contributing factors are: bacterial overgrowth and bile salt deconjugation, a pancreatic lipase insufficiency and a high turnover rate of intestinal epithelia.

Besides the hypochlorhydric conditions, some immunodeficiences are associated with a greater risk for giardiasis or a more prolonged and severe attacks of the parasite. In athymic mice, the incidence of giardiasis is greater than in normals. The restoration of thymus functions coincides with the dissappearance of the parasites without medical treatment. It has been found the association of hypogammaglobulinemia and asymptomatic giardiasis.

Clinical Features

The acute episode is characterized by diarrhea with loose stools with foul odor, abdominal cramps, flatulence, low-grade fever, nausea and vomiting. Usually the episode subsides in 3-5 days and in many cases the etiology was not known.

It is very frequent that the clinical condition evolves to a chronic or relapsing course. The main symptoms are: diarrhea bouts, flatulence, abdominal pain, malaise, loss of weight and malabsorption manifestations.

Morbidity and Mortality

The true incidence of giardiasis is not known, in different surveys a range from 2-6% was reported, (8) as well as several water and food-borne epidemics.

Giardiasis is not a lethal condition per se but it may be a contributory factor in severe immunodeficiences.

Diagnosis

The demonstration of cysts or trophozoites is duodenal or jejunal aspirates or in stools is a sine qua non condition to establish a diagnosis. The trophozoites are more frequent in loose stools and the cysts in formed feces.

It is recommended to realize 3 stools examination in alternate days by direct microscopic observation in saline suspensions. The concentration techniques destroy the trophozoites. The percentage of positive findings increase from 70% to 90 and 98% in 1,2 and 3 examinations respectively.

If the clinical diagnosis is under heavy suspicion but the stool samples are negative, the Enterotest capsule may be useful. A gelatin capsule in which a weight has been included is attached to a 1-meter long nylon string. The patient swallows the capsule and as the gelatin is dissolved, the string reaches the duodenum when is fully extended. If Giardia trophozoites are present, they attach to the nylon and after several hours the string is removed. The fluid absorbed is squeezed into a glass slide and a greater proportion of positives is found than in the direct examination.

Duodenal aspiration biopsy with Crosby's capsule is an useful resource in cases of diagnostic problems.

Differential Diagnosis

Giardiasis is not frequently considered among the possibilities in differential diagnosis of diarrhea and the demonstration of the parasite is frequently delayed. The symptoms and signs are non-specific. However, blood and mucus are never occur and may help to differentiate from shigellosis, salmonellosis or amebiasis.

Malabsorption conditions, disaccharidase insufficiencies and prolonged diarrhea are the most fequent reasons to include giardiasis in differential diagnosis of diarrhea.

Prevention and Therapy

Contamination of water and foods are the sources of infection and its avoidance is the most effective prevention.

Quinacrine, Furazolidone and Metronidazole has been used. Quinacrine 5-10 mg/kg per day x 5 results in 90% of successes. It produces yellow discoloration conjunctival. Furazolidone 7-10 mg/kg/day x 5 is equally effective. Metronidazole 25 mg/kg per day x 5 gives satisfactory results in 80% of the cases. In comparative simultaneous studies of the three drugs, all have been shown equally active. (9)

The treatment regimes may be repeated in case of failure. In children Furazolidone is preferred and in asymptomatic - adults Quinacrine is the drug of choice. Metronidazole is forbidden in pregnant women due to its potential mutagenic and teratogenic effects. (10)

Quinacrine is used as a therapeutic test due to its lack of antibacterial activity. In suspected cases without trophozoites, quinacrine administration may produce relief of symptoms.

III TRICHURIASIS

A soil-borne helminthiasis, with high prevalence among
school children in tropical areas whose clinical manifestations
are directly associated with the number of parasites.

Pathogenesis

The ova eliminated in feces mature in the soil under proper
conditions of moisture and temperature. The embryonated eggs
ingested in foods, beverages or in contaminated hands, reach
the small intestine. After ecdysis, the larvae are located in
the microvilli and move downwards until the cecal area and
ascending colon. In 90 days the females begin oviposition.

Clinical Features

Trichuriasis is asymptomatic in persons with less than 1,000
eggs/gram of stools (10). There is a direct relation between
the number of eggs in stools and the frequency and severity of
clinical manifestations.

In patients with 5,000 or more eggs/g, diarrhea was present
in 64.3%, abdominal pain in 58.9%, blood in feces in 39.3%,
rectal prolapse in 19.6% and marked skin pallor in 46.4%.

The most characteristic sign in heavy infections is rectal
prolapse in more than 50% in cases with 100,000 or more eggs/g.

The frequent association of protein-calorie malnutrition
and blood loss contribute to anemia which in severe cases may
mimic that seen in ancylostomiasis. There is no blood eosinphi-
lia.

Morbidity and Mortality

There is a great variability in the incidence ranging from
5% in dry and cool temperatures to more than 80% in tropical
regions. Trichuriasis is not a lethal disease.

Prevention and Therapy

There are no practical preventive measures besides the improvement of environmental sanitation and personal hygiene.

The drug of choice is Mebendazole, 100 mg twice a day, by
oral route x 3, irrespective of age or body weight. Its efficacy
varies from 80% in heavy infections and close to 100% in mild
conditions.

In patients heavily infected, especially with rectal prolapse and failures after repeated courses of Mebendazole, a
retention enema with Hexilresorcinol is recommended.

Rp:

Hexilresorcinol	3 g
Arabic Gum	100 ml
Water	900 ml

The patient receive an enema the night before and other
early in the morning. The perirectal skin is covered with vase-
line due to the caustic nature of the hexilresorcinol. The enema
volume is calculated as 25 ml/kg up to a maximum of 1,200 ml,
which should be retained for several minutes.

Diagnosis

Microscopic examination of recently emitted stools by concentration techniques and quantitation of eggs/gram of stools.

Rectal prolapse is very characteristic of trichuriasis but is absent in mild infections.

IV   ASCARIASIS

The most frequent of soil-borne helminthiasis, especially in tropical areas.   A nematode Ascaris lumbricoides the etiologic agent has intestinal and systemic phases.   It has tendency to produce obstructive conditions in the gastrointestinal tract.

Pathogenesis

Ova excreted in the stools after 2 weeks in the soil, become infective.   After ingestion and hatching in the upper small intestine, they invade the intestinal epithelium and via portal vein reach the broncho-pulmonary tree and are again ingested into the alimentary tract.

Clinical Features

The intestinal phase may be subclinical or there are non-specific symptoms as: abdominal cramps, flatulence, nausea or moderate diarrhea.   If the number of parasites is very great, i.e.: more than 50,000 eggs/gram of stools, some parasites leave occasionally through the nostrils or the mouth.   It is frequent the association of anorexia, mild anemia, weight loss and failure to thrive.

In patients with heavy infection, there may occur obstructive complications due to erratic migration of the adult parasites to bile and pancreatic ducts or to the hepatic parenchyma. In some cases a bolus of tangled Ascaris may block the intestinal lumen, provoke an intestinal intussuception or produce a perforation of the appendix.

In the systemic phase sometimes appears a neumonia episode which very frequently is misdiagnosed as bacterial. It is always accompanied by intense eosinophilia.

Morbidity and Mortality

A conservative estimation is 30% for children and even higher in pre-school age.   In tropical areas it may be more than 80% in children less than 5 years age.

Intestinal ascariasis is a benign condition and only in - cases of erratic migration there is a serious clinical condition. In many cases of intestinal obstruction, conservative management makes unnecessary a surgical intervention.

Diagnosis

The presence of eggs in the stools or the elimination of adult parasites in feces or through other orifices make the diagnosis.   There are no serologic tests available.

Prevention and Treatment

It is possible to cut the trasmission chain by giving treatment to the infected population during a year; however, the magnitude of the task makes it unpractical.

Mebendazole is the drug of choice at the dose of 100 mg every 12 hours during 3 days. An alternative is Tetramisol, a single dose of 150 mg in adults or 40-80 mg in children.

V   HOOKWORM

The infection produced by two nematodes, i.e.: Ancylostoma duodenale and Necator americanus. The infective larvae penetrate through the skin and reach the upper small intestine where they suck blood and may produce a severe anemia.

Pathogenesis

The eggs deposited in soil by defecation mature in 2 weeks to produce infective larvae which may penetrate the skin after 5-10 minutes contact. In the blood they pass through the lungs and end in the duodenum and jejunum where they fix and drain blood.

Clinical Features

The acute phase is completely unrecognized by the patient. The skin penetration is asymptomatic and the pulmonary stage is very mild in comparison with ascariasis. In the intestine the blood losses are subclinical.

When the blood losses are not restored due to malnutrition or a large number of parasites, there appear 3 clinical syndromes, i.e.: digestive, anemic and circulatory.

In the digestive tract we can recognize: nausea, vomiting, anorexia and abdominal cramps. Anemia due to iron deficiency which may be a severe one with tachycardia, edema,moon-face and cardiac murmurs. The cardiovascular manifestations may be cardiomegaly, cardiac insufficiency with hepatomegaly and edema.

Morbidity and Mortality

Very variable with a decreasing trend. In tropical areas in some places it may affect 20% of young population. (12)   In severe infections and lack or improper management it may be deaths, especially in infants and pre-school children.

Diagnosis

The examination of stools and demonstration of eggs which occasionally may be confounded with those of Trichostrongylus.

Prevention and Therapy

The avoidance of fecal contamination of the soil and the use of shoes are critical to prevent hookworm disease.

Mebendazole as in Ascariasis and Trichuriasis is the drug of choice. Equally or more important than the anti-helminthic treatment are: repositive therapy for anemia, i.e.: food, iron and transfusions.

VI   ENTEROBIASIS

The infection produced by pinworms, Enterobius vermicularis through the contamination of infective larvae excreted in the stools without soil hatching or systemic stage.

Pathogenesis

The adult parasites are fixed in cecum, appendix and adyacent areas of the small and large intestine. The gravid females migrate to the rectum with a circadian rythm by night and release eggs which mature to infective larvae in few hours.

Clinical Features

Anal pruritus which may be intense, tenesmus, insomnia and irritability. The migration of females may end in appendix or Fallopian tubes with clinical condition resembling appendicitis.

Morbidity and Mortality

Very variable with a higher incidence in urban areas due to overcrowding. In pre-school and school children of low socioeconomic condition it may be larger than 50%

Diagnosis

The celophan tape early in the morning is layered in the perianal region before defecation or bathing. In some cases it is necessary to practice multiple examinations.

Prevention and Therapy

Pirantel pamoate 10 mg/kg, a single dose. In cases of skin lesions of perianal region, local application of Thiabendazole cream is very helpful.

REFERENCES

1. Takeuchi, A., and Phillips, B.P. (1975) Am.J.Trop.Med.Hyg. 24:34
2. Sargeaunt, P.G., and Williams, J.E. (1978). Trans. Roy. Soc. Trop. Med. Hyg. 72:519
3. Sargeaunt, P.G., Williams, J.E., Kumate, J., and Jimenez, E. (1980). Trans. Roy. Soc. Trop. Med. Hyg. 74: 653.
4. Kumate, J. (1979). In "Enfermedades Diarreicas en el Niño" p.237. Ed. Med. Hosp. Infant. Mex., Mexico
5. Alvarez-Cordero, R. (1971). Presse Med. 48:2171.
6. Gutierrez, G. (1972). Gac. Med. (Mex.) 103:300
7. Duque, O. (1969). Bull. Int. Acad. Path. 10:9.
8. Meyer, E.A., and Radulescu, S. (1979) In: "Advances in Parasitology" (Lumsden, Muller and Baker, Eds.) 17:1 Academic Press, London
9. Botero, D. (1978). In:"Annual Rev. Pharmacol." Toxicol. 18:1 Annual Reviews Inc. Palo Alto.
10. Goldman, P. (1980). N. Eng. J. Med. 303:1212
11. Biagi, F. (1971) In:"Enfermedades Parasitarias". La Prensa Medica Mexicana, Mexico.
12. Neves, J. (1981). In:"Doencas Infectuosas a Parasitarias em Pediatria". Guanabara Koogan, Rio de Janeiro.

BIOLOGY OF PERITONITIS

Richard L. Simmons
David H. Ahrenholz

Department of Surgery
University of Minnesota
Minneapolis, Minnesota

Bacterial peritonitis is not simply the result of bacterial contamination of the peritoneal cavity. To establish this infectious process the local host defense mechanisms must be overcome either by the bacteria, by other adjuvant substances, or by the detrimental effects triggered by the inflammatory response. We shall examine the biologic properties of the peritoneal cavity and then examine the various factors which affect the development of intraperitoneal infection.

THE PERITONEAL DEFENSES

The peritoneum is a smooth layer of flat mesothelial cells resting on a basement membrane with a deeper layer of vascularized connective tissue. This covers the viscera as the visceral peritoneum and the abdominal cavity as the parietal peritoneum. In adults, it has a surface of about 1.7 m^2. Most of this surface behaves as a passive semipermeable membrane for the exchange of water and small molecular weight solutes. Peritonitis markedly increases the exchange rates of fluid and solutes presumably by means of local vasodilitation and increased vascular permeability. Fluid may be lost so rapidly into the peritoneal cavity that hypovolemia and shock results.

On the other hand, particulate matter up to about 10 microns in diameter is principally removed from the peritoneal cavity by lymphatics. Only the lymphatics of the diaphragm appear to

participate in this activity. Von Recklinghausen (1864) reported
that small openings called stomata connected the free peritoneal
cavity with the diaphragmatic lymphatics. Subsequent workers
denied this function and proclaimed that stomata were artifacts
of fixation. But Allen (1936) in a series of elegant papers has
shown that these are functional pores. He has shown that erythrocytes injected into the abdomen of rabbits are absorbed via the
stomata into the subdiaphragmatic lymphatics and then to the
retrosternal lymph nodes. Similarly, using polystyrene beads of
graded sizes, he has shown that particles of up to 10 microns in
size are rapidly absorbed into the lymphatics and particles up to
20 microns or greater are absorbed at a lesser rate (Allen and
Westerford, 1959). More recently scanning electrom micrographs
have demonstrated the presence of the stomata and shown that they
are anatomically limited to the peritoneal mesothelium overlying
diaphragmatic lymphatics (Tsilibary and Wissig, 1977). The
stomata are located between the boundaries of adjacent cells.

Allen (1936) has shown that passive stretching of the
diaphragm causes a rapid influx of fluid into the diaphragmatic
lymphatics. Thus respiratory cycles with contraction of the
diphragm continuously remove small amounts of fluid from the
peritoneal cavity, causing an upward circulation of peritoneal
fluid. As this fluid moves upward, any small particulate matter
present is sucked into the lacunae. Numerous investigators have
demonstrated that regardless of where particles are placed within
the free peritoneal cavity, they are rapidly swept upward by
normal respiratory movements and appear in the diaphragmatic
lymphatics within a few minutes.

Bacteria are cleared from the peritoneal cavity in a similar
manner. Steinberg (1944) showed that after intraperitoneal
injection of bacteria in dogs the organisms were recoverable from
the thoracic duct lymph within six minutes and from the blood
within twelve minutes. Similarly bacteria can be recovered from
the intrathoracic lymph nodes of patients who have died of
peritonitis. In the preantibiotic period, thoracic duct drainage
was used as a method for "preventing contamination of the blood
stream by bacteria". Similarly, Fowler (1900) reported a
decreased mortality from peritonitis when the patients were placed
in the semi-upright position, presumably because the rapid
absorption of toxins was prevented. Steinberg (1944) confirmed
the delay of bacterial absorption in dogs placed head up after
i.p. injection of bacteria.

A number of factors can influence the translymphatic removal
of bacteria from the peritoneal cavity. Florey (1927) noted
that increased intraperitoneal pressure accelerated the clearance
of particulate matter whereas Mengle (1937) reported that
depression of spontaneous respiration by general anesthetic agents
decreased this clearance. He was able to accelerate particulate
clearance from the peritoneal cavity using high concentrations of
CO_2 which increased the respiratory rate.

The classic studies of Autio (1964) showed that a similar upward circulation of fluid exists in man. He injected contrast material into the abdominal cavities of patients after routine appendectomy or cholecystectomy using a catheter left at surgery. Contrast material injected into the ileocecal area rapidly accumulated in the pelvis and to a lesser degree in the right pericolic and subhepatic areas. Lesser migration was found along the left pericolic gutter to the left subphrenic space. This upward movement of material may account for the high incidence of subphrenic abscess formation after peritonitis in man.

In the preantibiotic period when many patients were treated without operation, Fowler's position may actually have decreased the mortality of peritonitis. In more recent times, the treatment of choice for peritonitis is prompt operation, with elimination of the leak and removal of gross contamination. It is possible that Fowler's position, which interferes with rapid bacterial clearance, may actually increase the incidence of post-operative abscesses in these patients. Experimentally, we have found that survival of rats with $E.$ $coli$ peritonitis is increased if the rat is maintained in the head-down position for only four hours after intraperitoneal contamination. It is also possible that positive pressure ventilation, which decreases transthoracic lymph flow, may actually impair the clearance of bacteria from the contaminated peritoneal cavity. Experimentally, this has not been confirmed, however.

In summary, rapid physical absorption of bacteria from the peritoneal cavity may constitute the first line of defense against intraperitoneal infection. When bacteria are injected into the peritoneal cavity they begin to disappear rapidly, even before the appearance of phagocytic cells. Unaltered bacteria can be recovered from the right thoracic duct fluid within six minutes in dogs (Steinberg, 1944). The bacteria are filtered out in the retrosternal lymph nodes or passed into the systemic circulation where the reticuloendothelial system clears them from the blood.

Contamination of the peritoneal cavity results in a sterotyped inflammatory response, including degranulation of mass cells with release of histamine and other vasoactive substances. These chemicals cause a local vasodilatation and outpouring fluid, rich in antibodies and other serum proteins including fibrinogen. The fibrinogen is converted to solid fibrin by local tissue thromboplastin, trapping bacteria and often sealing hollow viscus perforations. The exact role of fibrin in the establishment of peritonitis is unknown. Trapping of bacteria may prevent rapid absorption and death of the host from endotoxic shock. However trapping of bacteria within fibrin ultimately leads to abscess formation unless the bacteria filled fibrin clot is removed (Ahrenholz and Simmons, 1980). Bacterial proliferation takes place rapidly within fibrin clots and neutrophils infiltrating into the fibrin mesh seems very inefficient.

The cellular defenses of the peritoneal cavity are mobilized within hours after bacterial contamination. A rapid influx of neutrophils occurs in response to a variety of stimuli including products of bacterial growth and C_5a fraction of serum complement. These neutrophils are extremely effective bacteriocidal agents. They may consume 30 to 50 bacteria during their limited life span outside the systemic circulation. In animals undergoing a single injection of intraperitoneal bacteria, the neutrophil response peaks within 24 hours. This is followed at about this time by an influx of mononuclear cells which scavage the cavity removing any remaining cellular debris. A number of substances which act to increase the lethality of peritonitis exert their action by blockade of this phagocytic system.

If these defense mechanisms are not able to rapidly control intraperitoneal bacteria, a number of changes take place. One of these is a marked depression of the fibrinolytic system of the peritoneal mesothelium (Hau, et al, 1978). Normal peritoneal tissue have measurable levels of plasminogen which becomes converted to plasmin and is rapidly able to lyse fibrin deposits in the peritoneal cavity. Numerous factors, including infection, trauma, and sterile irritants such as starch or barium, reduce these tissue plasminogen levels below detectable levels. As a result, fibrin deposits remain in situ for days or weeks. During this time, fibroblasts proliferate and grow into the fibrin strands. This results in intraperitoneal adhesions with their long-term adverse effects. The inflammation within the peritoneal cavity also usually results in reflex small bowel ileus. Experimental work indicates that this may have some protective effect in allowing fibrin to seal a perforation. In dogs undergoing cecal ligation, the resulting infection remained localized unless peristalsis was stimulated. Peristalic stimulation resulted in dissemination of the infection and death of the animals from generalized peritonitis (Mengle, 1937).

Ongoing peritonitis also commonly results in intermittent bacteremia. Saba (1978) has shown that the alpha-2 globulin is a nonspecific opsonin for the removal of particulate matter and fibrin monomers from the blood by the RES sytem. Prolonged bacteremia results in depletion of this opsonic protein so that the RES is unable to clear these materials from the blood stream. It has been proposed that the persistance in the peripheral circulation of fibrin split products results in organ dysfunction of the lungs, heart, and kidneys. This sequence of multiple organ failure is well documented in prolonged sepsis and Saba has documented markedly decreased levels of his opsonic protein in this condition. Further replacement of the opsonic protein was able to ameliorate or completely reverse organ dysfunction in some of his patients.

THE BACTERIOLOGICAL PROBLEM

Classically, surgeons for convenience have divided peritonitis into primary and secondary peritonitis. The former is caused by a single organism (e.g. pneumonococci, E. coli, etc.) in pure culture whereas characteristically the latter is a polymicrobial infection arising most often from the perforation of a viscus. When the perforation involves the GI tract, the level of the lesion can be used to predict the most probable bacterial flora involved (Stone, et al, 1975). For example, perforations of duodenal ulcers, usually associated with high gastric acid secretions, are very frequently sterile. Perforations of gastric ulcers, associated with lower gastric acid production, may release lactobacilli, candida and anaerobic gram positive oral organisms into the peritoneal cavity. Lactobacilli and streptococci are the only organisms characteristically found in the upper jejunum. As the terminal ileum is approached the lactobacilli decrease and colonic flora including bacteroides, enterobacteriaceae, enterococci and gram positive non-sporing anaerobes come to predominate. Within the colon, water is reabsorbed and bacterial counts with 10^{11} organisms per gram are achieved. The anaerobes characteristically outnumber the aerobic organisms by 10 to 1 or more.

When the colon is first perforated, feces containing 200 or more species of bacteria are released into the peritoneal cavity. Both clinical and experimental evidence indicates that the number of species in the bacterial inoculum is rapidly reduced when it is introduced into the peritoneal cavity. Onderdonk et al (1974) implanted pooled rat cecal contents mixed with barium into the rat peritoneal cavity; and serial quantitative bacterial counts were made. At least 27 species of bacteria were cultured from the implanted fecal inoculum. Initially, the disease was characterized by free peritonitis and cultures yielded 10^6 E.coli/ml, 10^5 enterococcae/ml, and 10^6 bacteroides/ml. There was a very high initial mortality and the animals that died usually yielded E. coli in blood cultures. The animals that survived all developed indolent abscesses, which consistantly yielded B. fragilis 10^9/ml, Fusobacterium 10^9/ml, E.coli 10^8/ml and enterococcus 10^6/ml. The majority of the bacterial species including those with the highest counts in the original inoculum were rarely found after implantation (eubacteria, streptococci, lactobacilli, micrococci, and diphtheroids).

It becomes apparent that the defense systems of the peritoneal cavity provide an inimical environment for majority of bacteria released. These are rapidly eliminated and only those organisms with the greatest virulence alone or in combination survive.

Meleney et al (1932) first documented that combination of bacteria may be more virulent than single bacterial species. He found that any combination of E.coli, Clostridium perfringens, and alpha streptococci were much more lethal than any of the organisms grown in pure culture. If all were pooled together, for example, only 1/24th of the LD_{100} of each was required to produce a fatal infection in mice and guinea pigs.

Onderdonk et al (1976) have studied the interactions between Bacteroides fragilis, Fusobacterium varium, E. coli and Streptococcus faecalis (enterococcus). No single organism was sufficient to produce an abscess when implanted in a barium-sterile feces-gelatin capsule in the peritoneal cavity. Similarly combinations of the aerobes only, or anaerobes only fail to produce an abscess. However, any combination of an aerobe and an anaerobe resulted in marked abscess formation within the rats.

The mechanisms by which bacteria interact in the peritoneal cavity have been little investigated. The majority of bacterial interactions are not cooperative, but are characterized by an intense competition for the available nutrients. Several synergistic mechanisms of bacteria can also be identified: (1) one bacteria may provide a growth of factor required for growth by another bacteria, (2) one bacteria may detoxify a waste product of another organism allowing both to survive, (3) one organism may alter the environment to allow the persistance of another organism i.e. acidifying the environment or lowering the oxygen tension, (4) one bacteria may block a specific host defense mechanism, either endogenous, such as blockade of the neutrophil phagocytosis, or exogenous, such as providing an enzyme which degrades antibiotics.

Some specific examples are available. E. coli is the most commonly isolated aerobe and Bacteroides fragilis, the most commonly isolated anaerobe from clinical peritoneal infections. Coliforms have been demonstrated to lower the oxygen tension or redox potential within the peritoneal cavity and allow the germination and growth of obligate anaerobes like bacteroides. Some bacteroides organisms require Vitamin K for growth which can be secreted by E. coli and other enterobacteraceae. In turn, bacteroides organisms have been shown to produce a wide variety of excellular enzymes such as penicillinases, deoxiribonucleases, alkaline phosphatases, proteases, and lipases which digest host tissue and release nutrients for bacterial growth (Rudek and Hoque, 1976).

Ingham, et al (1977) have shown that a variety of anaerobic organisms are capable of inhibiting the phagocytosis of Proteus mirabilis in vitro by normal neutrophils although aerobic organisms do not exhibit this ability. Bacteroides melanino-genicus and Bacteroides fragilis produce the greatest inhibition. This effect may be mediated by a capsule elaborated by the anaerobic organisms.

Microbiologists have in recent years documented that the survival of many microorganisms is dependent upon their ability to adhere to surfaces. Recently Onderdonk (1978) has demonstrated increased adherence for peritoneal mesothelium in Bacteroides fragilis strains which elaborate capsule compared to those which

do not. Since the B. Fragilis organisms are able to fix to
peritoneal mesothelium perhaps normal peritoneal clearance
mechanisms fail, allowing bacteroides to persist and cause intraperitoneal abscesses.

THE ROLE OF ADJUVANT SUBSTANCES

Large numbers of a single bacterial species can be cleared
from the peritoneal cavity without long term adverse effects.
However, the addition of many, but not all, foreign substances
will increase the lethality of a given bacterial inoculum. These
include increased necrotic tissue, Barium salts, gastric mucin,
bile and hemoglobin. Of these, hemoglobin has received the
greatest attention as an adjuvant substance.
Evidence strongly suggests that the bacterial inoculum and
the hemoglobin must co-exist within the peritoneal cavity for the
adjuvant effect of hemoglobin to be demonstrable, and that hemoglobin has no systemic toxic effect which makes the animals
susceptible to intraperitoneal bacteria. We have recently
reviewed this problem. Red cell stroma seem to inhibit neutrophil
motility, phagocytosis, and bacterial killing. The hemoglobin
released from lysed red blood cells is a potent adjuvant because
it can supply iron essential for bacterial proliferation (Lee and
Simmons, 1981).

DETRIMENTAL EFFECTS OF THE INFLAMMATORY RESPONSE

Phagocytosis and killing of bacterial organisms by neutrophils
is essential for host survival after any serious bacterial contamination of the peritoneal cavity. Neutropenic animals tolerate
intraperitoneal contamination poorly; but the neutrophil has
paradoxical effects in inflammation. The neutrophil is a fairly
efficient bactericidal machine but its capacities can be overcome
when the number of bacteria are too great or when conditions are
not favorable for bactericidal activity. Under these circumstances normal inflammatory defenses can be detrimental to the
host. For example, locomotion and phagocytosis by the neutrophil
is best accomplished on a surface, and floating bacteria are
difficult to engulf. Inflammation is, however, accompanied by
fluid influx and the surgeon may add fluid so that resident
bacteria cannot be efficiently killed.
Fluid accumulation in the peritoneal cavity is detrimental to
host defenses in other ways as well. The oxygen tension of the
fluid within the peritoneal cavity depends on close proximity to
peritoneal capillaries. When fluid accumulates in the peritoneal
cavity, the poor solubility of oxygen results in depressed redox

potential. Bacteria survive because neutrophils require oxygen
for their optimal killing. The peritoneal cavity becomes like a
huge abscess that is full of growing bacteria and dying neutrophils, isolated from a good blood supply.

Although the principal function of neutrophils is to kill
bacteria, neutrophilic enzymes are capable of digesting all
living tissue. A number of mechanisms release neutrophil enzymes
into tissue. Extracellular release of neutrophil granule enzymes
is exaggerated during the attempted phagocytosis of large
particles, such as particulate intestinal contents. Neutrophils
crawling along fibrin strands may release their enzymes either
because of a kind of frustrated phagocytosis, in an attempt to
engulf the fibrin, or because of activated complement in the
interstices of the fibrin web. Furthermore, factors in inflamed
areas such as leukocidin of Staph. aureus may kill neutrophils
and augment the autodigestion of normal tissue. Support for this
idea that autodigestion by neutrophilic enzymes may truly occur
in peritonitis has been shown by Ohlsson (1976) who found large
amounts of neutrophilic collagenase and elastase in the peritoneal
fluid of patients with diffuse peritonitis.

In short, the peritoneal cavity can itself become a virtual
abscess cavity if there is an imbalance between the number of
bacteria, the amount of fluid, local pH changes, hypoxemia, and
a balance between the activators and inhibitors of neutrophilic
enzymes. True abscess cavities develop necrosis of surrounding
tissue because of the activity of the neutrophilic enzymes; they
do not occur in the absence of neutrophils. Miles, Miles and
Burke (1957) showed the existence of a crucial period in the first
four hours of bacterial infection. If the bacteria are killed
within this 4-hour period the inflammatory response was aborted.
If the bacteria are killed after a large number of neutrophils
have been attracted to the area, however, an abscess still
develops. Operative debridement of the peritoneal cavity serves
to remove not only the bacteria, the necrotic material, fibrin,
and fluid, but also dead and dying neutrophils, which can
propagate abscess formation by themselves.

SUMMARY

We have seen that the normally sterile peritoneal cavity has
a number of defense mechanisms which serve to maintain this
condition. These include the upward circulation of peritoneal
fluid to the diaphragmatic lymphatics, where fluid and small
particulate matter can be removed. Fibrin, which can serve to
seal local luminal perforations, traps bacteria and impedes the
intraperitoneal circulation. Fibrin reduces the risk of
septicemia but the price of such a defense is abscess formation.
Opsonins such as complement serve to attract neutrophils and to

speed the engulfment of bacteria by these phagocytic cells. The
specific bacteria present to a large degree are determined by the
process which led to perforation and the organ perforated. Once
bacteria are released into the peritoneal cavity, however, only
a very few organisms (alone or in combination) survive. Certain
bacteria species commonly isolated from clinical human peritonitis
seem to undergo mutually beneficial interactions in the peritoneal
cavity which allow their proliferation. The presence of nonbac-
terial substances whether endogenous or exogenous within the
peritoneal cavity may be crucial in determining whether an
infection ultimately develops. Once the initial infection is
established, it is possible that a self-perpetuating process is
established, so that abscesses are not so much the result of
bacterial growth and digestion of host tissues, but the result of
continued neutrophil influx setting up an inflammatory process
resulting in tissue digestion, further neutrophil influx, and
abscess formation. Further work in these areas may delineate
other mechanisms in the pathophysiology of peritonitis and
ultimately reveal new modes of therapy in treating this very
serious disease entity.

REFERENCES

1. Ahrenholz, D.H., and Simmons, R.L. (1980). Surgery 88, 41.
2. Allen, L. (1936). Anat. Rec. 67, 89.
3. Allen, L., and Weatherford, T. (1959). Am. J. Physiol. 197,
      551.
4. Autio, V. (1964). Acta. Chir. Scand. Suppl. 321.
5. Florey, H. (1927). Br. J. Exp. Path. 8, 479.
6. Fowler, G.R. (1900). Med. Rec. 57, 617.
7. Hau, T., Hoffman, R., and Simmons, R.L. (1978). Surgery 83,
      223.
8. Hau, T., Payne, W.D., Simmons, R.L. (1979). Surg. Gynecol.
      Obstet. 148, 415.
9. Ingham, H.R., Sisson, P.R., Tharagonnet, D., et al. (1977).
      Lancet II, 1252.
10. Lee, J.T. and Simmons, R.L. (1981). Arch. Surg. (in press).
11. Meleney, F., Olpp, J., Harvey, H., and Zaytseff-Jem, H.
      (1932). Arch. Surg. 25, 709.
12. Mengle, H.A. (1937). Arch. Surg. 34, 839.
13. Miles, A.A., Miles, E.M., and Burke, J. (1957). Br. J. Exp.
      Pathol. 38, 79.
14. Ohlsson, K. (1976). Surgery 79, 652.
15. Onderdonk, A., Bartlett, J., Louie, T., et al. (1976). Infect.
      Immun. 13, 22.
16. Onderdonk, A.B., Moon, N.E., Kasper, D.L., and Bartlett, J.G.
      (1978). Infect. Immun. 19, 1038.
17. Onderdonk, A., Weinstein, W., Sullivan, N., et al. (1974).

Infect. Immun. 10, 1256.

18. Rudek, W., Haque, R. (1976). J. Clin. Microbiol. 4, 458.

19. Saba, T.M. (1978). Surgery 188, 142.

20. Steinberg, B. (1944). "Infections of the Peritoneum", Paul Hoeber, Inc., New York.

21. Stone, H.H., Kolb, L.D., and Geheber, C.E. (1975). Ann. Surg. 181, 705.

22. Tsilibary, E.C., and Wissig, S.L. (1977). Am. J. Anat. 149, 127.

23. Von Recklinghausen, F.T. (1863). Arch. f. Path. Anat. u. Physiol. 26, 172.

ANTIBIOTIC-ASSOCIATED (PSEUDOMEMBRANOUS) COLITIS:
DIAGNOSIS AND TREATMENT*

Robert Fekety

Division of Infectious Diseases
Department of Internal Medicine
University of Michigan Medical School
and University Hospital
Ann Arbor, Michigan

I. THE DISEASE ENTITY

A. Pathogenesis, Etiology, Incidence

Many hospitalized patients develop a mild and self-limited
diarrhea after being treated with antibiotics. The cause of this
benign diarrheal side effect is not known. Sometimes the diarrhea
is severe or persistent and the patient is found to have colitis.
Toxigenic Clostridium difficile is the most frequent cause of
antibiotic-associated colitis (AAC), the hallmark of which is
pseudomembranes. There are many mild cases of AAC in which pseudomembranes are either not present or evident only histologically.
Staphylococcus aureus is probably another cause of antibiotic-
associated enterocolitis; this entity is now rare, and characteristically effects the ileum and jejunum more than the colon.
The frequency of C. difficile colitis following treatment with
antibiotics has ranged from as low as one in ten thousand treated
patients to as high as one in ten in different reports. Recent
data suggest AAC may result from nosocomial cross-infection,
which may account for wide variations in incidence. C.
difficile colitis occurs at all ages, but is more frequent in
hospitalized patients, the elderly, in women, in patients with
cancer, in patients undergoing abdominal surgery and in intensive
care units. Cases have been reported following oral, intramuscular,
intravenous, topical, or prophylactic use of antibiotics.

*Supported in part by grant no. 1R01-AM21076-02 from the
National Institutes of Health and by grants from the Upjohn Co.
and the Frederick Novy Infectious Diseases Research Fund of the
University of Michigan.

In our hospital, approximately 90 percent of antibiotic-associated diarrhea is the benign type which is of unknown etiology; only 10 percent can be diagnosed as colitis.

A hamster model of the disease has provided important clues to the pathogenesis of AAC in man. Toxins produced by C. difficile cause the disease. Clostridium difficile is a spore-forming Gram-positive anaerobic bacillus that can be found in soil and in the intestinal tracts of healthy persons and some animals. Animals do not appear important in transmission of the organism to humans. The organism is not easily distinguished from other colonic organisms, and is frequently overlooked in routine stool cultures. George and his associates have developed a selective medium (CCFA) containing cycloserine (500 mcg/ml) and cefoxitin (16 mcg/ml) that is capable of detecting C. difficile when present in numbers as low as 100 CFU per gram. Using it, we found that four percent of healthy adults and six percent of 45 patients on a general medical ward were asymptomatic carriers. Three stool cultures were needed to detect all healthy carriers. The organism has been isolated from the vaginal or urethral secretions of a high proportion of men or women attending a venereal disease clinic, and from stools of up to 50 percent of healthy newborns.

Carriage of the organism seems the most important risk factor for colitis, and treatment with antibiotics is another, especially when the organism is resistant. Almost every antibiotic used for treatment of humans has been implicated in isolated cases. Cases are most often related to treatment with clindamycin (to which the organism is usually resistant), ampicillin (to which it is usually susceptible), or cephalosporins (which have variable activity against C. difficile).

Typically, the organism increases in numbers within the intestinal lumen because of the effects of antibiotics, and large amounts of the toxin are produced. Few if any cases have been related to vancomycin, which is widely used in treatment of the disease. However, administration of vancomycin to hamsters lowers their resistance to colonization with the organism to the point where only one or two ingested organisms are sufficient to cause enterocolitis. This suggests that the normal intestinal flora suppresses C. difficile and prevents colonization with it, and that antibiotics markedly interfere with the delicate ecologic balance maintained there. The number of organisms required to colonize humans treated with antimicrobials is not known, nor is the exact nature of the important microbial competitors.

Since antibiotic treatment can markedly lower resistance to colonization of hamsters with C. difficile, it has been suspected that outbreaks of the disease may occur in patients treated with antibiotics in hospitals because of cross-infection. The mode of transmission is not known. The environment (both in hospital and at home) of patients with AAC may be heavily contaminated with C. difficile. The organism can survive in spore form on hospital floors for long periods, and it can be found in small numbers on surfaces in the hospital even where there have been no known

cases.   Contamination is greatest when patients have diarrhea.
The organism has been isolated from the hands and stools of healthy
hospital personnel caring for cases. While isolation of infected
patients (using enteric or stool precautions) has not been shown
to prevent the spread of the organism, we recommend isolation of
patients with the disease, and stress the importance of careful
handwashing after contact with them.

Almost all isolates of C. difficile produce one or more toxins
that are detectable either by a cytopathic effect in cell culture
monolayers or by their lethality for small rodents. These toxins
are thought to cause the disease, but the pathogenetic mechanisms
are not defined. Many colonized newborns have large amounts of
the cytotoxin in their stools, and yet are well. This paradox
raises the possibility that their intestines are immune, immature,
or insusceptible to the toxin, or that the cytotoxin per se is not
responsible for the disease but merely a convenient marker for the
organism and other more pathogenic toxins. The toxins are proteins
with reported molecular weights as low as 50,000 and as high as
600,000. While Wilkins and associates have produced antitoxin to
partially purified C. difficile toxins, it is difficult to raise
antibodies to purified cytotoxin. Passive immunization of hamsters
with C. sordellii antitoxin, which cross-reacts with C. difficile
toxin(s), protects them against antibiotic-induced enterocolitis.
Immunity to the toxins or the disease in humans has not been
demonstrated.

C. difficile appears to produce and release toxin primarily
during growth; antibiotics do not seem to stimulate toxin production in the absence of growth. C. difficile does not adhere
well to colonic epithelium, so it is likely that toxin produced
intraluminally is bound to the mucosal epithelium, with production
of membrane damage leading to cell death and inflammation. In
man, the lesions of C. difficile colitis tend to be most numerous
in the distal colon, sigmoid, and rectum; in rare cases lesions
have been present only in the proximal colon. The diarrhea
associated with C. difficile toxin has been associated with mucosal
lesions; a purely secretory diarrhea of the sort caused by cholera
enterotoxin has been postulated but not documented.

B. Clinical Manifestations

The severity of the illness associated with C. difficile
intestinal intoxication is highly variable. Using non-invasive
tests for the organism and its toxin, it has been possible to
document many mild cases; in fact, they seem to be more numerous
than severe cases.

The disease typically begins about four to nine days after
starting antibiotics. About 25 percent of cases do not begin until
up to several weeks after antibiotics have been discontinued; in
these patients it seems either that the organism was inhibited by

the antibiotic used but survived and then multiplied after antibiotic concentrations declined, or that the organism was acquired after antibiotic therapy was discontinued. The effects antibiotics have upon resistance of the intestines to colonization persist for long periods.

The diarrhea associated with the disease is usually watery and profuse; bloody stools are rare. Abdominal tenderness and pain may be marked. Low grade fever is usual, but high fever (104-105°) is not rare. Occasionally the illness presents as unexplained post-operative fever with abdominal tenderness, but without diarrhea initially.

Clostridium difficile colitis may be fatal if it is unrecognized and untreated. The disease has a higher mortality rate in elderly and chronically debilitated patients. In one series the fatality rate was 19 percent (4/21) in patients over 50, while none of 8 patients under 50 died. Fatalities are usually related to hypovolemia, septic shock, toxic megacolon, perforation, or bleeding. Untreated cases usually resolve spontaneously in less than ten days if the inciting drug is discontinued, but some cases have a protracted course, with remissions and exacerbations over many months.

II. DIAGNOSIS

A. Key Diagnostic Tests

Patients with AAC often have leukocytosis (25-35,000/mm^3) and hypoalbuminemia. Fecal smears for leukocytes are positive in about 50 percent of cases. When present, these findings speak against a benign diarrhea. It is worth doing a fecal smear in patients with mild diarrhea, because a positive increases the index of suspicion of colitis and may lead to performance of proctosigmoidoscopy. Even though it is uncommon to detect large numbers of organisms resembling C. difficile when a Gram-stain of diarrheal stool is made, in those patients with staphylococcal enterocolitis the presence of large numbers of Gram-positive cocci in clusters may suggest that diagnosis.

Two laboratory studies of special importance in diagnosis of colitis are stool cultures for C. difficile on cycloserine-cefoxitin fructose agar (CCFA), and tests on stools for the presence of the cytotoxin of C. difficile.

CCFA is a very satisfactory selective medium for C. difficile, and is now commercially available. It can detect as few as 100 CFU of the organism per gram of stool. Patients with colitis usually have about 10^4-10^5 CFU or more per gram. Most laboratories with anaerobic capabilities can easily isolate the organism using CCFA. While healthy persons may carry the organism (4-5%), a positive culture may be useful in helping to decide whether to

perform sigmoidoscopy and whether treatment begun empirically
should be continued. In our hands, 81 percent of patients with
antibiotic-associated diarrhea and a positive stool culture for
C. difficile have had documentable colitis.
  Tests for the presence of the C. difficile cytotoxin in stools
have been even more specific than culture for colitis, but are not
widely available. A positive toxin test supports the diagnosis of
colitis, but does not establish this diagnosis with certainty.
Healthy infants often have toxin in their stools, but only rarely
is this the case with adults. We found that 91 percent of our
patients with antibiotic-associated diarrhea and a positive test
for toxin in stool had documentable colitis. Tests for toxin in
stools are usually done using cultured monolayers of fibroblasts,
but many other cell lines can be used. Special laboratory facilities are needed, and the test is expensive. A cytopathic effect
(CPE) is often evident within a few hours of testing, but more
often than not overnight incubation is needed. It is essential to
demonstrate that the CPE can be prevented by addition of C.
sordellii or C. difficile antitoxin to the stool extract being
tested. About 50 percent of stools from patients with antibiotic
diarrheal syndromes studied in our laboratory have been positive
for a cytopathic toxin, and about half of these were identifiable
as C. difficile toxin. All but a few toxin-positive stools from
patients with proven colitis contained C. difficile toxin in high
titer; a few contained what appeared to be a staphylococcus
enterotoxin or C. perfringens type C toxin. The remainder had
non-specific toxicity, usually at low titer.
  More practical tests for C. difficile or its toxin that utilize
fluorescent antibodies or ELISA techniques are under development
and appear promising. CIE is used, but false positives are seen.
It is unfortunately the case at present that there is no simple
non-invasive test that establishes the diagnosis of AAC and
supports the initiation of specific antibiotic therapy.
  The diagnosis of AAC is best established by proctosigmoidos-
copic or colonoscopic visualization of colitis, especially the
characteristic nodular inflammatory or pseudomembranous plaques.
Biopsy is confirmatory but not essential when typical lesions are
seen. If the mucosa appears abnormal and inflamed (friable,
edematous, congested), but no pseudomembranes are seen, a biopsy
is desirable and may reveal not only the typical histological
changes of colitis but also pseudomembranes not visible to the
naked eye. If the mucosa appears normal, but leukocytes, cytotoxin, or organisms are detectable in feces of a patient with
severe diarrhea, consideration should be given to colonoscopy
to detect lesions beyond reach of the sigmoidoscopy. These have
occurred in about three percent of cases.
  It is important to rule out infection with other recognized
intestinal pathogens in patients with antibiotic-associated
diarrhea. Staphylococcal enterocolitis is now uncommon and is

poorly defined, but tends to involve the small intestine
predominantly, with profuse watery diarrhea. Pseudomembranes
are uncommon in the rectosigmoid when staphylococci are causative.
It has been reported recently that C. difficile may be
responsible for 10-20 percent of relapses of chronic inflammatory
bowel diseases such as Crohn's disease or ulcerative colitis in
some cities. Some cases of C. difficile colitis have occurred in
patients who have not received any chemotherapeutic agents.
Similarly, it appears the gastrointestinal side effects formerly
attributed to cancer chemotherapy may be due in some cases to a
complicating C. difficile intoxication. Cases of pseudomembranous
colitis were diagnosed in the pre-antibiotic era, usually in
association with major abdominal surgery, and resembled so-called
ischemic colitis. Cases of AAC involving the cecum primarily
tend to occur in patients with leukemia or solid tumors, resemble
neutropenic typhlitis, and may be complicated by intestinal
perforation. Rare cases of pseudomembranous colitis (especially
if untreated) may be complicated by the megacolon syndrome and
require surgical intervention.

III.   THERAPY AND PREVENTION

A.   Non-specific Therapy

Many patients with this disease do not require specific
antibiotic therapy, but will respond in less than a week to
replacement of fluid losses and discontinuation of the inciting
drug. Toxic or elderly patients should be given specific therapy
without delay because of their higher mortality rate.

B.   Vancomycin

The treatment of choice for severe C. difficile colitis is
oral vancomycin. The organism is usually susceptible to vancomycin at concentrations of 5 µg or less per ml, and has never
been resistant to 20 µg per ml, even when patients have relapsed
after treatment. Dosages as low as 125 mg four times daily
routinely achieve concentrations of about 500 µg per ml in stools;
higher dosages have been used but do not appear more effective.
Since vancomycin is poorly absorbed when given orally, systemic
toxic reactions are expected to be rare, and in fact have not
occurred even in patients with inflamed colonic mucosa. The
efficacy of this condition has been proven in a controlled trial.
Patients treated with oral vancomycin usually show some sign
of improvement with 24 to 48 hours, and the amount of toxin in
stools starts to decline soon after treatment is started. Treatment should be continued for at least five days, but rarely is
needed for more than 10 days. Treatment should not be discontinued

if stools still contain detectable toxin, since such patients seem
more prone to relapse. Drawbacks to widespread use of vancomycin
are that the drug is expensive ($10 or more per day for 500 mg), is
in relatively short supply, and tastes very bitter. Vancomycin
should not be given to prevent diarrhea, and it does not appear to
ameliorate the antibiotic-associated diarrhea that is unassociated
with C. difficile (or S. aureus).

Patients who are too sick to be given vancomycin orally, even
via nasogastric tube, because of factors such as ileus still pose
a formidable therapeutic problem. When vancomycin is given intravenously, only relatively low concentrations are achieved within
the bowel lumen (10-80 µg/ml); sometimes none is detectable. No
form of parenteral therapy for this disease has been reliably
effective. Unpublished reports suggest intravenous metronidazole
may be useful in such patients. At present, it appears wise to
attempt to deliver vancomycin into the bowel lumen of critically
ill patients in whatever way feasible (via nasogastric tube, into
colostomies, by enema, etc.), and to supplement this with
intravenous vancomycin or metronidazole.

It is wise but probably not necessary to discontinue the
antibiotic that incited colitis when treatment with vancomycin is
given. The antibacterial effect of vancomycin on C. difficile has
not been antagonized by other antibiotics in vitro. Many antibiotics that have been substituted when continued therapy is needed
are themselves capable of inducing the disease. Probably the
major reason for changing antibiotics is medicolegal.

C. Bacitracin

A small number of patients have been treated with oral
bacitracin; most improve but some have relapsed and were then
treated with vancomycin. Bacitracin may be a useful alternative
to vancomycin, but costs about the same ($10/day). More experience
is needed to determine its place. Most isolates of C. difficile
are highly susceptible to bacitracin, but many require 32 µg per
ml for inhibition and some require more than 250 µg/ml. Very
little is known about the achievable stool concentrations when
bacitracin is given orally. We also need to determine the safety
of bacitracin in patients with an inflamed intestinal mucosa, as
well as the frequency of relapse with it.

D. Metronidazole

This antimicrobial drug is reportedly effective and inexpensive
in treatment of colitis in an oral dosage of 500 mg three times
daily. Pregnant women and children should not be treated with it,
because of fears of its potential mutagenicity. Only a handful
of treated cases have been reported, and it is usually reserved

for mild cases. One potential problem is that the fecal
concentrations achieved with oral therapy may not be adequate,
because its absorption in the small intestine is almost complete.
Intravenous metronidazole may be useful when oral therapy is not
possible, but is poorly studied so far.

E. Cholestyramine

This anion exchange resin was first used in treatment of
colitis when the cause of the disease was unknown. Patients
seemed responsive in uncontrolled studies. Subsequent experience
indicated that some patients respond slowly and that obstipation
may be a serious side effect when diarrhea subsides. Cholestyramine is able to absorb the toxin of C. difficile, and this is the
presumed mechanism of its action. It may also absorb vancomycin,
so simultaneous use of both drugs should be avoided. Since
cholestyramine does not appear to inhibit or kill C. difficile,
it is theoretically less desirable than antibiotic therapy. Its
primary usefulness is in mild cases. The usual dose is 4 gm three
times per day orally (approximate cost is $3-5/day).

F. Tetracycline and Erythromycin

In a few patients with antibiotic diarrhea, tetracyclines or
erythromycin derivatives have seemed beneficial. More study is
needed before assigning them a role. Many isolates of C.
difficile are resistant to these antibiotics.

G. Other Measures

Recent evidence suggests lactobacilli or other components of
the normal fecal flora may be important competitors or inhibitors
of C. difficile within the gut. Interest in using them in therapy
or prevention has increased. In the older literature, there are
fascinating reports of patients with refractory pseudomembranous
colitis who were given enemas of feces from normal persons in the
hope of restoring their normal flora, with apparent success.

H. Antidiarrheal Agents

Opiates and other antiperistaltic agents should be avoided in
patients with febrile diarrheal syndromes, including C. difficile
colitis. They tend to favor retention of toxins, continued mucosal
damage, and loss of fluid into the gut lumen, despite apparent
reduction of diarrhea.

I. Relapses and Recurrences

Recurrences of colitis have been reported in 10-20 percent of treated patients. They occur with all forms of specific therapy. The organisms from these patients have remained susceptible to vancomycin, and patients with relapses have usually responded to retreatment with oral vancomycin in ordinary doses. While some patients harbor the organism in feces after treatment, this is not always followed by relapse. Most relapses occur within a few weeks of treatment and are spontaneous. Some occur much later, usually after treatment with antibiotics. It is recommended that patients be treated for no more than 10 days for their first relapse. Most patients will have no further trouble. No good way to treat patients with multiple recurrences is known yet, although many things have been tried, including prolonged, intermittent, or gradually-tapered therapy. Some of these patients may reacquire the organism from their environment or asymptomatic contacts after treatment. Obviously, more research is needed in this area.

J. Prevention

Natural or artifically-induced immunity to C. difficile, its toxin, and the disease has not been demonstrated in humans. Since multiple attacks can occur, the disease does not appear to induce immunity. Avoidance of unnecessary use of antibiotics is obviously to be encouraged, but there is no convincing evidence that avoidance of any specific antibiotic will lower the risk of development of the disease in patients who are at high risk.

The immediate environment of patients with active colitis may be heavily contaminated with C. difficile. Air, walls, and food have not been positive so far, but floors, bedding, furniture, sinks, toilets, and bedpans have frequently been contaminated. The organisms may sporulate, resist disinfectants, and persist at these sites for months. Some hospitals experiencing a high rate of the disease have noticed that some rooms seem to have more cases of AAC than ought to occur by chance alone. Furthermore, hospital personnel caring for these patients may contaminate their hands, clothes, and equipment, and then transfer the organism to other susceptible patients, especially those receiving antibiotics that lower their colonization resistance.

While isolation of patients with colitis, using enteric precautions, has not been proven to prevent the spread of the organism in hospitals, it seems prudent at present to utilize it in the hope of doing so. Careful handwashing after contact with these patients is also strongly recommended.

SELECTED REFERENCES

Bartlett, J.G. (1979). Antibiotic-associated pseudomembranous colitis. Rev. Infect. Dis. 1, 530.

Chang, T.W., et al. (1980). Bacitracin treatment of antibiotic-associated colitis and diarrhea caused by C. difficile toxin. Gastroenterology 78, 1584.

George, W.L., et al. (1979). Selective and differential medium for isolation of Clostridium difficile. J. Clin. Microbiol. 9, 214.

Hafiz, S., et al. (1975). Clostridium difficile in the urogenital tract of males and females. Lancet 1, 420.

Kim, K.H., et al. (1981). Isolation of Clostridium difficile from the environment and contacts of patients with antibiotic-associated colitis. J. Infect. Dis. 143, 42.

Larson, H.E., et al. (1978). Clostridium difficile and the aetiology of pseudomembranous colitis. Lancet 1, 1063.

Lusk, R.H., et al. (1977). Gastrointestinal side effects following clindamycin or ampicillin therapy. J. Infect. Dis. 135, S111.

Lusk, R.H., et al. (1978). Clindamycin-induced enterocolitis in hamsters. J. Infect. Dis. 137, 464.

Rifkin, G.D., et al. (1977). Antibiotic-induced colitis. Implication of a toxin neutralized by Clostridium sordellii antitoxin. Lancet 2, 1103.

Tedesco, F.J., et al. (1974). Clindamycin-associated colitis. Ann. Intern. Med. 81, 429.

PART III
RESPIRATORY TRACT INFECTIONS

SINUSITIS

Isidro G. Zavala T.

Infectious Diseases Department
Autonomous University of Guadalajara
Guadalajara, Jalisco, México

INTRODUCTION

Sinusitis is an acute and/or chronic infection that involves
the para-nasal sinuses, usually being an extension or a complication of an upper respiratory tract viral infection. Other associated factors may include nasal allergy, peridontal infections or
dental manipulations which may produce fractures of the bony floor,
nasal anatomic defects which under special situations such as
the frequent practice of swimming disturb the normal muco-ciliary
function within the sinus cavity, and may render the cavities
highly susceptible to infections. Although sinusitis is a
common problem, its cause is very frequently undetermined, and
the treatment offered is essentially empiric, especially concerning the use of antibiotics. Sometimes, fortunately in a
very few cases, sinus infection may extend to the central nervous
system and give rise to acute and severe infections such as
bacterial meningitis, brain abscess, epidural and subdural
abscesses, osteomyelitis and spreading of the infection to the
orbit, with the potential danger of producing a retrobulbar
abscess or a cavernous sinus thrombosis.

PATHOGENESIS

Acute sinusitis is frequently considered a secondary
bacterial infection, or a complication of previous viral infection,
and in some cases it represents a primary infection caused by
bacteria, viruses and in a few cases by fungus (1). The paranasal sinuses under normal conditions are kept sterile by means
of the normal defense mechanisms, the most outstanding of which

are a continuous ciliary movement and the production of mucus, lysozyme and IgA. In some instances, small viral or bacterial particles are able to evade these defense mechanisms, and they adhere to the epithelial cells of the nasal mucosa. This phenomenon may be an important step in the pathogenesis of some infections of the upper respiratory tract related to this area. In some studies the adherence of bacteria such as *S. aureus, S. pneumoniae, H. influenzae* and *Group A streptococcus* has been demonstrated to be increased during natural or experimental viral infections (2,3).

Acute maxillary sinusitis may also have its origin in a dental infectious process which may be present in up to 10% of the cases. The floor of the maxillary sinus is located close to the roots of the molars, and an infection of this type frequently spreads to the sinus cavity.

Local conditions, not of infectious origin, but those that in a given moment may predispose to acute sinusitis include: septal deviation, foreign bodies, nasal tumors, turbinate hypertrophy, nasal polyps, adenoid enlargement, vasomotor rhinitis, drug induced rhinitis, trauma such as that caused by nasotracheal intubation, inhalation of excessively dry air, chemical irritation, edema and nasal obstruction (4,5). Occasionally, an allergic type of reaction may produce inflammation of the mucosa that covers the paranasal sinuses, allowing an inflammatory reaction and the formation of polyps. In the case of acute sinusitis, the mucosal layer is inflamed and edematous with a mucopurulent exudate containing polymorphonuclears in great numbers and bacteria in concentrations greater than 100,000 colony forming units/ml.

In prolonged sinusitis without proper management important changes may arise that favor the chronicity of the disease, such as, local inflammation, slight or absent drainage and decrease in arterial oxygen tension. The ciliary epithelium is then replaced by squamous stratified epithelium, losing in this manner an important mechanism for maintaining the sterility of the paranasal cavities. If to the above changes we add the prolonged use of nasal vasocontrictors, infections caused by anaerobic bacteria and gram-negative rods or mixed organisms frequently arise (6,7).

CLINICAL CHARACTERISTICS

In general, acute sinusitis develops during the course of a viral infection, such as the common cold, or during an infection caused by influenza viruses. At other times, sinusitis may be a consequence of an exacerbation of chronic sinusitis. The clinical manifestations simulate allergic rhinitis; however, in acute sinusitis the symptoms are more severe. There is headache, nasal obstruction, anterior and posterior mucopurulent secretions,

facial pain, disturbances of olfaction, sore throat, fever and
cough. The type of clinical presentation, severity, evolution
and presence of complications are determined in part by the
specific sinus(es) involved.

Acute frontal sinusitis may be a critical situation, because
the symptoms are variable and occasionally an emergency situation
ensues requiring immediate treatment. Most commonly, a frontal
headache develops which may spread to the roof of the ocular
orbit. Increasing body temperature is common. Fever may be
higher and more frequent in children and in those patients with
copious purulent material inside the sinus with scant drainage.
Also, frontal erythema and swelling may be observed as well as
tenderness in the involved area. When exudate is present, it is
usually purulent.

Acute ethmoidal sinusitis, more frequently observed in children than in adults, causes headache, inter- and retro-orbital
pain, edema of the eyelids and orbital cellulitis. Excessive
tearing may also be observed. The eye movements elicit significant pain. There is usually a moderate fever and purulent
nasal exudate. Often there is a history of a preceding upper
respiratory tract infection.

Acute maxillary sinusitis is usually present in older children
or adults, being commonly preceded by a dental process, but also
other situations may exist such as the presence of nasal polyps,
deviation of the nasal septum, allergic rhinitis, infections of
the upper respiratory tract or trauma. Tooth pain, the sensation
of having larger teeth, anterior and posterior rhinorrhea, and
voice tone changes are other findings. Fever is usually moderate.

Chronic sinusitis may go undetected by the patient even for
prolonged periods of time. However, sometimes there is posterior
rhinorrea which may be malodorous. In other patients the only
symptom may be a chronic non-productive cough and frequent lower
respiratory tract infections. Finally, as previously mentioned,
a chronic sinusitis with scarcity of symptoms may exacerbate and
present important signs and symptoms, such as, purulent anterior
and posterior exudate, fever, etc.

ETIOLOGY

Organisms responsible for paranasal sinus infections are
currently easy to isolate and recognize if two points are taken
into consideration: 1) enthusiasm and desire on the part of the
physician to know the responsible agent for the infectious process
and 2) availability of the means to achieve such a goal. The
lack of proper techniques to obtain samples uncontaminated by
normal flora, failure to isolate strictly anaerobic bacteria and
difficulty in documenting swelling of the sinus mucosa have been
reasons for misinterpretation in the past.

The infectious agents in most of the cases of acute maxillary sinusitis in children and adults are given in Table 1.

Table 1.   Isolated Strains in Patients with Sinusitis, Peri-pharyngeal Abscess, Otitis and Otomastoiditis[a]

Aerobic bacteria	No.	Anaerobic bacteria	No.
S. pneumoniae	21	Fusobacterium sp.	15
H. influenzae	12	Peptoestreptococcus sp.	14
Alpha-h. Streptococcus	3	B. melaninogenicus	7
Staphylococcus aureus	2	B. fragilis	3
Pseudomonas aeruginosa	2	Peptococcus sp.	2
Escherichia coli	1		
Klebsiella/Enterobacter	1		
T o t a l	42		41

[a] Values according to Mario Flores Salinas, M.D., Autonomous University of Guadalajara

All the samples in this study were obtained by direct puncture and aspiration of the sinus. Traditionally, *H. influenzae, S. pneumoniae, Alpha-hemolytic Streptococcus* and *S. aureus* have been the organisms predominantly isolated from inflamed sinuses (9). However, recent studies indicate that anaerobic bacteria such as *B. melaninogenicus, Peptococcus sp., S. microaerophilic, B. fragilis* and *Fusobacterium sp.* should be added to the list. Under special conditions, gram-negative rods are capable of inducing sinusitis, and the organisms isolated may be *Pseudomonas aeruginosa, K. pneumoniae* and *E. coli* (10).

With lesser frequency fungal organisms such as the agents of mucormycosis (*Phycomycetes*) may produce sinusitis. Involvement by these organisms is seen in special situations, such as, prolonged use of steroids (11,12,13). Aspergillosis of the sinuses is usually caused by *Aspergillus fumigatus*, although there are cases described due to *A. coryzae, A. flavus* and *A. niger*. The origin of the infection is by inhaling *Aspergillus* spores, which are found normally in spoiled food and plants and are mixed with dust. The infection occurs only in favorable conditions such as: local infection, retention of exudate and changes in the normal nasal flora by the prolonged use of antibiotics and immunosuppressive therapy (14–17). *Candida* may cause sinusitis also under special conditions such as in diabetic patients being treated with wide-spectrum antibiotics for another infectious process or after maxillary trauma involving the sinus (18).

EPIDEMIOLOGY

Infections of the paranasal sinuses have a peak incidence during autumn, winter and spring; the number of cases is highest during the days close to the change of season. The early presentation is similar to that of upper respiratory tract infections. Approximately 0.5% of common upper respiratory tract infections are complicated by acute sinusitis (19). Although it seems that adults suffer more frequent paranasal sinus infections, recent studies, using modern and appropriate techniques for taking and processing samples and better radiologic techniques, indicate that sinusitis may be as common in children as in adults. Sinusitis does occur more frequently in swimmers and excessive smokers.

DIAGNOSIS

As in all infectious disease problems, it is essential to completely evaluate each patient, paying special attention to physical examination of the upper respiratory tract.

The symptoms and clinical signs mentioned previously, i.e., headache, fever, cough, facial pain which increases when bending forward, nasal secretions, sinus "dullness" during transillumination, are not definitively diagnostic. There are published studies in which up to 75% of the patients with these findings and in whom a sinus puncture was performed, fluid levels were not found and the culture results were "sterile". Also, patients with diagnosed purulent sinusitis, established by study of samples obtained by sinus puncture and aspiration, were without symptoms (1). This is mainly because the complaints due to acute sinusitis are commonly mistaken for a common cold, and because it is extremely difficult to establish a definitive diagnosis of sinusitis based only on the clinical history, symptoms and physical examination of the patient.

Studies that may help us to establish the diagnosis of sinusitis are:

1) Transillumination (of relative and partial value) will have a high degree of diagnostic specificity if there is a complete dullness which is frequent in acute sinusitis. In chronic sinusitis the transmission of light is usually low or completely absent. Drawbacks of this technique include: the necessity of having a room with complete darkness to which the examiner must become adapted, which is time consuming; it is helpful only for frontal and maxillary sinuses; and, finally, it is a subjective study with a variable range of interpretation (1).

2)   Currently, radiologic studies are considered as the most
sensitive for establishing the diagnosis of sinusitis. When the
paranasal sinuses are radiologically examined, the degree of
mucosal thickness, the presence of an air/fluid level or complete
radiological dullness of one or more sinuses, are data with a
great diagnostic security index of active infection (20,21,22).
It appears that it is important to see mucosal thickening greater
than 9 mm, since lower figures have been seen in asymptomatic
patients and in children who without any treatment return to
normal (23,24). It is also important to point out that in
chronic sinusitis the value of radiography in establishing the
diagnosis of acute infections is limited, since the radiologic
changes usually are persistent. However, seeing an air/fluid
level, dullness and mucosal thickening greater than 8 mm in
the same patient almost always establishes the diagnosis of
sinusitis (certainty of 99.9%).

3)   In all infectious diseases the isolation of the causative
organism, its identification and susceptibility tests are very
important. Previous studies and more recent ones show that
*H. influenzae, S. pneumoniae, S. aureus, B. fragilis, B. melanino-
genicus, Peptococcus sp.*, and other anaerobic bacteria, are being
isolated in a high frequency. Currently there are different
strains of *H. influenzae* resistant to ampicillin and some to
chloramphenicol. Also, some strains of *B. melaninogenicus* and
most *B. fragilis* are reported as penicillin-resistant.

Under special conditions the gram negative rods and fungus
can be responsible for the infection. The only way of specifying
the microbial etiology of an acute and/or chronic sinusitis, is
by culture of the sinus exudate or material obtained by puncture
and aspiration of a sinus lavage. To obtain samples from the
frontal sinus we puncture under the infraorbitarium ocular ring
and for the maxillary antrum the puncture is done under the in-
ferior nasal turbinate. Previous to the puncture, a small quan-
tity of antiseptic like providone-iodine solution, is applied over
the area, with the objective of preventing or eliminating any
contamination due to the surface flora. However, Evans Jr. et al,
proved that the use only of 10% cocaine as anesthesic in the
nasal mucosa (site of puncture), was enough to prevent sample
contamination. For puncturing the sinus a needle is used,
passing a teflon catheter through it and aspirating with a sterile
syringe. Material obtained for culture via the sinus exudate
after a lavage or across the natural outflow meatus, like pus from
the nose, is contaminated and the information from these samples
lacks any diagnostic value. Samples obtained by puncture must
be cultured rapidly, using the following culture media: chocolate-
agar, blood-agar, MacConkey and pre-reduced brain-heart infusion
(BHI) supplemented with vitamin K and heme. It is important
to culture using the methods for anaerobic bacteria as the
Gas-Pack jar technic.

Also it has been proved that the total count of bacteria per ml of obtained material by puncture is important to distinguish from infection and contamination or colonization. It is considered a sign of infection if the bacterial titer is greater than 10^5 per ml and as colonization or contamination when the bacterial count is under 10^3 per ml. Another important factor in the study of material obtained by puncture, is the leukocyte count and the predominance of polymorphonuclear cells (PMN's). Greater than 5,000 leukocytes per ml is correlated with infection and under 100 per ml is considered normal, according to the studies of Evans Jr. et al, and Itzhak Brook et al.

The gram stain smear study of the material obtained by puncture has been shown to correlate with the presence of bacteria and leukocytes between 52 to 80 percent in patients with active infectious sinusitis and in some reports of chronic sinusitis. When these samples are inoculated in WI-38 human lung fibroblasts, we can isolate viruses.

TREATMENT

According to studies published before the 1970's, the most frequently isolated organisms from swollen sinuses were S. pneumoniae, S. aureus, Alpha-hemolytic Streptococcus and H. influenza. During the last decade, more specific techniques to document real cases of sinusitis, and methods to prevent sample contamination obtained by puncture and to facilitate isolation of anaerobic bacteria and virus, the use of antimicrobial drugs for treatment of sinusitis has become less empirical and more rational.

In careful studies done first at the University of Virginia School of Medicine and then at George Washington University, antibiotic use was guided by the organisms isolated and their in vitro susceptibility. It was shown by means of a second sample from the affected sinus, taken also by puncture after the completion of treatment, that the cultures were sterile and the mucosal thickness had diminished significantly.

The antibiotics most widely used are: ampicillin for H. influenzae or chloramphenicol in the case of resistant strains; penicillin G for S. pneumoniae, Alpha-hemolytic Streptococcus and anaerobic bacteria, like Peptococcus and Peptostreptococcus, and clindamycin for B. fragilis and some B. melaninogenicus strains; betalactamase-resistant penicillins or fosfomycin are excellent antibiotics with bactericidal effects against S. aureus and also H. influenzae. In some instances puncture drainage or surgery is required. Also, the use of nasal vasoconstrictives, topically or systemically, and of antihistamines are beneficial.

To prevent acute sinusitis, it might be of value to use vaccines against *H. influenzae* and *S. pneumoniae*; however, we do not know the results of such studies. In the case of an outbreak of viral influenza, the use of amantidine in high risk patients would be of great value, since the current vaccines do not have any proved efficacy in preventing sinusitis based on clinical studies.

We are currently attempting to improve diagnostic techniques in patients with previous treatment, and are developing a more rapid means of diagnosis using immunologic methods such as CIE, ELISA, etc. for *S. pneumoniae, H. influenzae, Alpha-hemolytic Streptococcus* and *Bacteroids sp.*

REFERENCES

1. Evans, F.O., Sydnor, J.B., Moore, W.E.C., et al. (1975). Sinusitis of the maxillary antrum. *N. Engl. J. Med. 293,* 735.
2. Fainstein, V., Muscher, D.M., and Cate T.R. Bacterial adherence to pharyngeal cells during viral infection.
3. Simpson, W.A., Brook, I., Sarasohm, C., Morrison, J.C., and Beachey, E. (1980). Characteristics of the binding of streptococcal lipoteichoic acid to human oral epithelial cells. *J. Infect. Dis. 141,* 457.
4. Quick, C.A., and Payne, E. (1972). Complicated acute sinusitis. *Laryngoscope 82,* 1248.
5. Rulon, J.T. (1970). Sinusitis in children. *Postgrad. Med. 48,* 107.
6. Barlett, J.G., and Gorbach, S.L. (1976). Anaerobic infections of the head and neck. *Otolaryngologic Clinics of North America 9(3),* 655.
7. Flores, M., Zavala, I.G., et al. (1980). Anaerobic infections in otolaryngology. *Actas de la Facultad de Medicina 3,* 172.
8. Finegold, S.M. (1977). Anaerobic Bacteria in Human Diseases. Academic Press Inc., New York.
9. Catlin, F.I., Cluff, L.E., and Reynolds, R.C. (1965). The bacteriology of acute and chronic sinusitis. *South Med. J. 48,* 1497.
10. Mandell, Douglas and Bennett. (1979). Principles and Practice of Infectious Diseases. Wiley's Medical Publication, New York.
11. La Touche, C.J. et al. (1963). Histopathological and mycological features of a case of rhinocerebral mucormycosis (phycomycosis). *Britain Sabouraudia 3,* 148.
12. Stephan T., et al. (1973). Rhinocerebral phycomycosis (mucormycosis). *Laryngoscope 83,* 173.
13. Parkhust, G.F., and Ulahides, G.D. (1967). Fatal opportunistic fungus diseases. *JAMA 202,* 279.
14. Hora, J.F. (1965). Primary aspergillosis of paranasal sinuses and associated areas. *Laryngoscope 75,* 768.

15. Mahgoub, S. (1971). Mycological and serological studies on
    Aspergillus flavus isolated from paranasal aspergilloma
    in Sudan. *J. Trop. Med. Hyg. 74,* 162.
16. Mislosheu, B., et al. (1966). Aspergilloma of paranasal
    sinuses and orbit in Northern Sudanese. *Lancet 1,* 746.
17. Rothfeld, I. (1972). Aspergilloma of sinus. *New York J. Med.
    72,* 493.
18. Gill, E.R. (1960). Mycotic infections in otolaryngology.
    Arch. Otolaryngol. 72, 321.
19. Dingle, J.H., Badger, G.F., Jordan, W.S., Jr. (1964).
    A study of 25,000 illnesses in a group of Cleveland families.
    Cleveland, Press of Western Reserve University.
20. Hamory, B.H., Sande, M.A., Sydnor, A., Jr. et al. (1979).
    Etiology and antimicrobial therapy of acute maxillary
    sinusitis. *J. Infect. Dis. 139,* 197.
21. Lusted, L.B., Keats, T.E. (1978). Atlas of roentgenographic
    measurement. (4th Edition). Year Book Medical Publishers,
    Chicago.
22. Wortzman, G., and Holgate, R.C. (1976). Special radiological
    techniques in maxillary sinus disease. *Otolaryngologic
    Clinics of North America 9(1),* 117.
23. Fascenelly, F.W. (1969). Maxillary sinus abnormalities:
    radiographic evidence in an asymptomatic population.
    Arch. Otolaryngol. 90, 190.
24. Szpunar, J., and Okrasinska, B. (1962). Sinusitis in children
    with bronchiectasis. *Arch. Otolaryngol. 76,* 352.

PNEUMONIA - NEW DIAGNOSTIC AND
THERAPEUTIC CONSIDERATIONS

Phillip K. Peterson

Department of Medicine
University of Minnesota
Minneapolis, Minnesota

INTRODUCTION

Although perhaps no longer the "captain of the ship of death",
pneumonia remains a major cause of morbidity and mortality. Only
cardiovascular disease and malignancy exceed pneumonia as causes
of death in the developed world. Over the past five years, major
strides have been made in defining the complex microbiology of
pneumonia. Newly recognized infectious agents have been characterized, such as *Legionella pneumophila* and other *Legionella* species.
The importance of opportunists, such as the enteric gram-negative
bacilli, fungi, and cytomegalovirus, has been clarifed by numerous
studies of pneumonia in immunocompromised patients. Our concepts
regarding the etiologic role of "old" agents, e.g., pneumococci,
meningococci, and *Mycoplasma pneumoniae*, have also changed
significantly.
But this plethora of etiologic agents is only one product of
the recent "opening of Pandora's box". The pharmaceutical industry has countered with a barrage of new antimicrobials with
increased or expanded spectra of activity. Additionally, multiple
new diagnostic methods have appeared on the scene.
Thus, it has become exceedingly difficult for the busy practitioner to assess the relative importance of each of these developments in the overall management of patients with pneumonia. The
goal of this chapter will be to put these advances in perspective
for primary care physicians. Given the constraints of space, it
is impossible not to oversimplify matters, and the reader is
referred to related chapters in this book as well as to the
bibliography for more in depth discussion.

THE PATIENT HISTORY - A KEY TO ETIOLOGIC DIAGNOSIS

Even though there has been a development of many new diagnostic methods and techniques, it is reassuring to most clinicans to realize that the taking of an accurate and detailed patient history remains the cornerstone of evaluating all patients with pneumonia. The major elements of the infectious disease history are listed in Table 1.

Table I. Patient History and the Etiologies of Pneumonia

History	Special etiologic considerations
Patient age	
Infants	Chlamydia trachomatis
Children	Respiratory syncytial virus
	Parainfluenza, influenza viruses
	S. pneumoniae, H. influenzae
Young adults	M. pneumoniae
Middle age - older adults	S. pneumoniae
Season	Many viral pneumonias, e.g.,
	influenza virus (fall, winter)
Exposure	
Animals	Psittacosis, Q fever, tularemia,
	histoplasmosis
Alcohol	Klebsiella pneumoniae, H. influenzae; aspiration pneumonia
Water	L. pneumophila
Travel	L. pneumophila (outbreaks); coccidioidomycosis (S.W. USA); paragonomiasis, melioidosis (Far East)
Hospital	Enteric gram-negative bacilli, Staphylococcus aureus
Nursing home	K. pneumoniae, S. aureus, influenza
Tuberculosis	Mycobacterium tuberculosis
Host defense abnormalities	SEE TABLE III.

Since antimicrobial therapy is initiated on the basis of which organism(s) is (are) considered the most likely cause of pneumonia, the importance of these historical data in this decision-making process cannot be overemphasized. Other historical features related to the rapidity of onset and pace of infection (bacterial pneumonias are generally more abrupt and rapidly progressive than are viral pneumonias or those caused by atypical or specialized bacteria such as *M. pneumoniae, Mycobacterium sp.* and *Nocardia*) and the type of sputum production (bacterial pneumonias are more commonly productive of copious, and often blood-tinged, sputum) are also helpful in thinking about an etiologic diagnosis. Of course, it must be remembered that there are non-infectious causes of fever and pulmonary infiltrates; the most important considerations here being pulmonary emboli, malignancy, drug reactions, and pulmonary edema.

THE PHYSICAL EXAM AND LABORATORY EVALUATION

The physical exam, although not nearly as helpful as the history in guiding the diagnostic work-up and therapy of pneumonia, nonetheless can provide important clinical clues. For example, a skin rash may suggest diseases such as atypical measles or Rocky Mountain spotted fever, and verrucous lesions may raise the possibility of blastomycosis or coccidioidomycosis. Neurologic abnormalities usually will dictate the performance of emergency neuroradiographic studies or lumbar puncture. Gram-negative sepsis or a fulminant gram-positive bacterial infection should be considered if hypotension is observed, and this finding generally necessitates the use of intravenous antibiotics, often given in combination until an etiologic diagnosis is established.

Although the value of the sputum Gram stain is still debated, this simple and rapid test can be helpful if a good *sputum* specimen is examined. The same can be said for sputum culture. In patients who are unable to provide a good sputum specimen, but who are nevertheless cooperative, sputum can be obtained by transtracheal aspiration (TTA). Specimens obtained by this technique can also be more reliably cultured for anaerobic bacteria. This procedure, however, should only be performed by those who are well-trained, and as a rule, TTA is not indicated in the management of most patients with pneumonia.

More invasive techniques, such as fiberoptic bronchoscopy or open lung biopsy, should generally be reserved for patients who have not responded to "appropriate" therapy where the etiologic diagnosis is still in question. Most patients in this category are immunocompromised, and consultation with infectious diseases and pulmonary specialists is desirable.

Blood culture should be routinely performed in all hospitalized patients with pneumonia prior to initiating therapy. A
positive culture result will not only establish an etiologic
diagnosis but will also be useful in reassessing therapy.
Of course, chest x-rays are essential in the management of all
patients with pneumonia. The extent of pulmonary involvement
can be better assessed by chest x-ray than by physical exam, and
the presence of pleural fluid can also be better defined. In
virtually all cases, pleural effusions should be evaluated by
thoracentesis. The type of pulmonary infiltrate seen on x-ray
can suggest a specific etiology, e.g., consolidation, nodular
or diffuse infiltrates, cavitation or air/fluid levels; however,
the radiographic findings taken alone can never establish an
etiology.
Peripheral blood white blood cell quantification with a
differential count should be performed in all patients, as clues
both to the etiology and prognosis may be obtained from this
simple test. In patients requiring hospitalization, tests of
liver and renal function, electrolyte determination, and arterial
blood gases are generally indicated. Serologic tests (acute and
convalescent phase samples) are potentially helpful in the
diagnosis of viral pneumonias, Legionnaires' disease, toxoplasmosis, rickettsial diseases and some of the fungal pneumonias.

SPECIAL DIAGNOSTIC CATEGORIES

Localized Pulmonary Infiltrates or Consolidation

S. *pneumoniae* is currently estimated to be the cause of about
75% of all community-acquired bacterial pneumonias, and this
organism is usually associated with relatively localized infiltrates on chest x-ray. The majority of patients with pneumococcal
pneumonia are not immunocompromised, although S. *pneumoniae* can
behave as an opportunist (agammaglobulinemia, splenectomy,
chronic obstructive pulmonary disease). Diagnosis can usually
be supported by analysis of sputum or blood culture. Penicillin
G remains the drug of choice, but treatment failures have been
linked with penicillin resistant organisms now seen throughout
the world, including the United States. Erythromycin or cefazolin
are alternatives in penicillin allergic patients. A polyvalent
vaccine, "Pneumovax", is recommended as prophylaxis for high
risk patients.
The differential diagnosis of localized pneumonia must also
include Legionnaires' disease. Some authorities estimate that
from 5%-10% of all pneumonias are caused by this gram-negative
aerobic bacillus. Although most commonly seen as the cause of
localized outbreaks of pneumonia, both in the community and in
hospitals, sporadic cases of Legionnaires' disease occur through-

out the United States. Although certain clinical features may
help distinguish Legionnaires' disease from pneumonia due to
other organisms, these findings are relatively non-specific, and
treatment with erythromycin should be used expectantly given the
right clinical setting. Some of the clinical characteristics
and diagnostic tests are listed in Table II.

Table II. Legionnaires' Disease*

Clinical features
> *Unproductive cough*
> *Diarrhea*
> *Mental status abnormalities*
> *Unresponsive to penicillin or cephalosporin therapy*

Laboratory findings
> *Abnormal liver function tests*
> *Renal failure*

Diagnostic tests
> *Direct immunofluorescent antibody staining (expectorated
> sputum, bronchoscopy specimens, etc.)*
> *Culture (TTA, bronchoscopy, lung biopsy, pleural fluid
> specimens)*
> *Serologies (may have to be monitored serially for up to 6
> weeks; not helpful in early management)*

---

*
*At least six different serotypes of L. pneumophila have been
described. Four additional species of Legionella that can cause
pneumonia have been characterized: L. micdadei (or pittsburgen-
sis; formerly called TATLOCK or HEBA), L. bozemanii, L. dumoffi,
and L. longbeachae. Erythromycin is used to treat pneumonia
caused by all of these agents; rifampin may be added in severe
cases.*

Other organisms to be considered in the differential diagnosis
of consolidating pneumonia include *S. aureus, K. pneumoniae, H.
influenzae* (increasingly recognized as a cause of pneumonia in
adults), and, less commonly, *C. psittaci* (psittacosis), *Yersinia
pestis* (plague), and *Francisella tularensis* (tularemia). Clearly
of major importance in the young adult population, *M. pneumoniae*
is estimated to cause up to 20% of all cases of pneumonia in the
general population. Over the past decade, our recognition of the
spectrum of disease caused by this bacterium has widened:
children and the elderly may be affected; the disease is usually
mild but can be fulminant and occasionally fatal; the upper and
lower respiratory tracts are most commonly involved, but hepatitis,
skin, and neurologic findings can develop. Diagnosis can be

established by serologic testing (cold agglutinin titers are usually >1:64, and there is a specific complement-fixing antibody test).

Pneumonia in the Compromised Host

The diagnostic and therapeutic considerations in managing patients with pneumonia who have compromised host defenses are dealt with in other sections of this book. However, several basic principles deserve re-emphasis: 1) opportunistic organisms are the most common etiologic agents in these patients, 2) the nature of the underlying host defense abnormality will pre-determine which organisms are most likely to cause pneumonia (Table III), 3) because of the multiplicity of possible organisms causing pneumonia in these patients, invasive diagnostic techniques are often indicated, and 4) antimicrobial therapy should generally be aggressive (high dose therapy given for more prolonged times than in patients with normal defenses).

Table III. Predisposition of Specific Host Defense Defects to Selective Groups of Opportunistic Organisms

Host defense abnormality*	Pneumonia commonly caused by
Neutrophil abnormalities	
Granulocytopenia	Escherichia coli, Pseudomonas aeruginosa, K. pneumoniae, S. aureus, Aspergillus, Candida
Chemotactic dysfunction	S. aureus
Microbicidal dysfunction	S. aureus, Serratia, Pseudomonas sp., Aspergillus, Candida
Agammaglobulinemia	S. pneumoniae, H. influenzae
Complement deficiency	Variety of gram-positive and gram-negative bacteria
Splenectomy	S. pneumoniae, H. influenzae
Cell-mediated immune disorders	Mycobacteria, Nocardia, Listeria, herpesviruses, Toxo-plasma, Pneumocystis, a wide variety of fungi
Cystic fibrosis (decreased mucociliary clearance plus other factors)	P. aeruginosa, S. aureus, H. influenzae

*Abnormalities may be either primary or secondary to cytotoxic drugs, immunosuppressive agents, etc.

Aspiration Pneumonia

The microbiology and approach to management of aspiration pneumonia is discussed in detail elsewhere in this book. It is important, however, to stress that whereas community-acquired aspiration is most commonly followed by infection with a poly-microbial oropharyngeal flora, predominantly comprised of anaerobic bacteria, aerobic gram-negative bacilli are an important component of the microbiology of hospital-acquired aspiration pneumonia. Antibiotic therapy should be selected accordingly. Also, evidence is lacking that either prophylactic antibiotics or corticosteroids are of any benefit when given immediately following the event of aspiration.

CONCLUSIONS

Treatment of pneumonia in 1982 has become considerably more challenging than it was only a decade ago. This is true not only because of the types of patients being treated, but because of our expanded understanding of the complex microbial flora that can cause pneumonia. Nonetheless, rational decisions regarding therapy, which potentially includes the use of many newer penicillins, cephalosporins, and aminoglycosides, can be based on data obtained from the patient history, physical findings, and simple laboratory tests. It is almost a certainty, that we can look forward to continued progress in the management of this important infectious disease.

ACKNOWLEDGMENT

I am greatly indebted to Jane Anderson for her assistance in the preparation of this manuscript.

REFERENCES

Special Etiologic Considerations

Center for Disease Control. (1978). Legionnaires' disease: diagnosis and management. *Ann. Intern. Med. 88,* 363.
Kirby, B.D., Snyder, K.M., Meyer, R.D., Finegold, S.M. (1980). Legionnaires' disease: report of sixty-five nosocomially acquired cases and review of the literature. *Medicine 59,* 188.
Meyer, R.D., Edelstein, P.H., Kirby, B.D., Louie, M.H., Mulligan, M.E., Morgenstin, A.A., Finegold, F.M. (1980). Legionnaires' disease: unusual clinical and laboratory findings. *Ann. Intern. Med. 93,* 240.

Aronson, M.D., Komaroff, A.L., Pasculle, W., Myerowitz, R.L. (1981). *Legionella micdadei* (pittsburgh pneumonia agent) infection in nonimmunosuppressed patients with pneumonia. *Ann. Intern. Med. 94,* 485.

Murray, H.W., Masur, H., Senterfit, L.B., Roberts, R.B. (1975). The protean manifestations of mycoplasma pneumoniae infection in adults. *Am. J. Med. 58,* 229.

Cassell, G.H., Cole, B.C. (1981). Mycoplasmas as agents of human disease. *N. Engl. J. Med. 304,* 80.

Hirschmann, J.V., Everett, E.D. (1979). Haemophilus influenzae infections in adults: report of nine cases and a review of the literature. *Medicine 58,* 80.

Simon, H.B., Southwick, F.S., Moellering, R.C., Sherman, E. (1980). Hemophilus influenzae in hospitalized adults: current perspectives. *Am. J. Med. 69,* 219.

Saah, A.J., Mallonee, J.P., Tarpay, M., Thornsberry, C.T., Roberts, M.A., Rhoades, E.R. (1980). Relative resistance to penicillin in the pneumococcus: a prevalence and case-control study. *JAMA 243,* 1824.

Diagnostic Techniques

Merrill, C.W., Gwaltney, J.M., Hendley, J.O., Sande, M.A. (1973). Rapid identification of pneumococci: gram stain vs. the Quellung reaction. *New Engl. J. Med. 288,* 510.

Thorsteinsson, S.B., Musher, D.M., Fagan, T. (1975). The diagnostic value of sputum culture in acute pneumonia. *JAMA 233,* 894.

Hahn, H.H., Beaty, H.N. (1970). Transtracheal aspiration in the evaluation of patients with pneumonia. *Ann. Intern. Med. 72,* 183.

Broome, C.V., Cherry, W.B., Winn, W.C. Jr., MacPherson, B.R. (1979). Rapid diagnosis of Legionnaires' disease by direct immunofluorescent staining. *Ann. Intern. Med. 90,* 1.

Light, R.W., Girard, W.M., Jenkinson, S.G., George, R.B. (1980). Parapneumonic effusions. *Am. J. Med. 69,* 507.

Special Categories of Patients

Gross, P.A., Neu, H.C., Aswapokee, P., Van Antwerpen, C., Aswapokee, N. (1980). Deaths from nosocomial infections: experience in a university hospital and a community hospital. *Am. J. Med. 68,* 219.

Garb, J.L., Brown, R.B., Garb, J.R., Tuthill, R.W. (1978). Differences in etiology of pneumonias in nursing home and community patients. *JAMA 240,* 2169.

Bartlett, J.G., Gorbach, S.L., Finegold, S.M. (1974). The bacteriology of aspiration pneumonia. *Am. J. Med. 56,* 202.

Lorber, B., Swenson, R.M. (1974). Bacteriology of aspiration pneumonia: a prospective study of community- and hospital-acquired cases. *Ann. Intern. Med. 81,* 329.

Murray, H.W. (1979). Antimicrobial therapy in pulmonary aspiration. *Am. J. Med. 66,* 188.

Williams, D.M., Krick, J.A., Remington, J.S. (1976). Pulmonary infection in the compromised host. Part 1. *Am. Rev. Resp. Dis. 114,* 359.

Williams, D.M., Krick, J.A., Remington, J.S. (1976). Pulmonary infection in the compromised host. Part 2. *Am. Rev. Resp. Dis. 114,* 593.

Pennington, J.E., Feldman, N.T. (1977). Pulmonary infiltrates and fever in patients with hematologic malignancy. Assessment of transbronchial biopsy. *Am. J. Med. 62,* 581.

Editorial. (1981). Indications for pneumococcal vaccine. *Lancet i,* 251.

ETIOLOGY AND DIFFERENTIAL DIAGNOSIS OF PHARYNGOTONSILLITIS

ERNESTO CALDERON
ROSA MARIA SANCHEZ

Infections of the upper respiratory tract are among the chief causes of absenteeism, loss of work energy, the reason for medical consultation and an enormous expenditure of money for antimicrobial drugs (1,2).

The inflammatory processes of the upper respiratory passages present a great variety of clinical pictures. Since the respiratory mucosa extends into numbers of neighboring structures as the ear, conjunctiva, paranasal sinuses, nasopharynx and larynx, the infection may manifest in different forms depending on the degree of damage it does. In these conditions one may see asymptomatic clinical pictures; others, the majority, with discreet signs; and still others, the minority, with serious pictures often complicating the lower respiratory passages.

The pharyngotonsillar area and several adjacent structures as the conjunctival mucosa, the middle ear, the oral cavity itself represent a diagnostic challenge since presenting manifestations of great variety are possible due to inflammation resulting from bacterial or viral infection.

The purpose of this paper is to present the clinician several perspectives that will aid in the establishment of a differential diagnosis during the acute phase as well as indicate possible complications and sequellae.

The etiology of pharyngotonsillitis is varied. Probably 95% of the responsible organisms are those in Table 1.

TABLE 1

PATHOGENIC ORGANISMS INVOLVED IN PHARYNGITIS, PHARYNGOTONSIL-
LITIS AND NASOPHARYNGOCONJUNCTIVITIS

Streptococcus pyogenes
Corynebacterium diphtheriae
Adenovirus
Epstein-Barr Virus
Kawasaki Disease
Mycoplasma pneumoniae
Herpes simplex
Coxsackie Virus
Candida Albicans

STREPTOCOCCAL PHARYNGOTONSILLITIS

(3-6) In no greater then 1% to 5% of apparently healthy
children under three years of age can the presence of Streptococcus pyogenes be demostrated. The illness presents with
specific characteristics in children of this age.

For five to ten days there are irregular elevations of
temperature. The dominant signs are of catarrh with a thick
mucopurulent drip accompanied by local irritation that increases
the patient's discomfort. The pharynx, palate and tonsils show
a homogeneous congestive erythema. The patient complains only
of local smarting. Extension into the middle ear is not uncommon.

The nasal discharge may continue for four to eight weeks
after abatement of the fever. Proof of etiology is possible only
on culture. Treatment with penicillin rapidly clears the
symptoms and pathogens. Treatment options are two: oral
penicillin V 25-50 mg/kg/day in equal divided doses at six to
eight hour intervals for ten days; IM penicillin G 50,000 U/kg
in one dose.

In children with streptococcal angina between three and six
years of age, the catarrhal manifestations and mucopurulent
discharge are prolonged. Fever from the onset is insidious and
irregular and continues for seven to ten days.

The mucopurulent nasal obstruction continues for two or
more months during which time middle ear and paranasal sinus
involvement is frequent. Temperature here may have peaks of
38-39°C indicative of complications, primarily otic. Confirmation of diagnosis is via culture of the nasopharyngeal secretions. In general, the patient's behavior is similar to that
seen in viral respiratory processes. Treatment is the same as
that for the yourger group.

Streptococcal pharyngotonsillitis is most common in the
six to twelve age group primarily during the spring and winter
months. Here it is characterized by sudden onset with 38.5-39°C

fever, intense headache, pharyngeal pain and burning, abdominal
pain occasionally with nausea and vomiting. Examination reveals
a diffuse redness of the pharyngeal mucosa, a few palatal
petechiae, edema of the peritonsillar mucosa with exudate or
purulent membrane formation. The cervical lymph nodes are
enlarged and painful on palpitation.

Frank improvement occurs within three to four days, the
temperature gradually descending to normal on the fourth to
sixth day.

This florid picture can be seen accompanying scarlet fever.
The oral mucosa here is more edematous; the tongue takes on a
violaceous appearance, "the raspberry tongue"; the tonsillar
lesions increase with zones of membranous ulcerations. The skin
shows an exanthem 24-72 hours after the appearance of fever.
This is erythematous in nature and on touch is like gooseflesh.

In the above conditions the diagnosis of streptococcal
angina is almost 100%. However, frequently the presenting
picture is only of fever, sore throat, discreet myalgias and
pharyngeal examination simply reveals an irregular redness and
a few nodular zones.

In non-florid conditions involving the pharyngotonsillar
area, the differential diagnosis may be difficult, streptococcal
involvement being ascertained in only 50-60% of cases.

Options, equally effective, for the clearing of streptococcal infections are:

a). Procaine penicillin G, 800,000 U IM/day for ten days.
Compliance is the problem here.

b). Procaine penicillin G, 800,000 U IM/day for three days.
On the fourth day penicillin G benzothine 600,000 U
for children under six years of age, 1,200,000 U for
those older.

c). Penicillin G benzathine in one dose of 600,000 U or
1,200,000 U depending on age. Improvement here is
delayed one to three days beyond that of b).

d). Penicillin V 250 mg (400,000 U) per every six to eight
hours for ten days. Here too, compliance is a problem.

Complications of Streptococcal Infections <u>Early</u>. During
the acute phase the patients may present with scarlet fever,
erysipelas or pyogenic dissemination to various anatomic areas
and systems, speticemia, meningitis, pneumonia. <u>Late</u>. Two or
three weeks later glomerulonephritis or rheumatic fever may
present. It is important to examine the patient two or three
weeks after the acute phase to determine wheter or not any of
these complications are present.

DIFFERENTIAL DIAGNOSIS

1).Diphtheric Angina. (7) In the prevaccination era this
was seen especially in the pre- and school-age children
regardless of time of year. Today it is infrequent,

nevertheless, it must be kept in mind. Onset is insidious with malaise, burning throath, low-grade and anorexia.

One to three days later, in the tonsillar area, a pseudo-membrane forms consisting of fibrin, b. diphtheriae, polymorpho-nuclear and mononuclear cells. This membrane is firmly adherent. Attempt to remove it causes bleeding. It is of a dark grey color and covers the pharynx, tonsils and part of the larynx. Fever is no more than 38-38.5°C and the pulse is rapid, not commensurate with the fever. The cervical nodes are conside-rably enlarged and painful due to periadenitis. It has been called "bull neck".

Progresses of the disease is variable depending on the degree of toxemia. In the mild cases cure occurs on an average within one week. In severe cases, the patient becomes prostrate on the third to fifth day, pallid, toxic or in comma with a serious risk of myocarditis, cardiac insufficiency and death.

The elements of importance in making a differential diagnosis are: previous vaccination; severity of the clinical picture; type of glandular response; fever curve; characteris-tics of the ischemic necrosis in the peritonsillar zones.

The etiologic diagnosis is via culture of b. diphtheriae in Loffler's medium and telurate. Toxin is present in those treated with or without dephtheria antitoxin. Those not immunized develop an inflamatory zone at the site of inoculation with toxigenic bacilli.

Complications of Diphtheria. Myocarditis appears in 10% to 70% depending upon the amount of toxin. Its onset is late, about the time when the pseudomembrane tends to disappear (5-7 days). Myocardial toxicity comes on at this time apparently due to the sudden onset of cardiac insufficiency. The preventive treatment of this complication is the early administration of diphtheria antitoxin.

The post-diphtheria neurologic lesions appear four to eight weeks after onset of the disease. The craneal nerves are those most frequently affected, the patient having difficulty swallowing and manifesting with salivation and nasal regurgi-tation.

The degree of nerve injury varies from mild paresis to frank paralysis. When the toxin has been matabolized, weeks or months later, resolution occurs.

2). Adenovirus Angina. (7-9) Upper respiratory tract infection occurs most frequently in the pre-school age children but may appear at any age. Children under three year of age present a catharral or nasopharyngoconjunctival picture with few systemic disturbances. They do manifest irregular tempera-ture elevations, nasoconjunctival secretion and membranous exudate of the pharynx which is reddened, edematous and mildly sore. This picture may continue for two to four weeks whether or not the patient is treated with antimicrobials. Clearing is spontaneous just as in any other non-specific respiratory condition.

In older children, the viral angina is similar to that due to the streptococcus. It can come on suddenly with fever of 38-38.5°C, pharyngeal discomfort, headache, malaise. The difference from streptococcal angina is subtle: less pharyngeal mucosal edema, less discomfort on opening the mouth or swallowing food, less marked glandular response (ordinarily the retroauricular glands are involved). Perhaps the most important aspect of the differential is that here, after five to seven days, the condition remains static and may go on for another week. Fever, no higher than 38°C, also continues for another week. The patient does not seem very seek unlike in the acute phase of streptococcal angina.

The condition clears spontaneously. It is therefore of little practical value to attempt a specific viral diagnosis.

Complications of Adenovirus Angina. During the infection, a viremia occurs. Coicident with the pharyngotonsillitis or a few days or weeks thereafter, one of the following conditions may appear: conjunctivitis, the pertussis syndrome, bronchitis, bronchiolitis, pneumonia, cutaneous exanthem, myocarditis, hepatitis, encephalitis and hemorrhagic cystitis.

3). Angina of Infectious Mononucleosis. (8-11) The manifestations of pharyngotonsillitis due to the Epstein-Barr virus are indistinguishable from those due to Streptocuccus pyogenes, particularly when the signs are minimal. When both conditions are florid, the extrapharyngeal signs of mononucleosis can be differentiated: fever of 38-39°C for more than a week, periorbital edema, marked cervical adenopathy, splenomeglay and occasionally jaundice.

Generally, monoculeosis is of longer duration than streptococcal angina (1-4 weeks). This most be taken into account since the persistence of the same signs after treatment with penicillin might be interpreted falsely as an antimicrobial failure. Keeping in mind the possibility of mononucleosis will sharpen the clinician's acuity and help to avoid overtreatment.

Complications of Mononucleosis Angina. The residual splenomegaly may result in mechanical splenic rupture. When this happens, the patient presents with sudden abdominal pain, peritoneal signs and shock.

4). Angina of Kawasaki Disease. (12) Etiology here is unknown. It occurs largely in children under three years of age. The onset is sudden with fever of 38-40°C or more and the patient is mildly or moderately ill. Fever dominates the picture lasting two to three weeks or more, temperature elevation being between 38 and 39°C, antimicrobials are ineffective.

Other signs appear twelve to twenty-four hours after onset

of fever. Non-suppurative bilateral conjunctival congestion occurs and several hours later the lips redden, dry and fissure. The oral mucosa is extremely reddened and edematous. The pharyngotonsillar area is homogeneously erythematous. The tonge shows prominent papillae with a raspberry appearance. The cervical nodes are palpable and accompanied by periadenitis. All of these signs may remain unchanged for three to five days. In addition there may appear an indurated edema with diffuse erythema of the palms and soles and also a polymorphic congestive exanthem.

At the beginning of the third week only the fever, indurated erythematous edema of palms and soles and the generalized maculopapullar exanthem persist. At this time a periungual exofoliative membranous desquamation appears.

No known treatment shortens the process.

Complications of Angina of Kawasaki Disease. It is possible that at the end of the first week the heart may be compromised by arrhythmia, myocarditis, pericarditis, ischemia, coronary thrombosis, aneurysmic arteritis and infarction. This may be the cause of early or late death in about 1.5% of patients.

With this syndrome there occasionally appears arthralgia, myalgia, diarrhea, meningitis, pneumonia, anterior urethral inflammation and other less frequent complications.

5). Mycoplasma pneumoniae Angina. (13-16) Infrequent in children under six years of age, it is more common in the six to twenty year age group. Depending on age, pharyngotonsillitis may appear. In those under six, the picture resembles mild catarrh. Here, the pharynx is diffusely reddened without exudate or membrane formation. Occasionally there is fever no higher than 38°C. The patient clears of signs and symptoms in the first week after onset. Differentiation from streptococcus angina is simple. Here the illness is shorter. There are no otic, nasal or conjunctival complications.

In shcool-age children and adolescents, the illness may be asymptomatic and manifest with a non-specific pharyngitis or irregular fever, burning throat with diffuse erythema, little or no mucosal edema, small plaques of pharyngotonsillar exudate and cervical adenopathy.

Generally, onset is insidious with headaches, irregular fever, shivering, malaise, anorexia followed by pharyngitis and cough that may be productive of a mucopurulent sputum.

If there is no pulmonary or pleuropulmonary involvement, complete clearing always occurs within one or two weeks.

It is important to keep this illness in mind since it may coexist with Streptococcus pyogenes in the pharyngotonsillar area. In general Mycoplasma pneumoniae infection acts in the manner of a spontaneous respiratory process of short duration in the upper passages.

Diagnosis by isolation of the organism is not practical. Immunoserologic tests and culture determine the presence or absence of Streptococcus pyogenes.

Treatment may be:

a) Erythromycin 30 mg/kg/day in divided equal doses at six to eight hour intervals per os for seven to ten days.

b) Optional. Tetracycline 25-50 mg/kg/day in divided equal doses at six to eight hour intervals for seven to ten days.

Complications of Mycoplasma pneumoniae Angina. Bronchiolitis, pneumonia, pleural effusion, aseptic meningitis, arthritis, hematologic changes.

6). Herpetic Gingivostomatitis. (17-19) May occur at any age but most frequently in those one to four years old. The clinical picture varies from mild manifestations of low fever, few vascular lesions to a florid picture with a severe systemic attack.

The basic difference from streptococcal angina is the presence of vesicular or ulcerated lesions.

The onset is sudden with fever that may be higher than 40°C The patient is anorexic, irritable with pain and burning in the affected areas of the oral cavity. The gums are markedly edematous, reddened, friable, bleeding easily with numbers of pale ulcers extremely painful surrounded by an erythematous areola. These same lesions are found disseminated in the labial mucosa, tongue, fauces, palate and posterior pharyngeal wall.

Depending upon the size and number of lesions, the illness courses toward complete cure without sequellae in one to two weeks.

A characteristic of this disease is recurrences due to a variety of stimuli.

There is no specific therapy for the condition or for prevention of recurrence.

Complications of Herpetic Gingivostomatitis. There are practically none. The risk of bacterial superinfection is minimal.

7). Herpangina. (20-21) This disease is caused by several types of Coxsackie A virus. It appears at any age more frequent in children under ten years old. It is characterized by small vesicular lesions or small ulcers surrounded by an erythematous halo. Signs are primarily in the fauces. It is differentiated from gingivostomatitis in that it does not involve the gums.

Onset is sudden with fever up to 39°C for three to four days, pharyngeal pain and burning, disseminated vesicles in the palate, anterior pillars, tonsils, uvula and posterior pharyngeal wall. The walls of the vesicles are fragile and break easily forming small greyish ulcers surrounded by an erythematous halo.

Herpangina has a shorter course that herpetic
gingivostomatitis. The lesions clear up in three to six days.
There is no specific treatment.
Complications of Herpangina. There are none. The
condition clears completely.

8). Candida Pharyngotonsillitis. (22-24) This is an
infrequent condition. Occasionally it may be confused with
streptococcal infection. It occurs largely in neonates,
nursing infants and in immunodeficient patients.
When lesions are florid, they are not ordinarily confused
with the above-mentioned conditions. The course is either
arebrile or with mild fever. The lesions organize in
confluent pale plaques that extend onto the tongue, fauces and
occasionally the posterior pharyngeal wall.
When small plaques are formed in the pharyngotonsillar
zone they are accompanied by an homogenous erythema especially
when the "cottony" plaque is removed leaving a bloody
reddened surface. The clinical impression made by this type of
lesion is that of pharyngitis.
Resolution, in general, is complete. There are practically
no complications.

REFERENCES

1. Greenberg, R.A., Wagner, E.H., Wolf, S.H. et al.
   (1978) J.A.M.A. 240: 650
2. Krugman, S., and Katz, S.L. (1981). Infectious Diseases of
   children. 7th. Ed., The C.V. Mosby Co. St. Louis.
3. Breese, B.B., and Breese, C. (1978). Beta hemolytic
   Streptococcal Diseases. Houghton Mifflin Professional
   Publishers, Boston.
4. Kaplan, E.L., Top. F.H., Jr., Dudding, B.A. et al.
   (1971). J. Infect. Dis. 123: 490
5. Wannamaker, L.W. (1972). Am. J. Dis. child. 124: 352
6. Calderón, J.E. (1981). Conceptos clínicos de infectología.
   7th. Ed. pag. 107. Méndez-Cervantes, Mexico
7. Van der Veen, J. (1963). Am. Rev. Respir. Dis. 88: 167
8. Evans, A.S. (1960). Am. J. Hyg. 71: 342
9. Epstein, M.A., and Achong, B.G. (1977). Lancet 2: 1270
10. Sumaya, C.V. (1977). Pediatrics 59: 16
11. Carter, R.L., and Penman, H.G. (1965) Infectious Mononucleosis
    Blackwell Scientific Publications, Oxford.
12. Yanagihara, R., and Todd, J.K. (1980). Am. J. Dis. child.
    134: 603
13. Levine, D.P., and Lerner, A.M. (1978). Clin. Med. North.
    Amer. 62: 967
14. Clyde, W.A., and Denny, F.W. (1967). Pediatrics 40: 669
15. Cherry, J.D., Hurwithz, E.S., and Welliver, R.C. (1975)
    Clin. Radiol. 28: 173

16. Dameron, D.C., Borthwick, R.N., and Philip, T. (1977) Clin. Radiol. 28: 173
17. Nahmias, A.J., and Roizman, B. (1973). N. Engl. J. Med. 289: 667
18. Schluger, S., Yuodelis, R.A., and Page, R.C. (1977) Periodontal Diseases. Lea and Febiger, Philadelphia.
19. Weathers, D.R., and Griffin, J.W. (1970) J.A.D.A. 81: 81
20. Magoffin, R.L., Jackson, E.W. and Lennette, E.H. (1961). J.A.M.A. 175: 441
21. Parrot, R.H. (1957). Ann. N.Y. Acad. Sci. 67: 230
22. Emmons, C.W., Binford, C.H., and Utz, J.P. (1963) Medical Mycology., Lea and Febiger, Philadelphia.
23. Myerowitz, R.L., Pazin, G.J., and Allen, C.M. (1977) Amer. J. Clin. Pathol. 68: 29
24. Grossman, M.E., Silvers, D.N., and Walther, R.R. (1980) J. Amer. Acad. Dermatol. 2: 111

ANAEROBIC PLEUROPULMONARY
INFECTIONS

Corando Sáenz[1]

Infectious Disease Service
Department of Internal Medicine
University Hospital, School of Medicine, U.A.N.L.
Monterrey, Nuevo León, México

Awareness of anaerobic infections involving the lung and pleura has been growing in the last few years. These diseases are still frequently overlooked because many clinicians lack knowledge about them, and because the characteristic foul odor of the sputum is missing in the first days of illness. Also, common media are unsuitable for culturing anaerobes.

While some anaerobic lung infections follow hematogenous dissemination (with or without clinical evidence of pulmonary emboli) from abdominal or pelvic abscesses, or by direct extension of subphrenic abscesses, most result from aspiration of oropharyngeal secretions containing oral bacterial flora. Severity of infection reflects host resistance factors, the level of tissue oxygenation, and the size of the bacteriál inoculum.

Pneumonitis, necrotizing pneumonitis, lung abscess and empyema are common clinical problems caused by one or more anaerobic bacterial species. Infections are usually polymicrobial, averaging three to four anaerobes. Aerobic bacteria are involved concurrently in nearly half of the patients. Penicillin G alone is the preferred therapy for all forms of anaerobic pleuro-pulmonary infections except for ones produced by some *Bacteroides fragilis*, and in patients allergic to penicillin, or with severe mixed aerobic and anaerobic infections.

[1]*Present address: Servicio de Infectología 2° Piso*
Hospital Universitario "Dr. José E. González"
Monterrey, Nuevo León, México

I. INTRODUCTION

Although anaerobic bacteria were first described by Pasteur
in 1861 and Guillemont (1904) established their pathogenic role
in lung infections (Rohini, L.A., 1978) at the beginning of this
century, it was not until recently, when technological advances
were applied to clinical laboratory isolation and identification
of these organisms, that their importance as a cause of lung
and pleural infections has become recognized among practicing
physicians. They should be considered in the etiological
diagnosis of cavitating lesions of the lung along with the other
well known pathogens.
    Anaerobic infections differ from the aerobic bacterial pneumo-
nias in several ways: (1) a majority of cases occur in men,
during the fourth and fifth decades of life; (2) onset usually is
insidious; (3) the degree of illness is often mild to moderate;
(4) almost all patients have episodes of altered consciousness;
(5) fever and leukocytosis are commonly mild to moderate; (6) the
roentgenographic picture is that of segmental pneumonia with
cavitation and an air-fluid level; and (7) response to therapy
is often protracted. In this chapter I will review the pathogenesis, clinical features, diagnosis, and treatment of these
infections.

II. PATHOGENESIS

Anaerobic growth depends primarily on a low redox-potential
of the bacterial environment, as occurs when tissue oxygenation
is impaired either by decreased blood supply or by tissue
destruction caused by trauma, tumor or infection. In this
setting anaerobic bacteria multiply freely. Moreover the
decreasing pH in areas of necrosis prevents proper action of
both polymorphonuclear leukocytes and antimicrobial agents.
    The routes by which anaerobic bacteria can arrive in the lung
are: (1) aspiration of oral secretions; (2) direct implantation;
(3) extension from contiguous infection; and (4) by the bloodstream, with or without clinical evidence of pulmonary emboli
from distant foci.
    The most common factor leading to the development of anaero-
bic pleuropulmonary infection is aspiration. Conditions carrying
a high risk of aspiration are listed in Table 1.

Table 1. *Major Risk Factors for Aspiration of Oral*
          Secretions into the Lung

Alcoholism	Head trauma
Cerebrovascular accident	Intestinal obstruction
Seizure disorders	Diabetic ketoacidosis
Esophageal disease	General anesthesia
Upper gastrointestinal bleeding	Drug overdose (suicidal)

Susceptibility to anaerobic lung infection increases in an already damaged lung, such as in bronchogenic carcinoma, bronchiectasis, pulmonary tuberculosis and pulmonary infarction due to pulmonary embolism. Important predisposing factors are poor oral hygiene and dental diseases, such as periodontitis and gingivitis, and also the intra-abdominal and pelvic suppurative diseases, like subphrenic abscess and acute pelvic infections complicated by suppurative thrombophlebitis and septic pulmonary emboli (Bartlett, J.G., 1974).

Proper techniques for obtaining samples for culture require the bypassing of oral secretions, and these techniques have made it possible to determine the true bacteriology of anaerobic pleuropulmonary infections. Percutaneous transtracheal aspirates and thoracentesis specimens are the most reliable, but there are other means of obtaining adequate material for bacteriological studies, e.g., blood culture, direct lung puncture, thoracotomy, puncture of metastatic abscess and autopsy.

Unlike aerobic pneumonias, usually more than one pathogen is isolated. In Finegold's experience (Finegold and Bartlett, 1975), an average of three or four different organisms were recovered from each patient. We found a mean of 2.7, as is shown in Table II.

Table II. *Bacteriology of Anaerobic Pleuropulmonary*
           Infections in 35 Patients[a]

	isolates %		isolates %
Gram-negative bacilli		*Gram-positive cocci*	
Bacteroides spp.	26	Peptostreptococcus	21
Bacteroides melanino-		Peptococcus	15
genicus	15		
Fusobacterium spp.	13	*Gram-positive cocci*	
Bacteroides fragilis	7		
		Eubacterium	12
		Clostridium	1

[a]*Infectious Disease Service, University Hospital School of Medicine, Nuevo León, México*

When the host defenses fail, a liquefactive necrosis with abscess formation develops. Following bronchial wall destruction, the abscess may spill and disseminate to other pulmonary segments. The inflammatory process can affect the pleura with empyema formation. Eventually a bronchopleural fistula can develop allowing air into the pleural space.

Several lung segments are usually involved. Aspiration usually occurs in the recumbent position, and the most frequently affected areas of the lung are those that are gravity-dependent, especially in the posterior segments of upper lobes, and the superior segments of lower lobes, the right greater than the left. It is unusual to see anaerobic infections in other pulmonary segments and, in such cases, a careful search for an obstructing endobronchial carcinoma or an abscess below the diaphragm should be undertaken.

III. CLINICAL FEATURES

According to Bartlett and Finegold (1974) anaerobic pleuropulmonary infections have several clinical patterns: (1) pneumonitis (pulmonary infiltrate with no evidence of cavitation); (2) necrotizing pneumonia (multiple small areas of cavitation within one or more pulmonary segments or lobes); (3) lung abscess (defined as a solitary or dominant cavity measuring at least 2 cm in diameter); (4) empyema (infected pleural exudate). Any combination of the parenchymal lesions with or without pleural fluid can be present. The severity of these infections ranges between a benign pneumonitis to indolent progressive necrotizing pneumonia, referred to in the past as pulmonary gangrene. The severity depends on the virulence of the bacteria involved, the size of inoculum and host response. The clinical features are summarized in Table III.

IV. DIAGNOSIS

The diagnosis of anaerobic pleuropulmonary infection rests on clinical, radiologic and bacteriologic clues (see Table IV).

Table III. Clinical Features of Anaerobic Pleuropulmonary Infection

CLINICAL CLUES	Types of Anaerobic Infection			
	ASPIRATION PNEUMONITIS	NECROTIZING PNEUMONIA	LUNG ABSCESS	EMPYEMA
Onset	Fairly acute	Insidious (one week)	Insidious (2-3 weeks)	Insidious (2-3 weeks)
Predisposing	Periodontal disease Altered consciousness	Altered consciousness Periodontal diseases Aspiration	Altered consciousness Aspiration Abdominal anaerobic infection (20%)	Aspiration Periodontal diseases
Symptoms	Fever, cough, mild chest pain	Severe pleuritic chest pain, fever and cough	Moderate fever, anorexia and weight loss	Low grade fever, anorexia, weight loss, pleuritic pain
Sputum	Rarely putrid	Putrid	Putrid	Foul smelling, also pleural fluid
Peripheral WBC and RBC	Relatively normal	Moderate increase and anemia	Mild increase and anemia	Mild increase and moderate anemia
Chest X-ray	Patchy infiltrate	Abscess, empyema or bronchopleural fistula	Cavitation (right upper lobe), air fluid level	Massive or loculated pleural fluid, air fluid level
Response to treatment	Quick	Slow	Slow	Slow

Table IV. Clues to the Diagnosis of Anaerobic
Pleuropulmonary Infections

Clinical	Radiologic	Bacteriologic
Putrid sputum or empyema fluid Mild and insidious course Suspected aspiration	Lung parenchymal cavitation with air-fluid level Massive or loculated pleural fluid	Polymicrobial and typical forms on Gram stain. Negative aerobic culture.

Clinical Clues

    With the exception of aspiration pneumonitis, the hall-
mark of these infections is sputum or pleural exudate of
putrid character. Anaerobes produce foul smelling organic
acids, short-chain fatty acids and volatile amines. But not
all patients with this type of infection have a fetid odor
to their bronchopulmonary secretions. This is especially
true with aspiration pneumonitis (Bartlett, J.G., 1979).
Therefore, the absence of this sign should not deter one from
suspecting an anaerobic infection. On the other hand, it
is well recognized that *K. pneumoniae, S. aureus,* and
Mycobacterium tuberculosis can produce fetid pulmonary
exudates.
    A second important clinical clue is the subacute course
of the infection. The natural history of patients with lung
abscess, empyema and necrotizing pneumonia due to anaerobes
is characteristically one of symptoms for more than one or
two weeks before medical attention is sought (Tillotson, J.R.,
1968).
    The final important clinical clue is an episode of
bronchial aspiration. Altered states of consciousness
or esophageal diseases are reported in the clinical history
of more than 75% of patients. Among the causes predisposing
to aspiration, alcoholism is the single most important in the
adult patients, but in children convulsive disorders take
the lead (Brook, I., 1979). Poor oral hygiene, gingivitis
and periodontitis are important bacterial sources in
aspiration cases, but in contrast with past experience
(Brook, R.C., 1952), Bartlett and Finegold (1974) and Brook
and Finegold (1979) found lung abscesses in edentulous
adults and children, respectively, in their series. In
edentulous patients with confirmed anaerobic lung disease

a meticulous search should be made for evidence of carcinoma causing bronchial obstruction and of subdiaphragmatic foci of infection.

Radiological Clues

Radiologic findings are not pathognomonic of any form of anaerobic pleuropulmonary infection. Cavitary lesions with fairly thick walls and shaggy margins, air-fluid levels, massive or loculated empyemas with air fluid levels or bronchopleural fistula are frequently present. The most commonly affected sites are the posterior segment of the right upper lobe and the superior segment of the right and left lower lobes. The predilection for these areas is explained by their anatomical situation. It has been well demonstrated that gravity causes contrast material instilled into the trachea to flow to these most dependent pulmonary segments when a person is in a recumbent position. Thus, they receive the greatest load of the infective aspirated material (Brook, R.C., 1952) (Berkman, Y.M., 1980).

When anaerobic infections develop in other pulmonary segments, an underlying process other than aspiration, such as bronchial occlusion from tumor or metastatic infection, should be suspected.

Bacteriological Clues

The Gram stain is the most useful tool for rapid assessment. Appropriate material for staining can be obtained from percutaneous transtracheal aspiration or from thoracentesis if empyema is present. Sputum and bronchoscopy specimens should not be used for these purposes, since such material is contaminated by oral microbial flora, and it very seldom correlates with culture results, even when a quantitative culture technique is done (Guckian, J.C., 1978).

Transtracheal aspiration should be performed only by physicians well trained in the procedure and should be avoided in patients who are uncooperative, in respiratory distress syndrome, with bleeding disorders, or in those with goiter or severe pathological changes of the neck.

On the Gram stain the polymicroflora and the morphology of anaerobes set them apart from aerobic infections. Metachromatic granules occur along the length of the rod in certain anaerobic species like Bacteroides melaninogenicus.

Fusobacterium appears as slender Gram-negative rods with sharply pointed ends. *Bacteroides* are seen as irregularly staining, pleomorphic Gram-negative rods. Anaerobic Gram-positive cocci may be difficult to distinguish from their aerobic counterparts, staphylococci and streptococci, but the presence of anaerobic Gram-negative rods may reveal their anaerobic nature.

Because *Mycobacteria* and some fungus infections may mimic bacterial process it is mandatory that acid-fast and potassium hydroxide preparations should be routinely done and carefully examined. Culture for these organisms is indicated in any purulent lung material that fails to grow in aerobical and anaerobical media.

Blood and material from percutaneous transtracheal aspiration, thoracentesis and direct lung aspirates (Wimberly, N., 1979) are best suited for the recovery of anaerobes. Proper collection, transportation and processing of these materials are of paramount importance for anaerobic bacterial isolation, since these microorganisms are quite sensitive to oxygen.

Use of a syringe for collection of purulent material is helpful in that all air can be immediately expelled after collection. For transportation, a pre-reduced anaerobic medium may be available that allows for inoculation at the bedside. If this is not possible, the syringe specimen must be transported without delay to the microbiology laboratory for immediate processing. The specimens are planted on various selective media such as Schaldler broth, Brain-heart infusion, Brucella agar or broth and Wilkins-Chalgren agar, and the cultures placed into an oxygen-free environment such as Gas-Pack jar, an anaerobe glove box or a roll tube system. Several recent studies comparing the relative efficacy of these three systems for isolation of anaerobic bacteria showed that they are equal in yield of clinically important anaerobes.

Growth of anaerobic bacteria on a culture medium usually takes several days. Therefore, cultures must not be discarded as negative before at least one week.

Choice of the appropriate medium is a critical factor in the recovery of anaerobes. The use of selective agar media, such as those containing kanamycin and vancomycin to inhibit growth of facultative bacteria, is very helpful in isolating anaerobic Gram-negative rods. Phenylethyl-alcohol or colistin-nalidixic-acid blood agar plates are similary helpful for isolation of Gram-positive anaerobes. Many clinical laboratories still rely exclusively on thioglycolate broth medium for recovery of anaerobes. This is to be condemned since many anaerobes fail to grow in it (Bartlett, J.G., 1972).

There is not a unanimous opinion regarding whether it is necessary to routinely test anaerobes for susceptibility to antimicrobial agents. However, susceptibility patterns for some anaerobic bacteria do change, as has happened with *Bacteroides* and tetracycline in the past, and *Bacteroides* and clindamycin at present. If the tests are not routinely done, they should at least be tried on those anaerobes isolated from treatment failures, and periodically on stored isolates, to determine if susceptibility patterns are changing in any particular institution. The Kirby-Bauer disk diffusion technique is not to be used with anaerobes, because this technique is intended only for rapidly growing aerobic and anaerobic facultative bacteria, and has not been useful for slow growing bacterias like the strict anaerobes.

V. DIFFERENTIAL DIAGNOSIS

Tuberculosis, aerobic necrotizing pneumonia (due to type 3 pneumococci, *S. aureus, K. pneumoniae, E. coli, Legionella pneumophilia)*, fungal infection, carcinoma, infected bullae or bronchogenic cysts must be carefully searched for in every patient since any one of these lesions may mimic or actually coexist with anaerobic pleuropulmonary infections.

VI. MANAGEMENT

Drug Therapy

Patients with anaerobic infections such as aspiration pneumonia, necrotizing pneumonia, lung abscess or empyema, can usually be treated with a single antibiotic. During the initial toxic phase of the disease, parenteral penicillin G (12 to 24 million units/day, I.V., divided in four hourly doses) can be used. Simple pneumonitis can usually be treated with a 10 to 14 day course of therapy, but the more suppurative processes, such as lung abscess, empyema and necrotizing pneumonia, may require a 4 to 12 week treatment. An alternative regimen, particularly for patients with penicillin allergy, would be clindamycin administered intravenously at a dosage of 300-600 mg diluted in 30-50 ml of 5% dextrose in water administered during 15 minutes every six hours.

Many other antimicrobial drugs are now available for the treatment of anaerobic infections, and each one has its own indication. Table V lists antibiotics currently in use for anaerobes, mainly against *B. fragilis* and other potential anaerobes resistant to penicillin, such as *B. melaninogenicus* and *Cl. ramosum.*

Table V. Antimicrobial Agents Other Than Penicillin G[a]
          Used for Anaerobic Pleuropulmonary Infection
          Therapy

Antimicrobial Drug	Doses	
	I.V.	Oral
Clindamycin	600-900 mg q/6 hrs	300 mg q/4 hrs
Chloramphenicol	1 gr q/6 hrs	500 mg q/4 hrs
Metronidazole[b]	15 mg/kg over 1 hr Then 7.5 mg/kg q/ 6 hrs	250-750 q/8 hrs
Cefoxitin	2 gr q/4 hrs	- - -
Carbenicillin	5 gr q/4 hrs	- - -
Lincomycin	600-1,200 mg q/6 hrs	500 mg q/4 hrs
Tetracycline; Doxycycline[c]	100-200 mg q/24 hrs	100 mg q/12 hrs (the first day), then 100-200 mg q/24 hrs
Minocycline	- - -	200 mg initially, then 100 mg q/ 12 hrs
Erythromycin	1-2 gr q/6 hrs	0.5-1 gr q/6 hrs

[a]Penicillin G is the drug of choice for initial therapy of all the anaerobic pleuropulmonary infections, but it should be exchanged with other drugs when B. fragilis, Cl. ramosum or B. melaninogenicus or other penicillin resistant strains are isolated.

[b]It has not been approved by the FDA to be used for anaerobic infection. The I.V. administration is in 250 WD 5% volume.

[c]100-200 mg/day should be administered in 400 ml WD 5% during a 4 hr period once a day.

Hospital acquired aspiration pneumonia, as it occurs in postoperative patients or in intensive care units, deserves special consideration. In addition to its own flora, the oropharyngeal cavity is rapidly colonized by Gram-negative bacterial hospital flora, often antibiotic resistant, including *Pseudomonas, Serratia, Providentia,* and indole-positive *Proteus* strains. In this setting an aminoglycoside, such as amikacin 500 mg I.V. every 6-12 hrs; isomycin 1 mg/kg/day, divided in 3 daily doses; or gentamicin 5-7 mg/kg/day divided in 3 daily doses, may be added to the regimen (Murray, H.W., 1979).

Drainage

Mechanical drainage procedures play a critical role in many patients. Empyema caused by anaerobes is usually not successfully treated with even repeated needle aspiration; our practice is to insert a thoracostomy tube as soon as empyema is established on the basis of grossly cloudy fluid and the presence of organisms on smear. With a pH lower than 7.2 empyema is rarely successfully treated without tube drainage (Light, R.W., 1973) (Potts, D.E., 1976). If the patient with empyema does not defervesce after 7 days of tube drainage and antimicrobial therapy, additional procedures are indicated. The options include: (1) insertion of multiple chest tubes; (2) rib resection for better drainage, and (3) decortication. In our experience the latter procedure is preferable in patients who are otherwise reasonable surgical candidates; prolonged tube drainage is reserved for those patients at greater surgical risk.

Fiberoptic bronchoscopy plays an important role in the ruling out of causes of bronchial obstruction, such as tumors or foreign bodies. Although these techniques are of little diagnostic benefit early in the course of anaerobic infection, since purulent material obstructs the endoscopist's view, they can add to treatment by allowing instrumented drainage.

Postural drainage is also a very important adjunct in the treatment of lung abscess.

Surgery

The current indications for surgery are summarized in Table VI. In general, a conservative approach to the management of anaerobic pleuropulmonary infections is preferred, since a 25% incidence of morbidity is associated with surgery (Bartlett, 1975).

Table VI. Surgery Indications in Pleuropulmonary Anaerobic Infection

- *Life threatening hemorrhage*
- *Bronchial obstruction with poor drainage*
- *Lung cancer*
- *Symptomatic bronchiectasis*

ACKNOWLEDGMENTS

I wish to thank Dr. Rodrigo F. Barragán for his help in preparing this manuscript, and Mrs. Guadalupe Pérez for her secretarial skill.

REFERENCES

Bartlett, J.G., Finegold, S.M. (1972). *Medicine 51,* 413.
Bartlett, J.G., et al. (1973). *Ann. Intern. Med. 79,* 535.
Bartlett, J.G., Finegold, S.M. (1974). *Amer. Rev. Resp. Dis. 110,* 56.
Bartlett, J.G., Gorbach, S.L. (1975). *JAMA 234,* 935.
Bartlett, J.G. (1979). *Amer. Rev. Resp. Dis. 119,* 19.
Berkman, Yahya M. (1980). *Seminars in Roentgenology:XV (1).*
Briggs, D., Jr. (1977). *Med. Clinics of North Amer. 61(6).*
Brock, R.C. (1952). "Lung Abscess". Charles C. Thomas Publisher, Springfield, IL, p. 8.
Brook, I., and Finegold, S.M. (1979). *J. of Pediatrics 94,* 10.
Finegold, S.M., Bartlett, J.G., Chow, A.W., et al. (1975). *Ann. Intern. Med. 83,* 375.
Gonzalez, C.L., and Calia, F.M. (1975). *Arch. Intern. Med. 135,* 711.
Green, G.M., Jakab, G.J., Low, R.B. et al (1977). *Amer. Rev. Resp. Dis. 115,* 479,
Guckain, J.C. and Christensen, W.D. (1978). *Amer. Rev. Resp. Dis. 118,* 997.
Hoeprich, P.D. (1970). *Calif. Med. 112,* 18.

Holdeman, L.V., Moore, W.E.C. (1972). Anaerobe Laboratory
    Manual, the Virginia Polytechnic Institute and State
    University, Blacksborg, Va.
Johanson, W.G., Jr., and Harris, G.D. (1980). *Clin. Med. of*
    North Amer. 64(3), 379.
Light, R.W., MacGregor, I., Bill, W.C. Jr., et al (1978).
    Chest 118, 997.
Murray, H.W. (1979). *Amer. J. of Med. 66*, 188.
Potts, D.E., Levin, D.C., and Sahn, S.A. (1976). *Chest 70*, 328.
Rohini, L., Abeysundere, E., Hudson, M., Szawatkowski, P.
    (1979). *Br. J. Dis. Chest 72*, 187.
Tillotson, J.R., Leaner, M.A. (1968). *Ann. Intern. Med. 68*,308.
Wimberly, N., Faling, L.J., and Bartlett, J.G. (1979). *Amer.*
    Rev. Resp. Dis. 119, 337.

TUBERCULOSIS - NEW THERAPIES OF AN OLD PROBLEM

Publio Toala
Edgardo Fernández
Enrique Diaz

University of Panama Medical School
Complejo Hospitalario Metropolitano del
Seguro Social and Hospital Santo Tomás
Panama City, Panama

The discovery of streptomycin, the use of a combination of drugs to prevent emergence of resistant bacteria, the discovery of isoniazid, the ambulatory management of tuberculosis, the introduction of supervised intermittent chemotherapy and finally the data on short-course chemotherapy for pulmonary tuberculosis are six major developments that have affected the direction of treatment of tuberculosis.

The primary antituberculosis drugs are highly effective, relatively simple to take, need not be parenteral and are usually tolerated well. Hospitalization of newly diagnosed cases is not necessary and in the few cases where it becomes necessary for diagnostic purposes or because of incapacitating illness, care now takes place within a community hospital.

It is necessary to emphasize that tuberculosis still occupies an important position among the 21 communicable diseases considered as priority problems by the World Health Organization. In the Americas tuberculosis was sixth in order of importance despite the fact that information is sometimes incomplete and that only in a few countries are morbidity rates based on bacteriologically-confirmed new cases. In the Americas, case rates did not exceed 200 per 100,000 (Bolivia), but the lowest rates were under 20 per 100,000 in only a few countries (Cuba, U.S.A., Jamaica, etc.). By some calculations the estimated worldwide incidence of tuberculosis was over 3.5 million in 1971, or 96 per 100,000 (1).

Even before the discovery of the tubercle bacillus, there
was already a marked decline in mortality from tuberculosis.
Thus, in England and Wales the decrease was more than 80 percent
between 1900 and 1950. In the Americas, despite the availability
of potent drugs, tuberculosis still ranks among the most important causes of death. Even in Canada, in 1974, deaths from
tuberculosis accounted for 62 percent of all deaths due to
notifiable diseases.

Failure of chemotherapy is due to: 1) prescribing inadequate
regimens, 2) drug toxicity, 3) patients discharging themselves
from treatment prematurely, 4) patients attending treatment
services, but a) stopping taking drugs, or b) becoming irregular
in taking drugs, and 5) drug-resistant infection at the start of
chemotherapy. It is now known that the main reasons for failure
of treatment regimens are patients who either stop taking drugs
or who do so irregularly. There is now sufficient evidence to
support this thesis. Primary drug-resistance at the start of
chemotherapy is not that important, as we have learned from
studies in Hong Kong. On the other hand, in several studies done
in Africa, treatment failure using so-called standard chemotherapy was 15%; of this figure between 7-9% was due to
insufficient duration of the prescribed regimen and 3% was
accounted for by primary resistance to isoniazid. This problem
was also analyzed in Scotland where of the overall failure rate
(11.4%), patients who either refused therapy or defaulted perman-
ently accounted for 8%. It is interesting to note that only 0.9%
of failure was due to primary drug resistance. In a cooperative
study reported by Jorge A. Pilheu, of 145 patients from four
South American countries they found only one case with resistance
to isoniazid and four other cases with resistance to isoniazid
plus ethambutol; all five cases were from Bogota, Columbia (2).

The main standard daily regimens, prescribed for 18 months to
two years, and the dosages of the drugs, are summarized in Table 1.
The daily triple drug phase is usually continued for up to three
months. A major development in chemotherapy has been the finding
that "pulse therapy" could be useful in treating patients with
tuberculosis, either with standard duration or with so-called
short course chemotherapy.

Efforts have been directed toward ensuring that patients
actually receive the full course as prescribed with supervision
of intermittent therapy and short-course chemotherapy.

Table 1. *Tuberculosis Chemotherapy Standard Regimens*

	Regimen		Dosages
	Initial	*Continuation*	*Dosages*
Daily	SPH	PH	S - 0.75-1 G
	SRH	RH	P - 10-12 G
	SEH	EH	R - 450 or 600 mg
	STH	TH	E - 15 mg/kg
			T - 150 mg
Intermittent[a]	SPH	SH	S - 0.75-1 G
	SRH	SH	H - 15 mg/kg
	SEH	EH	E - 50 mg/kg
	STH	SH	

S = streptomycin   P = para-aminosalicylic acid (PAS)
H = isoniazid   R = rifampin   E = ethambutol   T = thiacetazone

[a] *Twice-weekly*

SUPERVISED INTERMITTENT CHEMOTHERAPY

The standard most widely used intermittent regimen is a twice-
weekly combination of streptomycin, 1 G or 0.75 G, plus isoniazid,
15 mg/kg, per dose. This regimen should be preceded, whenever
possible, by a daily intensive phase of three drugs for up to
three months. A combination particularly used in the U.S.A. is
ethambutol plus isoniazid twice a week. Therapeutic results
with this regimen in a number of controlled clinical trials
are summarized in Table II. All the data from studies done in
several developing countries using the once a week regimen have
shown an overall failure rate (failures during chemotherapy
and bacteriologic relapses after stopping chemotherapy) of 66% or
slightly less; but it is of interest to mention here the data
from Singapore that gives only a 7% overall failure rate using
isoniazid and rifampin once a week. The organization of intermittent chemotherapy must be designed to meet the convenience of
patients. The patients should be able to receive chemotherapy at
facilities near their home, place of work or en route to work.
These might include community health centers, dispensaries,
hospitals, factory clinics, rural health units, etc. It is
important to emphasize that the responsibilities for these
programs should remain in the hands of the physician.

The main advantages of supervised intermittent chemotherapy are: it is therapeutically highly effective, it has lower chronic toxicity than daily regimens, the cost is lower and it avoids the undetected irregularity inherent in the self-administration of daily regimens.

Table II.   Intermittent Chemotherapy. Streptomycin
plus Isoniazid Twice-Weekly

Study	Initial phase (mo.)	No. of Patients	Results (%)
Madras, 1964	0	72	94
Madras, 1970	0	117	91
WHO, Prague 1971	3	233	100
1976	1½	85	99
1976	3	96	98
Singapore, 1972	3	168	98
British Medical Research Council, 1973	3	95	99

SHORT COURSE CHEMOTHERAPY

Because of the problems created by the so-called standard duration chemotherapy (18 to 24 months), namely poor patient compliance, high costs and logistic difficulties in delivery of services, several developing countries undertook clinical trials with drug regimens that might permit shorter duration of treatment and still be satisfactory as far as high rates of cure are concerned. Great Britain and France have been involved in these trials and they applied their experience in more technologically advanced countries. Great Britain shortened the treatment of previously untreated pulmonary tuberculosis to a period of nine months, provided that isoniazid and rifampin are used; ethambutol, in a dose of 25 mg/kg, is added during the first two months of therapy. On the other hand, Fox (4) has stated that the third drug (ethambutol or streptomycin) adds nothing to the efficacy of isoniazid and rifampin and Stead and coworkers in Arkansas, U.S.A., confirmed this data (5).

The American Thoracic Society (ATS) has recently given limited sanction to this short-course chemotherapy of tuberculosis (6). Essentially the statement takes notice of all the experience from Asia, Africa and recent data from Arkansas, U.S.A. (7).

We would like to point out certain conditions stated by the
ATS that are important in evaluating short course chemotherapy,
and we quote: "In choosing a short course chemotherapy regimen,
considerations must be given to: 1) assuring overall therapeutic
success comparable to conventional duration therapy, 2) avoiding
any significant increase in drug toxicity, and 3) keeping the cost
of such a drug program within an acceptable range". Finally, the
ATS, the U.S. Center for Disease Control, and the U.S. Public
Health Service issued the following recommendations for short-
course chemotherapy in the United States. Whether these recommendations are applicable to the rest of the Americas must be a
decision made by each country which knows best its own logistical
problems and the state of development in the control of tuberculosis. We find these guidelines adequate for the Republic of
Panama and are now recommending: 1) A chemotherapy regimen
using a "core" of isoniazid and rifampin for a minimum of nine
months' duration is an acceptable alternative to regimens now
being used for adults with uncomplicated pulmonary tuberculosis.
Although extensive data are not available for children, the
regimen would probably be suitable for children as well. At
this time, recommendations for shortened treatment cannot be
made for patients with extrapulmonary tuberculosis, for drug-
resistant cases or for patients with complicating medical
conditions (diabetes, silicosis, immunosuppressive drugs of
diseases); 2) For the initial phase of treatment, the patient may
or may not be hospitalized, depending on the severity of symptoms,
public health considerations of infectiousness, and the ability
to ingest medications and provide self-care; 3) The data
on drugs, dosages, duration of initial treatment, etc., are
summarized in Table III; 4) Patients should remain under surveillance for 12 months after completion of therapy.

Table III. Short-Course Chemotherapy of Tuberculosis

| Drug | Dosage | |
	Initial Daily (Self-given)	Intermittent (Supervised)
Isoniazid	A^a: 300 mg	15 mg/kg
	C^b: 10 mg/kg (300 mg)	?
Rifampin	A^a: 600 mg	
	C^b: 10-20 mg/kg (600 mg)	?
Ethambutol^c	A^a: 15 mg/kg	

^{a}Adults ^{b}Children ^{c}If resistance is suspected

SPECIAL THERAPEUTIC SITUATIONS

Pregnant women, patients with impaired renal function, drug side effects, drug interactions and patients with suspected isoniazid-resistant bacilli, deserve special attention. Isoniazid and ethambutol are well tolerated by both mother and fetus. Rifampin is relatively safe but we need more data to confirm this. Streptomycin should be avoided due to ototoxicity. Ethionamide has been reported as possibly teratogenic. We must consider also that isoniazid, rifampin and streptomycin are secreted in breast milk.

In patients with impaired renal function, ethambutol and the aminoglycosides need reduction of the dose. If it is possible, periodic measurement of serum concentrations should be performed to avoid toxic levels. Recent data show an increased incidence of tuberculosis among patients with end-stage renal disease. We have to remember that isoniazid, ethambutol and the aminoglycosides are dialyzable. If ethambutol must be used, a dose of 9 mg/kg appears to be safe. In general, therapy with these products should be given immediately after dialysis.

Antituberculosis chemotherapy may produce well-recognized side effects and it is important to know how to monitor patients for these untoward effects. Table IV summarizes data for the most important side effects of the so-called first line drugs. The reader is referred to a review by Addington (8) for more detailed information. As far as the use of large doses of rifampin in the so-called "pulse therapy" a word of caution is given because isoniazid and rifampin have been demonstrated to participate in important drug interactions. Rifampin, and hepatic mixed-function-oxidase inducer is particularly likely to interact with other drugs. Since the oxidase enzyme system participates in the clearance of many drugs, a wide variety of rifampin interactions might be expected. To date, rifampin has been reported to accelerate the metabolisms of corticosteroids, oral hypoglycemic agents and digitoxin. The management of patients taking one or more of these drugs in combination with rifampin can be difficult. In some instances, it is best to avoid rifampin, but when necessary, doses must be adjusted to accomplish proper effects. Women on oral contraceptives and rifampin should be made aware of the increased risks of pregnancy.

It is highly undesirable to treat patients with isoniazid and rifampin when there is a suspicion of isoniazid resistance, e.g., cases of failure or relapse from previous treatment, patients from countries with high prevalence of tuberculosis and isoniazid resistance. Such patients should be given two additional bactericidal drugs (streptomycin and pyrazinamide) for four to eight weeks at the outset or until susceptibility studies have been reported. Thereafter, patients in whom the organisms are fully susceptible to both drugs may be continued on twice

Table IV. Side Effects of Antituberculosis Drugs

Drug	Side Effects	Monitoring	Comments
Isoniazid	Peripheral neuritis		Pyridoxine: 10 mg for prophylaxis; 50–100 for treatment
	Hepatitis	SGOT, SGPT	Discontinue if symptomatic or liver enzymes more than twice normal
	Central nervous system: convulsions optic neuritis with atrophy muscle twitching dizziness ataxia toxic encephalopathy hypersensitivity: fever, rash		
Ethambutol	Optic neuritis	Visual acuity and red-green color discrimination	Occurs at 25 mg/kg
	Skin rash		

Table IV. Continued

Drug	Side Effects	Monitoring	Comments
Streptomycin	8th cranial nerve damage	Audiogram Vestibular function	
	Nephrotoxicity	BUN, creatinine	
	Neuromuscular junction blockade		Seen in patients also receiving muscle relaxants
	Hypersensitivity: rash, dermatitis, anaphylaxis		
Rifampin	Orange urine, tears, saliva, flu-like syndrome		
	Hepatitis	SGOT, SGPT	Discontinue if jaundice or liver enzyme more than twice normal
	Thrombocytopenia	Platelet count	Discontinue
	Hemolysis		Discontinue
	Renal failure		

weekly therapy with only rifampin and isoniazid. Those with isoniazid resistance should be continued on twice weekly streptomycin, pyrazinamide, and rifampin (usually also isoniazid for its effect on susceptible organisms in closed lesions and macrophages). Where such bactericidal therapy is continued for the full course of therapy, nine months is generally adequate to assure success with little chance of relapse. On the other hand, Moulding considers that data on this matter are conflicting and suggests further study in controlled trials (9).

REFERENCES

1. Bulla, A. (1977). Tuberculosis patients. WHO Chronicle 286.
2. Pilheu, J.A. (1970). Ambulatory treatment of pulmonary tuberculosis with ethambutol-isoniazid. Chest 58, 497-500.
3. Fox, W., and Mitchison, D.A. (1975). State of the art short course chemotherapy for pulmonary tuberculosis. Am. Rev. Resp. Dis. 111, 325-353.
4. Fox, W. (1979). The chemotherapy of pulmonary tuberculosis: A review. Chest (Suppl) 76, 785-796.
5. Stead, W.W., and Good, W.E. (1980). Contribution of a third drug to various two-drugs regimens in the treatment of tuberculosis (Abstract). Am. Rev. Resp. Dis. (Suppl) 121, 463.
6. American Thoracic Society and the Center for Disease Control. Guidelines for Short-Course Tuberculosis Chemotherapy. Am. Rev. Resp. Dis. 121, 611-614, 1980.
7. Dutt, A.K., Jones, L., Stead, W.W. (1979). Short-course chemotherapy for tuberculosis with largely twice-weekly isoniazid-rifampin. Chest 75, 441-447.
8. Addington, W.N. (1979). The side effects and interactions of antituberculosis drugs. Chest (Suppl) 76, 782-784.
9. Moudling, T.S. (1981). Should isoniazid be used in retreatment of tuberculosis despite acquired isoniazid resistance? Am. Rev. Res. Dis. 123, 262-264.

PART IV
CARDIOVASCULAR INFECTIONS

INFECTIVE ENDOCARDITIS--NEW CONCEPTS IN THERAPY

Walter R. Wilson
Joseph E. Geraci

Department of Infectious Diseases
Mayo Clinic
Rochester, Minnesota

In the preantibiotic era, the mortality of patients with infective endocarditis (IE) was virtually 100%, and the majority of these patients died from sepsis. With the advent of antimicrobial therapy, the majority of deaths occur as a result of heart failure. At least 75% of all cases of IE are caused by streptococci or staphylococci. Host defenses play a minimal role in the control of IE and in no other infectious disease is cure so dependant upon administration of bactericidal antimicrobial therapy. An understanding of the use of antibiotics and the treatment of heart failure assoicated with IE is essential in the management of these patients.

I. PENICILLIN-SENSITIVE STREPTOCOCCAL IE

Approximately 50% of all cases of IE are caused by penicillin-sensitive viridans streptococci or Streptococcus bovis--minimum inhibitory concentration (MIC) ≤ 0.1 μg/ml of penicillin. The optimal antimicrobial therapy of these patients has been controversial. Recently published studies have confirmed earlier observations that the majority of these patients may be treated successfully with two weeks rather than four weeks of antimicrobial therapy (1-3). The therapeutic regimens which are now considered to be appropriate therapy for patients with penicillin-sensitive streptococcal IE are shown in Table 1.

The relapse rate and mortality associated with each of the threee regimens is approximately 1%. The major advantage of the two-week regimen is that short-term therapy is more cost effective than the four-week regimens. The major disadvantage of short-term therapy is the risk of streptomycin-associated vestibular toxicity which occurs in approximately 2% of patients (1). This risk is presumably the same for the four-week regimen which includes streptomycin. The risk of streptomycin-associated toxicity is highest in patients greater than

TABLE 1. Antimicrobial Therapy for Patients with Penicillin-
Sensitive Streptococcal IE[a]

Therapeutic Regimens	Duration of Therapy (Weeks)
Penicillin 10-20,000,000 units IV daily (4)	4
Penicillin 10-20,000,000 units IV daily plus streptomycin[b] 7.5 mg/kg IM b.i.d. (5)	4 2
Procain penicillin 1.2 mu IM q.i.d. or penicillin 10-20,000,000 units IV daily plus streptomycin[b] 7.5 mg/kg IM b.i.d. (1-3)	2 2

[a]Dosages suggested are for patients with normal renal function
[b]Dosage of streptomycin not to exceed 500 mg per dose

65 years old and in those with abnormal renal function. These
patients should be treated with penicillin administered intravenously for four weeks.

Procaine penicillin should not be administered to patients
with shock or decreased peripheral perfusion due to IE. In these
patients, cardiac valve replacement is more important than control
of infection, and intravenously administrated penicillin is
preferable to the use of intramuscular administration because of
poor peripheral perfusion. Patients with central nervous system
mycotic aneurysm should be treated with intravenous penicillin
rather than intramuscular penicillin. The relatively low serum
and cerebral spinal fluid concentrations achieved with intramuscular procaine penicillin may not be sufficient to permit
successful therapy of these patients. Two-week antimicrobial
therapy should not be administered to patients with prosthetic
valve endocarditis caused by penicillin-sensitive streptococci.
These patients should be treated with penicillin administered
intravenously for four weeks combined with streptomycin for the
first two weeks of therapy.

Patients who are allergic to penicillin may be treated with
vancomycin 7.5 mg/kg intravenously every 6 hours for four weeks,
or vancomycin in the same dosage together with streptomycin
7.5 mg/kg intramuscularly twice daily for two weeks. The dosage
of vancomycin and streptomycin must be adjusted in patients with
abnormal renal function. Patients at increased risk of streptomycin-associated eighth cranial nerve toxicity should be treated
with vancomycin alone.

TABLE 2. Antimicrobial Therapy of Patients with Enterococcal IE[a]

Streptomycin Susceptibility	Antimicrobial Therapy	Duration of Therapy (Weeks)
Streptomycin-susceptible (MIC < 2,000 µg/ml)	Penicillin 20,000,000 units IV daily or ampicillin 2 g IV q 4 H plus streptomycin[b] 7.5 mg/kg IM b.i.d.	4-6 4-6
Streptomycin resistant (MIC > 2,000 µg/ml)	Penicillin or ampicillin in the same dosages as above plus gentamicin[b] 1 mg/kg IV q 8 H	4-6 4-6

[a]Dosage suggested are for patients with normal renal and hepatic function.
[b]Dosage of streptomycin should not exceed 500 mg per dose, and peak one hour serum concentration should not exceed 20 µg/ml. Dosage of gentamicin should not exceed 100 mg per dose and peak one hour serum concentration should be adjusted to achieve a concentration of approximately 3 µg/ml.

II. THERAPY OF ENTEROCOCCAL IE

Infection caused by enterococci accounts for 10-15% of the
total number of cases of IE and the majority of these are caused
by Streptococcus faecalis. Enterococci are inhibited but not
killed in vitro by penicillin. Penicillin combined with an aminoglycoside (streptomycin or gentamicin) acts synergistically in
vitro to kill enterococci, and successful therapy of patients with
enterococcal IE requires the use of penicillin or ampicillin combined with streptomycin or gentamicin (6,7). Enterococci are
relatively resistant in vitro to streptomycin (MIC > 2,000 µg/ml
streptomycin). Approximately one-third of enterococci isolated
from patients with IE are highly streptomycin-resistant (MIC >
2,000 µg/ml) (7). These microorganisms are resistant in vitro
to the combination of penicillin and streptomycin and may be
killed by the synergistic action of penicillin together with
gentamicin. The suggested antimicrobial therapeutic regimens for
patients with enterococcal IE are shown in Table 2.

The serum bactericidal titer (SBT) should be determined in
patients with enterococcal IE on the second day of antimicrobial
therapy. A peak SBT of ⪰ 1:8 is considered satisfactory. In
patients with SBT < 1:8, adjustment of dosages of antimicrobial
therapy may be necessary. It is desirable to determine serum
concentration of antimicrobials using the same serum specimen
obtained for the SBT. A low SBT may be secondary to inadequate
concentration of drug rather than failure of bactericidal activity. The frequency of streptomycin-associated eighth cranial
nerve toxicity is approximately 20% in patients with enterococcal
endocarditis and patients should be monitored closely for signs
of vestibular abnormalities. Serum creatinine should be measured
frequently in patients treated with gentamicin. Patients who are
allergic to penicillin may be treated with vancomycin 7.5 mg/kg
intravenously every 6 hours plus streptomycin or gentamicin for
4-6 weeks in the same dosages outlined in Table 2.

III. THERAPY OF STAPHYLOCOCCAL IE:

The large majority of strains of Staphylococcus aureus isolated from patients with IE are resistant in vitro to penicillin
(MIC > 0.1 µg/ml). These patients may be treated with nafcillin,
2 g intravenously every 4 hours or a cephalosporin such as cefazolin (1.5 g intravenously every 8 hours) for 4-6 weeks. The
use of combined antimicrobial therapy in patients with S. aureus
IE is controversial. Nafcillin, together with gentamicin, acts
synergistically in vitro against S. aureus, and the combination
is more effective in the treatment of experimental animal IE than
either drug administered alone (8,9). However, the outcome of
patients with S. aureus IE was the same in patients

treated with nafcillin alone compared with those treated with
nafcillin plus gentamicin (10). The duration of bacteremia was
shorter among patients treated with combined nafcillin-gentamicin
than among those treated with nafcillin alone, but the frequency
of nephrotoxicity was higher among patients in the gentamicin-
treated group. If combined nafcillin-gentamicin therapy is used,
gentamicin should probably not be administered for longer than
5-7 days following initiation of therapy.

Some S. aureus are "tolerant" in vitro to nafcillin or oxacillin and exhibit a high minimum bactericidal concentration (MBC).
Tolerance is defined as MBC/MIC ratio of $\geq$ 32 (11). The management of these patients is controversial. In our experience, these
patients may be treated successfully with nafcillin or oxacillin
alone, provided that the SBT is satisfactory. If the SBT is < 1:8,
vancomycin alone or in combination with gentamicin or rifampin is
often active in vitro against tolerant strains. The selection of
single-drug or combination-drug antimicrobial therapy should be
based upon the results of in vitro susceptibility and synergy tests.

Patients who are allergic to penicillin may be treated with
vancomycin 7.5 mg/kg intravenously every 6 hours for 4-6 weeks.
Rarely, isolates of S. aureus are resistant in vitro to nafcillin
or oxacillin. Vancomycin administered alone or in combination
with rifampin may be useful in these patients.

IV. MANAGEMENT OF HEART FAILURE CAUSED BY IE

Heart failure is the most common serious complication of IE
and is the leading cause of death among these patients. Patients
with heart failure caused by IE who are treated medically have a
higher mortality than patients treated surgically. The mortality
associated with aortic valve infection and moderate or severe
heart failure was 100% (18/18) among patients treated medically
compared with 18.5% (5/27) of patients who underwent cardiac valve
replacement P = < 0.001 (12,13).

The hemodynamic status of the patient is the most important
factor in the decision to proceed with cardiac valve replacement
and in the timing of surgery. In patients with severe heart
failure unresponsive to medical therapy after 24-48 hours of
treatment, consideration should be given to prompt cardiac valve
replacement, irrespective of the duration of preoperative antimicrobial therapy. In these patients, procrastination in cardiac
valve replacement in an attempt to stabilize heart failure by
medical therapy and to complete a course of antimicrobial therapy
preoperatively usually results in death from heart failure.

The operative mortality of patients who undergo cardiac valve
replacement because of heart failure caused by IE is directly
related to the functional class of heart failure present at the
time of surgery. During a 13-year period at Mayo Clinic among

TABLE 3. Number of Patients and Mortality (%) by Valve Replacement and Functional Classification with and without Infective Endocarditis (IE)[a]

Valve	Class II		Class III		Class IV	
	No IE	IE	No IE	IE	No IE	IE
Aortic	100 (5)	65 (6)	100 (7)	11 (0)	100 (19)	23 (22)
Mitral	100 (11)	8 (0)	100 (14)	1 (0)	100 (18)	7 (0)
Multiple	25 (16)	15(20)	25 (12)	3 (33)	25 (36)	5 (20)
TOTAL	225 (9)	88 (8)	225 (11)	15 (7)	225 (20)	35 (17)

[a]From Wilson, W. R. et al, Mayo Clinic Proceedings. 54:223, 1979.

4,238 patients who did not have IE, we determined the operative mortality in 100 patients with aortic, 100 patients with mitral, and 25 with multiple cardiac valve replacement with class II, class III, and class IV functional disability, respectively (14). The mortality by valve replacement in these patients was compared with the operative mortality in patients with IE matched according to age (decade), valve, and functional class heart failure present at the time of surgery (Table 3). Patients with functional class IV heart failure had the highest surgical mortality. The operative mortality was remarkably similar in patients with or without IE when the degree of heart failure was the same for both groups of patients at the time of cardiac valve replacement.

Cardiac valve replacement may be performed successfully in patients with active IE and severe heart failure, even in patients with blood cultures positive within 48 hours preoperative (15). The risk of valve dehiscence and prosthetic valve endocarditis may be slightly higher in patients with active IE than in those who complete a course of antimicrobial therapy preoperatively, but these risks are justified by the excessively high mortality in patients with class IV disability who are not subjected to early cardiac valve replacement. In patients with severe, sudden-onset aortic insufficiency, urgent cardiac valve replacement offers the only hope for survival.

REFERENCES

(1) Wilson W. R., Thompson R. L., Wilkowske C. J.,
     Washington J. A. II, Guiliani E. R., Geraci J. E.: Short-
     term therapy for streptococcal infective endocarditis:
     combined intramuscular administration of penicillin and
     streptomycin. JAMA, 245:360, 1981.
(2) Wilson W. R., Geraci J. E., Wilkowske C. J.,
     Washington J. A. II: Short-term intramuscular therapy with
     procaine penicillin plus streptomycin for infective endo-
     carditis due to viridans streptococci. Circulation, 57:1158,
     1978.
(3) Geraci J. E.: The antibiotic therapy of bacterial endocar-
     ditis: therapeutic data on 172 patients seen from 1951
     through 1957; additional observations on short-term therapy
     (two weeks) for penicillin-sensitive streptococcal endocar-
     ditis. Med Clin North Am, July 1958, p 1101.
(4) Karchmer A. W., Moellering R. C. Jr, Maki D. G., Swartz M.N.,
     Single-antibiotic therapy for streptococcal endocarditis.
     JAMA, 241:1801, 1979.
(5) Wolfe J. C., Johnson W. D. Jr.: Penicillin-sensitive
     streptococcal endocarditis: in vitro and clinical observa-
     tions on penicillin-streptomycin therapy. Ann Intern Med,
     81:178, 1974.

(6)   Mandell, G. L., Daye, D., Levison, M.E., Hook, E. W.:
      Enterococcal endocarditis: an analysis of 38 patients
      observed at the New York Hospital-Cornell Medical Center.
      Arch Intern Med, 125:258, 1970.

(7)   Moellering, R. C. Jr, Wennersten, C., Weinberg, A. N.:
      Synergy of penicillin and gentamicin against enterococci.
      J. Infect Dis, 124(Suppl):S207, 1971.

(8)   Sande, M. A., Courtney, K. B.: Nafcillin-gentamicin
      synergism in experimental staphylococcal endocarditis.
      J. Lab Clin Med, 88:118, 1976.

(9)   Watanakunakorn, C, Glotzbecker, C.: Enhancement of the
      effects of anti-staphylococcal antibiotics by aminoglycosides.
      Antimicrob Agents Chemother, 6:802, 1974.

(10) Sande, M. A., Korzeniowski, O. M., Endocarditis Collaborative
      Group: Comparison of nafcillin with nafcillin plus genta-
      micin in the treatment of addicts with S. aureus endocarditis.
      11th International Congress of Chemotherapy--19th Inter-
      science Conference on Antimicrobial Agents and Chemotherapy.
      Boston, Massachusetts. October 1979. Abstract No. 362.

(11) Sabath, L. D., Wheeler, M., Laverdiere, M., Blazevic, D.,
      Wilkinson, B. J.: A new type of penicillin resistance of
      Staphylococcus aureus. Lancet, 1:443, 1977.

(12) Griffin F. M. Jr, Jones G, Bobbs C. G.: Aortic insufficiency
      in bacterial endocarditis. Ann Intern Med, 76:23, 1972.

(13) Snow R. M., Cobbs, C. G.: Treatment of complications of
      infective endocarditis. In Infective Endocarditis, Kaye D.
      editor, University Park Press, Baltimore, 1976, p 213.

(14) Wilson, W. R., Danielson, G. K., Giuliani, E. R.,
      Washington, J. A. II, Jaumin, P. M., Geraci, J. E.: Cardiac
      valve replacement in congestive heart failure due to infective
      endocarditis. Mayo Clinic Proceedings, 54:223, 1979.

(15) Wilson, W. R., Danielson, G. K., Giuliani, E. R.,
      Washington, J. A. II, Jaumin, P. M., Geraci, J. E.: Valve
      replacement in patients with active infective endocarditis.
      Circulation, 58:585, 1978.

PART V
CENTRAL NERVOUS SYSTEM INFECTIONS

BACTERIAL INFECTIONS
OF THE CENTRAL NERVOUS SYSTEM

Carlos H. Ramirez-Ronda
Jose J. Gutierrez-Nuñez

Infectious Disease Program
University of Puerto Rico School of Medicine
and Affiliated Hospitals
Departments of Research and Medicine
V. A. Medical Center and
University of Puerto Rico School of Medicine
San Juan, Puerto Rico

INTRODUCTION

Bacterial meningitis continues to be an important clinical problem. With the availability of effective antibiotic therapy the mortality has been reduced to 10-20%, where it has remained essentially unchanged during the past 20 yrs. This mortality rate, together with the occurrence of serious neurological seque-lae in a number of survivors, underscores the continuing challenge of bacterial meningitis. Because appropriate antibiotic therapy is most important in the treatment of bacterial meningitis, rapid and accurate identification of the infecting agent is of the greatest importance in the management of patients. This paper attempts to summarize for the practitioner the highlights of cur-rent knowledge in this area and to outline certain areas in which recent advances can be anticipated.

I. EPIDEMIOLOGY

The incidence of bacterial meningitis has remained nearly the same over the past 40 yrs, affecting approximately 5 individuals per 100,000 population. Its highest incidence is observed in the winter, but occurs throughout the year. There is no recognized racial predilection and the sex difference is not remarkable. The majority of the patients are children less than 15 yrs of age; approximately 15% of cases occur under 1 mo of age, 37% before 1 yr of age, and 75% before 15 yrs of age. Mortality also varies with age, being highest in the first year of life, decreasing during the middle years and rising again after the age of 50-60 yrs. A number of factors predispose individuals to bacterial meningitis. These include respiratory infection and otitis media, mastoiditis, head trauma, recent neurosurgical procedures, sickle cell anemia, agammaglobulinemia, and immunosuppressed patients.

The incidence of the various bacterial etiologies varies in different age groups. Gram-negative bacilli and Group B streptococci are responsible for the majority of the cases in the neonate. Haemophilus influenzae is the most common etiology in the child 6 mo to 5 yrs of age, and Neisseria meningitidis and Streptococcus pneumoniae cause most diseases in older children and in adults.

Many other organisms may cause bacterial meningitis with perhaps the most important ones being the S. aureus especially in conjunction with brain abscesses, paranasal sinusitis, endocarditis, trauma, postneurosurgical procedures, or severe staphylococcal septicemia; Listeria monocytogenes mostly causing meningitis in the neonate, in the aged, or immunosuppressed patients, and a scattering of gram-negative bacilli characteristically present in the neonate and in posttraumatic or postneurosurgical patients. Infections have been reported with more than one organism, but mixed infections are very rare. At least 10-15% of cases of purulent meningitis are of unknown etiology. In a significant number of cases the diagnosis is unknown because patients have been treated with antibiotics before cultures of blood and cerebrospinal fluid were taken.

II. CLINICAL MANIFESTATIONS AND INITIAL EVALUATION

The patient with bacterial meningitis usually presents with fever and some combination of neurologic symptoms and signs. Certain aspects of the history are especially important. They include the patient's age, his host-defense status against potential infecting microorganisms, and the epidemiology of any infectious central nervous system disorder in the patient's close contacts or in the community.

The onset is abrupt, with fever, headache, vomiting, and pain in the neck and back. The patient is restless and irritable and resents examination. As the infection advances, headache becomes constant and severe and is aggravated by movement or coughing. Localizing signs of meningeal irritation are revealed by the development of reflex muscle spasm of the neck and back. As muscle spasm develops nuchal rigidity becomes marked, Brudzinski signs are elicited by attempting to flex the head, whereupon flexion of the thighs and knees occurs. Kerning's sign, like nuchal rigidity, is most constant when the thigh is flexed at right angles on the abdomen, spasm of the hamstrings makes exten-

sion of the knee joint impossible, thus preventing pulling on the
inflammed spinal meninges. Signs of increased cerebrospinal fluid
pressure are manifested by excruciating headache, projectile
vomiting, seizures and slow pulse. The temperature ranges from
37°C-40°C. There may be associated pneumonia or gastroenteritis.
As the infection advances, restlessness and mental irritability
increase and the patient may become delirious; later coma
supervenes and then death.

In the neonate the diagnosis is often difficult since the
child may present with only nonspecific signs, such as irritability, poor feeding, lethargy, respiratory difficulty, or jaundice.
Bulging fontanelles and fever are not always present and meningismus is usually absent. High index of suspicion leading to early
diagnosis and treatment is extremely important.

Atypical presentations may be seen in elderly or debilitated
patients. In older patients confusion may be the only clue that
a patient with fever has a bacterial infection of the central
nervous system.

Physical examination may suggest a specific bacterial etiology
for meningitis when the examination uncovers disease in cranial
structures. Sinusitis and otitis predispose to pneumococcal
meningitis; staphylococcal disease in frontal sinuses may result
in erosion of frontal bone and spread of the inflammatory process
into subdural space causing subdural empyema. Occasionally,
patients with chronic external otitis may develop gram-negative
bacillary meningitis due to resistant species such as Pseudomonas
aeruginosa. When there is a cerebral spinal fluid leak, sometimes
manifested as rhinorrhea or otorrhea, and this is complicated by
bacterial meningitis, the pneumococcus, staphylococcus and gram-
negative bacilli are commonly responsible. Following severe head
trauma or extensive neurosurgical procedures, the most common
early cause of bacterial meningitis is the pneumococcus. Staphylococci and gram-negative bacilli are the predominant pathogens
when the onset of meningitis is delayed.

Clues to the etiology of meningitis may be found as one
examines other organ systems. Purpura suggests meningococcal
disease or may suggest pneumococcal bacteremia. One may visualize
the characteristic gram-negative diplococcus in material obtained
directly from a skin lesion. Purpura is not pathognomonic of
meningococcal disease and has been noted in patients with overwhelming pneumococcal bacteremia as well as in a variety of other
disseminated infectious disorders. A petechial rash is also seen
in infections with echovirus type 9 and in that situation may
accompany aseptic meningitis. Antecedent cellulitis suggests
staphylococcal or group A beta-hemolytic streptococcal meningitis.
Pneumonia is present in about one third of patients with pneumococcal meningitis.

There are some diagnostic steps in the evaluation of a patient
with fever and neurological disorders. First, we have to assess
if the patient has meningitis or encephalitis with or without

focal neurological localizing signs. If the patients have focal
localizing signs then we should consider if these neurological
signs are of upper motor neuron or lower motor neuron.

In those patients with meningitis or encephalitis without
focal neurologic signs, lumbar puncture should be performed.
Centrifuged CSF should be gram-stained and examined for bacterial
forms. In addition, an India ink preparation and acid fast smear
should be prepared (M. tuberculosis may gravitate to the top of
centrifuged CSF because of its buoyancy). In addition to these
routine studies, physicians should save an aliquot of CSF in case
special serologic studies (i.e., the cryptococcal antigen
determination) are later deemed necessary.

A CSF with a predominance of polymorphonuclear leukocytes,
elevated protein, and depressed glucose out of proportion to the
serum glucose, should suggest pyogenic meningitis or meningeal
tuberculosis and appropriate antimicrobial therapy should be
started. The specific antimicrobial regime will depend on the
predisposing factors such as patient's age, underlying anatomic
and host defense circumstances and, most important, findings on
the stained preparation of the spinal fluid itself.

In those patients with meningitis or encephalitis with focal
neurologic signs of upper motor neuron, one must consider the
possibility of a mass lesion, i.e., a brain abscess that has
ruptured into the ventricular system. In such situations there is
a significant risk from lumbar puncture and it is appropriate to
proceed with special studies to rule out a mass lesion such as the
echoencephalogram, radioisotopic brain scan, and Computerized
Axial Tomography (CAT) scan with contrast media injection. If a
mass lesion is identified, neurosurgeons should be consulted. In
addition, the physician should consider the possibility of Herpes
virus hominis encephalitis in the patient with an encephalitis
picture and focal signs, especially if they involve the temporal
lobe. If special studies do not delineate a mass lesion, the
physician may want to reconsider a lumbar puncture. It is
important to appreciate that papilledema is not always present in
the patient with brain abscess even when there is a marked
increase in intracranial pressure.

In those patients with meningitis or encephalitis with focal
neurologic signs of lower motor neuron, it is important to rule
out an inflammatory process in the spine or epidural space.
Vertebral osteomyelitis, Pott's Disease, and epidural abscess are
particularly noteworthy. The latter is often manifested by back
pain, point tenderness over the involved area, and rapidly
progressive neurologic deficit below the level of the lesion. It
is a neurosurgical emergency. X-ray examination of the spine may
reveal osteomyelitis, narrowing of the intervertebral disk space,
or paraspinal soft tissue swelling. When there is no evidence of
focal inflammatory disease near the spinal cord in the patient
with encephalitis and lower motor neuron signs, the presumptive
diagnosis is the poliomyelitis syndrome.

III. DIAGNOSIS

Bacterial meningitis is a medical emergency. The single most important test in the diagnosis of bacterial meningitis is gram staining. In the CSF of bacterial meningitis, organisms range from 4.5×10^3 to 3×10^8/ml in previously untreated cases and from 4×10^1 to 1.4×10^6/ml in partly treated cases. In the latter cases, the gram-stained smear is much less frequently positive than in those who have not received prior antibiotic therapy, notably in patients with H. influenzae type B and N. meningitidis infections. In the aggregate, the gram stain of the sediment is positive in about 80% of the proven cases; the remaining 20% being falsely negative because too few organisms are present to be recognized by microscopy or because ordinary laboratory centrifugation does not provide the 10,000 g necessary to bring some bacteria, notably H. influenzae, down into the sediment. In either event, the gram stain may well be negative even in the presence of clinically apparent or subsequently proven bacterial meningitis.

In some centers fluorescent antibody stains are applied directly to smears of the sediment when organisms have been noted in gram-stained smears. Immunofluorescence of the organisms may provide rapid identification of H. influenzae, S. pneumoniae, and N. meningitidis, among others, with a high degree of specificity. While its sensitivity is 80-90%, the procedure is time consuming and poorly adapted to screening.

When the gram stain is negative and the results of culture are pending, strong supportive evidence for bacterial infection may be provided by WBC and differential counts. In bacterial meningitis the initial WBC count may range from slightly increased to 20,000/ cu mm. In a recent series of pneumococcal meningitides the mean count was 4,500/cu mm. The total WBC count is especially helpful when it exceeds 1,000/cu mm since this rarely happens with viral meningitis.

On occasion when the gram stain is negative the cell count is in the tens or hundreds and no other investigative methods are available, the CSF glucose determination may play a role in the diagnosis of bacterial meningitis. CSF glucose concentration less than 40 mg/ml support the clinical diagnosis of bacterial infection. Concentrations less than 10 mg/ml are even more characteristic of bacterial meningitis. However, low CSF glucose concentrations occur in only about 50% of proven cases of bacterial meningitis. Therefore, normal glucose levels do not exclude the diagnosis.

Fortunately, some newer diagnostic methods have recently been proposed as rapid methods for the diagnosis of bacterial meningitis. Of these, the most important at present is the counter-immunoelectrophoresis (CIE). The object of this process is to demonstrate soluble bacterial capsular antigens in CSF.

The major advantage of CIE is that it provides a specific diagnosis as to type of organism often in less than 1 hr and, when patients are already being treated with antimicrobial drugs as in partially treated meningitis, can detect antigens from bacteria that may not grow on culture. It appears to be at least as sensitive as gram staining in detecting bacterial disease. Occasionally, false positive results can occur due to a cross-reaction between antigens, the antiserum to N. meningitidis group B, i.e., can react with capsular polysaccharide of certain E. coli strains that frequently cause neonatal meningitis. False negative results, which can have more serious clinical consequences than false positives, occur more commonly. If the body fluid contains fewer than 10^4 bacteria per ml, the amount of antigen may be too small to produce a positive CIE test. Sometimes in an early infection, even when a large number of bacteria are present, not enough time may be elapsed for the antigen to dissolve off the bacterial surface; in such cases, a markedly positive gram stain may be accompanied by a negative CIE test. False negative reactions can also occur if the antibody is of poor quality; this happens particularly with group B meningococci. Some antigens, particularly those of pneumococcal types 7 and 14, often give false negative results unless the laboratory adjusts the conditions of the test.

There is now evidence that determination of CSF lactic acid levels may be useful in distinguishing between bacterial or fungal meningitis from viral meningitis. In both bacterial and fungal meningitis, levels are increased (above 35 mg/dl in 1 report). In viral meningitis, levels are lower (below 35 mg/dl). In patients with bacterial meningitis who have taken antibiotics for 1 or 2 days, CSF lactic acid levels are still elevated in most cases; a major advantage when the question of bacterial vs viral meningitis has not yet been resolved.

Two to three blood cultures should be obtained from every patient because of the high incidence of associated bacteremia; up to 65-70% are positive in H. influenzae type B meningitis. In a recent series 71% of the blood cultures in S. pneumoniae meningitis were found positive, 53% in N. meningitidis meningitis and 45% in H. influenzae meningitis. Occasionally, the blood culture is positive whereas CSF cultures fail to yield an organism.

Radiographic study of the skull, mastoid processes and sinuses may be helpful, especially if trauma or paracranial infections are suspected.

A. Partially Treated Meningitis

One of the major problems in diagnosis is that of differentiating aseptic meningitis from partially treated bacterial meningitis, since up to 50% of these patients receive some form of antimicrobial therapy before a diagnostic lumbar puncture is

performed. It has long been taught that partial treatment with
antimicrobial drugs may change cerebrospinal fluid findings. The
content of the CSF sugar and protein may be modified and CSF
cultures may be less likely to be positive for bacteria.

When the initial CSF evaluation leaves some doubt as to the
accuracy of the diagnosis of aseptic meningitis, the physician
should re-examine the CSF after a 6-12 hr period. After this
interval, the CSF findings in aseptic meningitis will frequently
show a shift toward mononuclear cells, whereas in bacterial
meningitis the preponderance of polymorphonuclears will persist,
and the concentration of CSF glucose and protein may change
sufficiently to leave little doubt about the correct diagnosis.
Obviously, if the patient's clinical condition deteriorates before
the 6-12 hr period has elapsed, repeat examination of the CSF
should be undertaken without delay.

In the adult patient with meningitis that received antibiotics
for 48 hrs or less prior to evaluation, the finding of a CSF
glucose of 40 mg/dl or less or a protein of 150 mg/dl or greater
or a WBC count of 1200 or greater point toward partially treated
bacterial meningitis. If the patient is alert and the CSF shows
none of the above criteria, the CSF can be re-examined in 6-12
hrs.

The CIE is especially helpful in this circumstance. CIE is
routinely used in many hospitals and may detect antigens of
pneumococci, meningococci, and H. influenzae in spinal fluid when
gram stain and culture have been rendered negative prior to
therapy. The test is not sensitive enough to exclude bacterial
etiology when a negative result is obtained.

The decision to continue treatment for unproven bacterial
meningitis remains a matter for fine clinical judgment.

B. Recurrent Meningitis

Recurrent bacterial meningitis most often signals the presence
of a communication of the subarachnoid space with the paranasal
sinuses, nasopharynx, middle ear, or skin. Communications with
the paranasal sinuses, nasopharynx and middle ear are usually the
result of fractures of the paranasal sinuses, cribriform plate, or
petrous bone, respectively. Communications with the skin are
usually associated with midline dermal sinuses, dermoid cyst or
myelomeningoceles. The causative agent in over 80% of such
instances is S. pneumoniae. If the patient has received antimicrobial prophylaxis, especially with ampicillin, gram-negative
bacilli are the more likely causative organisms. The value of
such antimicrobial prophylaxis in skull fractures associated with
CSF leak is not clear. The occurence of meningitis in any patient
with a history of head trauma, even years previously, should
prompt a search for CSF rhinorrhea or otorrhea. This can be done
by injecting a radioactive tracer into the lumbar CSF and monitor-

ing its appearance in the nose or ear. Testing for rhinorrhea can be done by measuring the glucose content of nasal secretions which should be low relative to CSF.

The defects of the immune system most frequently associated with recurrent meningitis include splenectomy, hypogammaglobulinemia, leukemia, and lymphoma, sickle cell anemia and other hemoglobinopathies. Recently, it has been reported of patients with recurrent N. meningitidis and N. gonorrhoeae bacteremia associated with C_6, C_7, or C_8 deficiency.

In some patients with recurrent meningitis no anatomic or functional defects can be found.

IV. THERAPY

Management of bacterial meningitis involves a number of considerations other than selection of the proper antimicrobial drug. Some of these include administration of intravenous fluids and electrolytes, and treatment of shock, seizures, or cerebral edema.

The keys to successful antimicrobial therapy are prompt administration, proper route, and adequate dosage with minimal toxicity of an antibiotic which penetrates the blood brain barrier. Although therapy often must be instituted empirically, the choice of drugs should be influenced by the history, knowledge of epidemiologic factors, the age of the patient and presence of underlying disease. Obviously, the antimicrobial therapy should be as specific as possible and this will depend on the accurate identification of the causative organisms.

In all patients with culture or gram stain proven pneumococcal or meningococcal meningitis, the antibiotic of choice is penicillin G, with chloramphenicol an effective alternative drug for patients who cannot tolerate penicillin. In all patients with culture or gram stain confirmed meningitis due to H. influenzae type B, treatment should be initiated with both ampicillin and chloramphenicol until either sensitivities or assays for beta-lactamase have been performed. Thereafter, therapy can be continued with the single most appropriate agent.

In all patients with suspected but unconfirmed purulent meningitis (initial gram stain is negative) due to the 3 major pathogens, treatment should be initiated with ampicillin and chloramphenicol in children; and penicillin G alone in adults in view of the rarity of H. influenzae type B in adults. All penicillin-allergic patients should receive chloramphenicol.

The cephalosporins should be avoided as substitutes for penicillin in the treatment of purulent meningitis because of its poor penetration into the CSF.

The initial therapy of suspected bacterial meningitis in the neonate should include ampicillin (directed against group B streptococci, Listeria and enterococci) and gentamicin, tobramycin or amikacin (directed against gram-negative bacilli). If the gram stain or culture verify group B streptococcal meningitis, crystalline penicillin G is the drug of choice. Recent studies suggest that the addition of intraventricular aminoglycosides is detrimental to the outcome of gram-negative bacillary meningitis.

The optimal antimicrobial route of administration and duration of therapy of gram-negative bacillary meningitis have never been defined in a systematic trial. If the patient is not severely ill, therapy for meningitis can be begun with chloramphenicol 25 mg/kg IV q 6 hrs. If the organism is initially resistant or becomes resistant to chloramphenicol during therapy, one should consider either intralumbar or intraventricular administration of an aminoglycoside. A trial of intralumbar aminoglycoside 0.03 mg/ml of estimated CSF volume of gentamicin or tobramycin or 0.1 mg/ml of estimated CSF of amikacin every 24 hrs. The total CSF volume has been estimated to be 40-60 ml in infants, 60-100 ml in young children, 80-120 ml in older children, and 110-160 ml in adults with hydrocephalus. If the patient is critically ill, has altered sensorium or is in coma, an Ommaya or Rickhan reservoir should be put in place immediately and intraventricular therapy should be begun in the operating room with gentamicin, tobramycin or amikacin in the doses suggested above. After the first dose of aminoglycoside into the ventricle, the concentration should be monitored in the lumbar CSF to assure adequate distribution of the drug throughout the CSF space. In addition, ventricular levels of aminoglycoside should be measured just before the next intraventricular dose every 2 or 3 days, and the dose altered to maintain trough level in an approximate range of 2-10 µg/ml. Regardless of the drug chosen for treatment of the meningitis per se, the patient should also be treated intravenously with antimicrobials appropriate for gram-negative bacteremia which is present in 70% or more of the patients with gram-negative meningitis. Therapy should be maintained for 7-10 days after cultures of CSF become sterile. In the near future, newly developed β-lactam antibiotics like moxalactam may become the drug of choice for gram-negative bacillary meningitis since it appears to penetrate well into CSF avoiding the administration of intraventricular or intralumbar aminoglycosides.

The management of the patient with partially treated meningitis presents a problem. In patients ages 12 and over, the following criteria can be utilized for management. All patients that received antimicrobial agents for longer than 48 hrs prior to evaluation and having the clinical diagnosis of meningitis should be managed as bacterial meningitis. Patients with pretreatment for 48 hrs or less and not alert should also receive therapy like bacterial meningitis. Patients alert and who were pretreated for 48 hrs or less and whose CSF demonstrates a glucose <40 mg/dl or protein 150 mg/dl or WBC count >1200 should be treated as

bacterials; the rest should be observed and a CSF exam repeated in
8-12 hrs. If there is a tendency for reversal toward bacterial,
then they should be treated.

V. COMPLICATIONS

A. Persistent or Recurrent Fever

If fever persists beyond the fourth or fifth day of therapy or
if it recurs after a satisfactory initial response, the patient
must be re-evaluated carefully. The most common causes include
brain abscess, lateral sinus thrombosis, phlebitis, urinary tract
infection, subdural effusion and drug fever. In order to differentiate among them, it may be necessary to perform angiography or
computerized tomography.

B. Seizures

Seizures occur in up to 30% of cases and are most common in
meningitis due to H. influenzae. Three basic kinds of seizures
can be recognized: 1) Intermixed focal and generalized seizures
of short duration and low frequency are usually not a clinical
problem; 2) Recurrent and prolonged seizures of varying focality
are very difficult to control and have a poor prognosis; and
3) Focal recurrent seizures should bring to mind the possible
complication of subdural effusion or venous or arterial thrombosis
with infarction. The first consideration in treating seizures
should be the maintenance of a clear airway, administration of
oxygen, suction, and aids to metabolic homeostasis. Diazepam,
phenobarbital and diphenylhydantoin are the agents usually
employed to control seizures in patients with bacterial
meningitis.

C. Subdural Effusion and Subdural Empyema

The incidence of subdural effusions in some series of
meningitis in children has been as high as 50%. This frequency is
related to the diligence of the physician and the age of the
patients, being most common in infants under 18 mo of age.
Despite this high incidence, only 10-15% of effusions are symptomatic. Persistent or recurrent fever, lethargy, coma, increasing
head size, an area of transillumination, and persistent focal
seizures should suggest subdural effusions and diagnostic and
therapeutic tap should be done removing 15-20 ml/side/day until
dry. Reaccumulation of subdural fluid beyond 2 wks may require
neurosurgical intervention.

Empyema is very rare and usually the patient presents predisposing factors in conjunction with meningitis, especially sinusitis and otitis media and is associated with the same signs as significant subdural effusion but correlates with hectic fever. In suspicious cases, skull x-rays and CAT scan are needed to evaluate the cases. The treatment is surgical and prolonged administration of antibiotics.

D. Abscess

Its appearance resembles that of subdural empyema secondary to a parameningeal focus, such as otitis, mastoiditis, sinusitis, and osteomyelitis. Clinically, late focal signs and increased intracranial pressure appear and may be associated with papilledema. Positive Technetium[99] brain scans or CAT scanning prove especially helpful in early diagnosis. Treatment consists of surgical evaluation and prolonged antibiotics.

E. Late Complications, Sequelae and Prognosis

Communicating and, occasionally, noncommunicating hydrocephalus occurs in a small number of cases, most commonly infants. If such a complication occurs, signs will become apparent, usually within approximately 3 mo. Deafness occurs in up to 2-3% of these cases. This complication is important to recognize as it may mimic retardation. Transient vestibular disturbance can also occur, manifested as ataxia. Mental retardation with overt neurological abnormalities (with or without seizures) can occur in up to 29% of survivors. Subtle perceptual difficulties with features (commonly lumped under the catch phrase "minimal cerebral dysfunction"), or else, lowered IQ's compared to siblings, occur in up to 20% of "normal" survivors. These may or may not have an abnormal EEG which in turn may or may not be associated with seizures. Obviously, long-term follow-up of children who have recovered from meningitis is important, even in those children who seem to have made a successful recovery.

Several factors predispose to a poor prognosis. These are extremes of age, delay in initiation or inadequate duration of therapy, underlying illness such as diabetes, agammaglobulinemia, or sickle cell disease, and seizures, coma, bacteremia during the course of illness, and causative organism. Of all these, the severity at time of admission appears to be the most consistent determinant of survival and residual. Mortality and residual are highest in the neonatal group. Case fatality rates decrease with maturity and remain low in adults until cardiovascular disease or other intercurrent debility intervenes.

Pneumococcal meningitis carries a more adverse prognosis than other meningitides with comparable clinical presentation. The overall mortality rate is 10-20%; that associated with the meningococcus is approximately 6-7%, with pneumococcus 15-20%, and with H. influenzae 7-9%. Sequelae in patients exclusive of the neonate include deafness, hydrocephalus, mental defects, ataxia, epilepsy, and cranial nerve paresis. The overall rate of sequelae is estimated to be 15-20% but in most studies these are very gross estimates. As far as sequelae with specific organisms are concerned, it is estimated that meningococcus carries a 4% rate, pneumococcus about 25%, and H. influenzae about 22%. In the latter regard, retrospective studies tend to indicate that less than half of the victims of H. influenzae meningitis escape sequelae. These depressing findings await corroboration by more detailed prospective studies.

VI.   PROPHYLAXIS

Prophylactic administration of antibiotics to contacts of patients with pneumococcal meningitis is not indicated. The change in the sulfonamide sensitivity pattern of the meningococcus has removed the best prophylactic drug against meningococcal infection. Penicillin and chloramphenicol which are very effective in treating meningococcal infections do not eliminate the carrier state, possibly because they do not appear in high concentrations in saliva. Rifampin and minocycline have been demonstrated to be highly effective in eradicating meningococci from carriers being active against sulfadiazine resistant and susceptible strains, possibly because they achieve bactericidal levels in saliva. One of the most difficult questions about prophylaxis is how far it should be extended when a case or a larger outbreak of meningococcal disease occurs. Household contacts of patients with meningococcal disease have a much higher risk than the general population of developing meningococcal disease and certainly should be treated. How far to go with classmates, medical personnel and other contacts is not well established. Culturing contacts for meningococcal carriage in the nasopharynx has no value in identifying those at risk. The Public Health Service states that, in addition to household contacts, persons at highest risk are day-care center contacts, medical personnel who resuscitated, intubated or suctioned the patients before treatment was begun, and others who had contact with the patient's oral secretions either through or from sharing of food or beverages. Rifampin is recommended as a two-day regime of 600 mg twice a day for adults, 10 mg/kg twice a day for children 1 mo to 12 yrs old and 5 mg/kg twice a day for newborn infants. Regardless of whether or not a prophylactic antimicrobial is administered, surveillance of all close contacts of patients with meningococcal disease for early symptoms is mandatory.

A polysaccharide vaccine that protects against infection with meningococcal groups A and C is available from Merck Sharpe & Dohme (Meningovax-AC) and from Connaught Laboratories (Menomune). The vaccine causes only mild erythema and tenderness at the site of injection and no serious adverse effects, and begins to protect against meningococcal disease within a week after vaccination. Of meningococcal isolates in recent years, however, only about 15-20% have been group C, and less than 1% group A, limiting the usefulness of the vaccine.

The conventional view that H. influenzae type B meningitis is a noncontagious disease of children has been seriously questioned by various major studies. A secondary attack rate of 1.9% was reported for children less than 5 yrs of age from a large retrospective study. This high secondary attack rate documented by these investigators has stimulated efforts to identify an antibiotic regimen which might interrupt transmission of H. influenzae type B among close contacts. Sulfa-methoxazole-trimethoprim, ampicillin, and cefaclor have not been consistently useful in eradicating nasopharyngeal carriage. Rifampin has been used successfully to eradicate carriage, it is recommended 20 mg/kg once daily for 4 days for close contacts less than 6 yrs of age, maximum dose of 600 mg.

The capsular polysaccharide, polyribophosphate, of H. influenzae type B is probably critical to the invasive potential of this organism. A polyribophosphate vaccine has been developed, but presents its limitations being nonimmunogenic for the youngster at greater risk and in older children does not produce protective antibodies in concentration in the first days after inoculation.

SELECTED REFERENCES

Artenstein, M. (1975). J.A.M.A. 231, 1035

Baker, C., Barrett, F., Gordon, R., et al. (1973). J. Pediatr. 82, 724

Benson, P., Nyhan, W., and Shimizu, H. (1960). J. Pediatr. 57, 670

Berk, S., and McCable, W. (1980). Ann. Intern. Med. 93, 253

Biegeleisen, J., Mitchell, M., Marcus, B., et al. (1965). J. Lab. Clin. Med. 65, 976

Brook, I., Bricknell, K., Overturf, G., et al. (1978). J. Infect. Dis. 137, 384

Bruce, H., Terrence, J., Snyderman, R., et al. (1979). Ann. Intern. Med. 90, 917

Carpenter, R., and Petersdorf, R. (1962). Am. J. Med. 33, 262

Chernik, N., Armstrong, D., and Posner, J. (1973). Medicine 52, 563

Clough, J., Clough, M., Weinstein, A., et al. (1980). Arch.
    Intern. Med. 140, 929
Cox, F., Trincher, R., Rissing, J., et al. (1981). J.A.M.A. 245,
    1043
Feigin, R., and Shackelford, P. (1973). N. Engl. J. Med. 289, 571
Feldman, W. (1976). J. Pediatr. 88, 549
Feldman, W. (1978). Am. J. Dis. Child. 132, 672
Filice, G., Andrew, J., Hidgins, M., and Fraser, D. (1978).
    Am. J. Dis. Child. 132, 757
Geiseler, P., Nelson, K., Levin, S., Reddi, K., and Moses, V.
    (1980). Rev. Infect. Dis. 2, 725
Guttler, R., Counts, G., Avent, C., et al. (1971). J. Infect.
    Dis. 124, 199
Hand, W., and Sanford, J. (1970). Ann. Intern. Med. 72, 869
Horner, D., McCracken, G., Jr., Ginsburg, C., et al. (1980).
    Pediatrics 66, 136
Iwarson, S., Liden-Janson, G., and Svensson, R. (1977).
    Infection 5, 204
Jenson, K., Ranek, L., and Rosdahl, N. (1969). Scand. J.
    Infect. Dis. 1, 21
Jonsson, M., and Aluin, A. (1971). Scand. J. Infect. Dis. 3, 141
LeBeau, J., Creissard, P., Harispe, L., et al. (1973). J.
    Neurosurg. 38, 198
Lewin, E. (1974). Am. J. Dis. Child. 128, 145
Mangi, R., Quintiliani, R., and Andriole, V. (1975). Am. J.
    Med. 59, 829
Overturf, G., Steinberg, E., Underman, A., et al. (1977).
    Antimicrob. Ag. Chemother. 11, 420
Rytel, M. (1975). Hosp. Pract. 10, 75
Sanders, E., and Deal, W. (1970). J. Infect. Dis. 121, 449
Schwartz, J. (1972). Neurology 22, 1071
Sell, S., Merrill, R., Doyne, E., and Zimsky, E. (1972).
    Pediatrics 49, 206
Smith, D., Ingram, D., Smith, A., Gilles, F., and Bresnan, M.
    (1973). Pediatrics 52, 586
Swartz, M., and Dodge, P. (1965). N. Engl. J. Med. 272, 725;
    272, 779; 272, 842; 272, 898
Underman, A., Overturf, G., and Leedom, J. (1978). Disease-A-
    Month 24, 7
Ward, J., Fraser, D., Baraff, L., and Plikaytis, B. (1979). N.
    Engl. J. Med. 301, 122
Weiss, W., Figueroa, W., Shapiro, W., et al. (1967). Arch.
    Intern. Med. 120, 517
Wirt, T., McGee, Z., Oldfield, A., et al. (1979). J. Neurosurg.
    50, 95

PART VI
SKIN INFECTIONS

DERMATOLOGIC MANIFESTATIONS OF
SERIOUS INFECTIONS

Phillip K. Peterson

Department of Medicine
University of Minnesota
Minneapolis, Minnesota

INTRODUCTION

A great variety of bacterial, viral, fungal, and parasitic
infections become manifest in the skin. Careful examination
of this readily accessible organ system can yield the key to a
specific diagnosis of many of these infections. Primary
infection of the skin by certain groups of microorganisms
may result in truly life-threatening illnesses, and secondary
involvement of the skin may provide clues to the nature of
more deep-seated, serious infections.

Such life-threatening or serious infections are the main
focus of this chapter. Several of these infections are covered
in greater detail in other chapters but yet deserve re-emphasis and will therefore be mentioned summarily. Diseases are
also discussed that are rarely, if ever, fatal, but may nevertheless cause considerable morbidity and not infrequently will
lead to hospitalization.

The purpose of this chapter is to aid clinicians in the
early recognition of serious infectious diseases. Emphasis is
placed on the dermatologic findings in these diseases, and
only brief reference will be made to other clinical features,
diagnosis, and therapy. A morphologic classification is used
since categorization of skin findings into such a scheme is
generally the starting point in the clinical evaluation of
these patients.

HEMORRHAGIC LESIONS (PETECHIAE, PURPURA, ECCHYMOSES)

The febrile patient with signs of bleeding into the skin (petechiae, purpura, or ecchymoses) is always cause for great concern. Although diseases other than infections are in the differential diagnosis, e.g., leukemia, collagen vascular diseases, hypersensitivity reactions, and rarely, idiopathic thrombocytopenia, the febrile patient with hemorrhagic skin lesions deserves a prompt and thorough work-up for treatable infections. The most important infectious diseases to be considered under this category of skin findings are listed in Table 1.

Rocky Mountain Spotted Fever (RMSF)

Although a skin rash may go undetected in RMSF, cutaneous lesions are a hallmark of this rickettsial disease. The initial rash usually appears by the third day of illness, and begins on the wrists and ankles as small red macules. When organisms multiply in the endothelial cells of small vessels, leakage of red blood cells and thrombosis occur thus producing petechiae, purpura, ecchymoses, and, rarely, gangrene. Involvement of palms and soles is a key feature of RMSF; however, petechial lesions in these areas can be seen in measles, atypical measles, meningococcemia, and dengue. Salient clinical features include fever, severe headache, myalgias, and confusion. In the U.S., most cases occur in the spring and summer in the Southeast, and exposure to ticks is a helpful part of the history (Hattwick et al, 1976).

The diagnosis of RMSF can be made either by serologic tests (Weil-Felix or complement fixation tests) or immunofluorescent antibody staining of skin biopsy material. However, most importantly, therapy should be initiated on clinical grounds, before the diagnosis is established. Chloramphenicol is the drug of choice. Untreated, RMSF is associated with a mortality of about 20%.

Meningococcemia

Meningococcemia is regularly associated with hemorrhagic skin lesions. *N. meningitidis* causes an acute vasculitis or local Schwartman-like reaction producing petechiae, purpura, and/or ecchymosis. Frank gangrene of the distal extremities, with resultant need for amputation, is not uncommon. The rash of meningococcemia often begins on the

Table 1. Infections with Hemorrhagic Skin Lesions

Disease[a]	Etiology	Exposure history	Key findings	Diagnostic tests	Therapy
Rocky Mountain spotted fever	Rickettsia rickettsii	Ticks; spring, summer	Petechiae palms, soles	Serology; biopsy	Chloramphenicol[b]
Meningococcemia	Neisseriae meningitidis	May be epidemic	Purulent meningitis	Culture (blood, CSF)	Penicillin G[b]
Disseminated gonococcal infection	Neisseriae gonorrhoeae	Sexual contact	Pustule on red base; arthritis	Culture (blood, genital, etc.)	Penicillin G[b]
Infective endocarditis	Many organisms	Dental work, etc.	New heart murmur	Culture (blood)	According to etiology[b]
Epidemic hemorrhagic fever	Many viruses	Endemic area	Bleeding	Serology; culture	Supportive
Plague	Yersinia pestis	Endemic area; rodents	Buboes	Culture; special stains	Streptomycin, tetracycline[b]

[a]Other infectious diseases with hemorrhagic skin lesions
include: gram-negative septicemia; pneumococcal, staphylococcal, clostridial septicemia; atypical measles, measles,
some enterovirusal infections, colorado tick fever; rat-
bite fever.

[b]Treat expectantly, before diagnosis established.

trunk or legs in areas where pressure is applied. Fever, malaise, hypotension, headache, and meningeal signs are associated clinical findings in acute meningococcemia. Recurrent bouts of arthralgias or arthritis are a feature of chronic meningococcemia.

Blood culture will confirm the diagnosis. The finding of purulent cerebrospinal fluid in the proper clinical setting is also virtually diagnostic. Again, treatment should be initiated expectantly, before diagnosis is established. Penicillin G is the drug of choice; however, if there is a question about possible RMSF, chloramphenicol is a good alternative.

Disseminated Gonococcal Infection (DGI)

Some strains of *Neisseria gonorrhoeae* have the capacity to disseminate from anogenital or pharyngeal sites to the skin. A common picture in patients with DGI is the "dermatitis-arthritis" syndrome. Skin lesions begin as tiny red papules or petechiae that may evolve into pustules, vesicles, or bullae. Pustules on an erythematous base are characteristic skin lesions. Skin lesions are typically few in number (usually less than 40) and are distributed primarily over the distal extremities. Fever, chills, polyarthralgias, and monoarticular arthritis are components of the syndrome (Holmes, et al, 1971).

Culture of blood, synovial fluid, skin lesions, or secretions from the anogenital area or pharynx will establish the diagnosis. Once again, therapy should be initiated on clinical grounds, and penicillin G remains the drug of choice.

Infective Endocarditis (IE)

Petechiae, most commonly seen in the conjunctivae, the buccal or palatal mucosa, and the upper chest, occur in up to 40% of patients with IE. Given the proper clinical setting, these lesions can provide helpful clues to the diagnosis of IE. Subungual "splinter" hemorrhages can also be a valuable finding; however, these lesions may also be related to trauma, and they can occur in certain types of hypersensitivity vasculitis. Osler's nodes (wheal-like tender nodules) and Janeway's lesions (painless macules or plaques) are found in the hands and feet of some patients.

The reader is referred to Walter Wilson's chapter in this book for a detailed discussion of the clinical features, diagnosis, and therapy of IE.

Epidemic Hemorrhagic Fevers

A number of life-threatening viral illnesses are associated with hemorrhagic skin lesions as well as with bleeding into other organ systems, especially the gastrointestinal tract. These infections are epidemic in specific countries through-out the world, e.g., Lassa fever (Lassa virus; West Africa), Argentine hemorrhagic fever (Junin virus; Argentina), Bolivian hemorrhagic fever (Machupo virus; Bolivia), and dengue hemorr-hagic fever (dengue virus; Southeast Asia, and Cuba). With the ease of international travel, these diseases may be seen anywhere in the world.

In addition to hemorrhagic fever, dengue virus can cause "classic dengue fever" which is a benign disease characterized by severe headache, backache, and muscle pain ("break-bone fever"), and lymphadenopathy. The skin rash of classic dengue fever is morbilliform or scarletiniform in the early stages of disease; petechiae develop during the last few days of illness. This viral disease occurs world-wide and is epidemic in the Caribbean. Increasing numbers of travelers to this area have returned to the U.S. with this illness. Diagnosis can be established serologically or by virus isolation. Treatment is largely symptomatic.

Plague

Yersinia pestis, a gram-negative baccillus maintained in nature by a rodent-flea infection cycle, is the etiologic agent of plague. Only about 10% of patients develop cutaneous lesions; petechiae and erythematous papules are most common. Purpura and ecchymoses are seen in septicemic plague. Fever, chills, headache, myalgias, arthralgias, painful and enlarged lymph nodes (bubonic plague) are common clinical manifestations. Travel to or residence in an endemic area, e.g. New Mexico or California in the U.S., and exposure to rodents are help-ful historical clues. Diagnosis can be established by culture (blood, purulent material) or by special antibody staining of a bubo aspirate. Rapid initiation of antibiotic therapy, before the diagnosis is established, is critical. Streptomycin is the drug of choice, and is often used in combination with tetracycline. If untreated, mortality is between 60%-100%, depending on the form of disease.

NECROTIZING CELLULITIS AND ULCERATION

Necrotizing (gangrenous) cellulitis is discussed in detail by Richard Simmons in another chapter of this book. Because of the importance of this group of infections in the context of the current chapter, a few points deserving of re-emphasis are summarized in Table II.

Table II. Necrotizing (Gangrenous) Cellulitis

Disease (etiology)	Skin	Other tissues involved	Gas	Pain	Systemic toxicity	Therapy
Clostridial myonecrosis (clostridial sp.)	Yellow-bronze; bullae	Muscle	++	++++	++++	Emergency surgery; penicillin
Clostridial cellulitis (clostridial sp.)	Minimal discolor-ation	Sub-cutaneous	++++	+	+	Emergency surgery; penicillin
Synergistic necrotizing cellulitis (anaerobes + aerobes)	Scattered areas of necrosis	Deep compart-ments	++	++++	++++	Emergency surgery; anti-biotics
Necrotizing fasciitis (aerobes +/or anaerobes)	Erythema	Fascia	++	+++	+++	Emergency surgery; anti-biotics
Non-clostridial anaerobic cellulitis (anaerobes + coliforms)	Minimal discolor-ation	Sub-cutaneous	++++	+	++	Surgery; anti-biotics

The most dramatic and serious of these diseases is clostridial myonecrosis (gas gangrene). Several other forms of necrotizing cellulitis, however, are associated with an almost equally high mortality. Anaerobes are of major etiologic importance in all these diseases, either acting alone or in a synergistic manner with aerobic organisms. Gas in tissues is another feature they have in common, and gas is actually most abundant in some of the non-clostridial infections. Key clinical features are pain and systemic toxicity. The mainstay of treatment is urgent surgery with extensive debridement of devitalized tissue. Antibiotics, appropriate for the antici-pated microbial flora, should be started immediately.

Non-gangrenous forms of cellulitis can, of course, also be potentially life-threatening. Although group A streptococci and *Staphylococcus aureus* are the most common causes of cellu-litis, in the immunocompromised host, a variety of gram-negative aerobic bacilli, and even fungi, can cause cellulitis.

Necrosis of the skin may also be well-localized, and when the epidermis or dermis is lost, skin ulcers are produced. Ecthyma gangrenosum is an example of skin ulceration associated with a serious infection. Although most commonly related to *Pseudomonas aeruginosa* bacteremia, ecthyma gangrenosum can be produced by a variety of other gram-negative bacterial species, and rarely, even by disseminated candidiasis. Most patients who develop this skin lesion are immunocompromised. The lesions are usually multiple and commonly occur on the extre-mities or lower trunk. They begin as painful, red macules that evolve into hemorrhagic bullae or frank necrosis. A characteristic picture is that of central purple then black necrosis with sharply defined, geographic margins. Diagnosis is established by culture. Antibiotic treatment should be started expectantly and, generally, is directed at gram-negative aerobic bacilli, especially *Pseudomonas*.

Bacillus anthracis is a gram-positive bacillus that can produce localized skin necrosis, i.e., cutaneous anthrax. This skin infection begins as a red, painless macule or papule that enlarges to form a hemorrhagic ulcer covered by a black eschar ("malignant pustule") on a brawny, edematous base. Cutaneous anthrax usually remains localized, but bacteremia can ensue, and this is a potentially lethal development. A history of exposure to contaminated wools, hides, or bone meal are helpful clues to the diagnosis. Systemic penicillin is the treatment of choice.

A variety of other infectious diseases may be associated with skin necrosis or ulceration. These diseases are listed in Table III. Skin biopsy for culture (bacterial, mycobacter-ial, fungal) and histopathologic study with special stains (gram, acid fast, methenamine silver) is often necessary to establish an etiologic diagnosis.

Table III. Infections Producing Skin Ulcers

Gram-negative bacilli (ecthyma gangrenosum)	*Sporotrichosis*
Anthrax ("malignant pustule")	*Histoplasmosis*
Impetigo	*Blastomycosis*
Tularemia	*Coccidioidomycosis*
Atypical mycobacterial infection	*Chromomycosis*
Tuberculosis	*Leishmaniasis*
Nocardiosis	*Venereal disease*

MACULOPAPULAR RASHES

At some stage, virtually all skin eruptions are either
macular and/or papular. A febrile patient with a maculopapular skin eruption poses a difficult diagnostic problem
because of an extensive list of possible etiologies. Fortunately, many of these rashes are due to benign viral infection
or hypersensitivity reactions. Morbilliform and scarletiniform eruptions are two types of maculopapular rash which
deserve special attention since they can be caused by serious
infections and there are important developments in understanding the etiologic nature of these rashes.

Morbilliform Eruptions

Morbilliform eruptions are measles-like, erythematous
rashes with elevated portions assuming a net-like configura-
tion. Measles (rubeola) and German measles (rubella) are
classic morbilliform eruptions. In many countries, due to
active vaccination programs, these diseases have become
considerably less common, and now are seen primarily in seas-
onal epidemics among unprotected adolescents and young adults.
Clinical features which can help to distinguish these two
viral diseases include: the enanthem of measles (pathognomonic
Koplik spots); coryza, conjunctivitis and cough in the prodromal phase of measles; and the arthritis and lymphadenopathy
(posterior auricular, cervical, and suboccipital) of rubella.
Other than for its well-established consequences for the fetus
when contracted during pregnancy, rubella is not a serious
infection. Rubeola, however, is associated with an incidence
of encephalitis of about 1/1500, and can cause a serious form
of pneumonia, especially in the immunocompromised host. Diagnosis of both diseases is usually confirmed by serologic tests.

Treatment is symptomatic. Enteroviral infections, infectious mononucleosis, toxoplasmosis, and the scarletiniform eruptions (scarlet fever, toxic shock syndrome) are among the infections in the differential diagnosis.

A hypersensitivity response may occur in persons vaccinated with killed measles virus (used before 1968 in the U.S.) upon exposure to wild measles virus, and these individuals will develop atypical measles (Hall and Hall, 1979). The skin rash of atypical measles begins peripherally as an erythematous maculopapular eruption and characteristically progresses into protean skin lesions including vesicles, urticaria, petechiae, and/or purpura. Interstitial pulmonary infiltrates develop in the majority of patients with atypical measles. Although there have been no deaths reported as yet, patients with atypical measles often require hospitalization, and pose great difficulties in diagnosis (Table IV). Diagnosis is established by serologic testing (the virus cannot be isolated).

Table IV. Differential Diagnosis of Atypical Measles

Rocky Mountain spotted fever	*Varicella*
Scarlet fever	*Enteroviral infection*
Meningococcemia	*Mycoplasma pneumoniae*
Gonococcemia	*infection*
Infective endocarditis	*Coccidioidomycosis*
Typhoid fever	*Disseminated intravascular*
Typhus	*coagulopathy*
Secondary syphilis	*Drug eruption*

Scarletiniform Eruptions

Two relatively newly recognized syndromes - Kawasaki syndrome and toxic shock syndrome - are characterized by the development of more-or-less confluent maculopapular rashes which are virtually indistinguishable from the rash of scarlet fever. The rash of scarlet fever is caused by an erythrogenic toxin produced by group A streptococci; the rash of toxic shock syndrome is caused by a similar toxin produced by *Staphylococcus aureus* (Schlievert *et al*, 1981). A scarletiniform rash can also be seen in the early stages of staphylococcal scalded skin syndrome, a disease characterized by bullous skin lesions produced by epidermolytic toxin (Melish *et al*, 1974). The etiology of Kawasaki syndrome has thus far eluded intensive investigation (Bell *et al*, 1981). The

clinical features, diagnostic criteria, and the therapy of
these serious infections are discussed in detail in another
chapter of this book by Walter Wilson.

PLAQUES AND NODULES

Plaques are raised, palpable skin lesions greater than one
centimeter in diameter. Nodules are more deep-seated sphere-
like lesions of the dermis or subcutaneous tissue. A number
of potentially serious infections are characterized by the
development of these types of skin lesions.

Erythematous and Hypopigmented Plaques

Given the increased mobility of the world population,
patients with skin diseases that were previously rarely seen
in some areas, are now appearing throughout the world.
Leprosy is a good example of such a disease. Patients with
this infection, caused by *Mycobacterium leprae,* usually
present with dermatologic manifestations. Because leprosy
is a great imitator of other skin diseases, the diagnosis is
often overlooked. Erythematous or hypopigmented plaques are
the predominant skin lesion in each of the major forms of
leprosy - tuberculoid, borderline, and lepromatous. Whereas
in tuberculoid leprosy skin lesions are often subtle and few
in number and symptoms and signs of peripheral neuropathy
are prominent, in lepromatous leprosy one finds numerous
plaques and lesser neuropathy. Thickened facial skin (leonine
face), enlarged ears, and loss of eyebrows are additional
features of lepromatous leprosy.
Important clues to the diagnosis of leprosy include a
history of residence in an endemic country and the development
of numbness, cutaneous anesthesia, or enlarged peripheral
nerves. Diagnosis of leprosy is established by skin biopsy
with special acid fast stains (bacilli are sparse in tuberculoid but abound in lepromatous leprosy). Therapy of
leprosy is guided by classification into one of the major
forms of the disease. In general, tuberculoid leprosy is
treated with dapsone alone, and in other forms, rifampin is
added to the regimen.
Erythema nodosum leprosum may develop in some patients
after the initiation of therapy, and this nodular skin lesion,
i.e., erythema nodosum, is a hypersensitivity reaction also
associated with a wide variety of other infections (Table V).

Table V.   Infections Associated with Erythema Nodosum[a]

Leprosy	*Coccidioidomycosis*
Tuberculosis	*Histoplasmosis*
Group A streptococcal	*Influenza*
infection	*Measles*
Psittacosis	*Orf*
Lymphogranuloma venereum	*Cat-scratch disease*
Syphilis	*Pertussis*

[a]*Tender, red, warm, confluent, ill-defined nodules,
occurring predominantly on the anterior lower legs; also
precipitated by drugs, foods, and inhalents, and associated with other diseases, e.g., sarcoidosis, collagen
diseases, dysproteinemias, and inflammatory bowel disease.*

Verrucous Plaques

The surface of nodules or plaques may assume a very rough,
rugated, or wart-like appearance, and several serious infections may be characterized by the development of such verrucous lesions. The most important, and potentially serious of
these, are North American blastomycosis, coccidioidomycosis and
chromomycosis. These fungal infections are discussed in other
chapters of this book by John E. Bennett. Tuberculosis
verrucosa cutis, a form of primary inoculation tuberculosis,
and cutaneous leishmaniasis are also in the differential
diagnosis.

Annular Plaques

Another morphologically distinctive type of skin lesion
is the annular plaque. This lesion is characterized by its
more-or-less round shape with an area of central clearing
(ring-like). Annular plaques are a hallmark of erythematous
multiforme, a hypersensitivity skin reaction associated with a
large number of infections, as well as with certain drugs,
chemicals, and other factors (Table VI).

Table VI. Infections Associated with Erythema Multiforme[a]

Streptococcal, staphylococcal, salmonella, pseudomonas, mycobacterial infections	Herpes simplex, herpes zoster, echovirus, coxsackie B5 virus, poliovirus, influenza B virus,
Syphilis	adenovirus, mumps virus
Lymphogranuloma venereum	infections
Coccidioidomycosis	Orf
Histoplasmosis	Milker's nodules
Trichomoniasis	Vaccinia

[a]Annular plaques with "target lesions"; also associated with certain drugs, chemicals, and other factors.

Erythema multiforme begins with the sudden appearances of symmetric urticarial papules, predominantly found on the extremities, and commonly affecting the palms and soles. The papules enlarge into annular plaques creating classical "target" or "iris" lesions. Mucous membrane involvement heralds Stevens-Johnson syndrome. Conjunctivitis, stomatitis, urethritis, and bronchitis are additional features of this syndrome which can result in significant morbidity, and when serious complications ensue, rarely death.

The diagnosis of erythema multiforme can be confirmed by skin biopsy (the histopathology is relatively specific). The disease will resolve as the underlying inciting etiology is cleared. Treatment is largely symptomatic. Systemic corticosteroids are recommended for serious forms of the disease.

Erythema chronicum migrans (Lyme disease) is a newly recognized disease characterized by the striking development of annular plaques which slowly enlarge to form bright red rings up to 50 cm in diameter. The Ixodes dammini tick appears to act as a vector of an as yet unidentified infectious disease agent. A small puncta may be present at the center of the annular plaque, and patients can develop multiple secondary lesions. Skin findings last from a few days up to several months.

Lyme disease occurs in the summer months, and, although endemic in areas such as New England, cases have been seen in many geographical areas. Recurrent arthritis (often mistaken for rheumatoid arthritis) and neurologic or cardiac abnormalities are common features of the disease. Treatment is symptomatic. Currently, penicillin or tetracycline are recommended for patients with erythema chronicum migrans (Steere, et al, 1980).

ACKNOWLEDGMENTS

I am indebted to Mark Dahl, associate professor of dermatology at the University of Minnesota, for his invaluable advice and to Jane Anderson for her assistance in the preparation of this chapter.

REFERENCES

Bell, D.M., Brink, E.W., Nitzkin, J.L., et al (1981). N. Engl. J. Med. 304, 1568.

Hall, W.J., Hall, C.B. (1979). Ann. Intern. Med. 90, 882.

Hattwick, M.A.W., O'Brien, R.J., Hanson, B.F. (1976). Ann. Intern. Med. 84, 732.

Holmes, K.K., Counts, G.W., Beaty, H.N. (1971). Ann. Intern. Med. 84, 979.

Melish, M.E., Glasgow, L.A., Turner, M.D., Lillibridge, C.B. (1974). Ann. N.Y. Acad. Sci. 236, 317.

Schlievert, P.M., Shands, K.N., Dan, B.B., Schmid, G.P., Nishimura, R.D. (1981). J. Infect. Dis. 143, 509.

Steere, A.C., Malawista, S.E., Newman, J.H., Spieler, P.N., Bartenhagen, N.H. (1980). Ann. Intern. Med. 93, 1.

LIFE-THREATENING SOFT TISSUE INFECTIONS

Richard L. Simmons

Department of Surgery
University of Minnesota
Minneapolis, Minnesota

PATHOGENESIS OF SOFT TISSUE INFECTIONS

Experimental Skin Infections

Normal skin is extremely resistant to infection, and few
pathogenic organisms are capable of penetrating and invading
intact epidermis. Topical application of even high concentrations
of pathogenic bacteria does not result in infection. The
requirements to produce infection include: (1) a high concentration of microorganisms, (2) occlusion, which both prevents
desquamation and provides a moist environment in which the
bacteria can proliferate, (3) nutrients in the area, and
(4) sufficient damage to the corneal layer for the organisms to
penetrate. Corneal layer damage can be achieved by repeated
stripping of the skin with cellophane tape, by plucking hair, by
incision, or by occlusive dressings which result in skin
maceration. In addition, a foreign body within the skin will
potentiate most infections and is required for the production of
infections from a small inoculum. Experimental folliculitis or
impetigo results when Staphylococcus, Streptococcus, or Candida
is applied in combination with these factors. In this sense,
skin infections are usually opportunistic, i.e. caused by normal
skin flora, transient residents, or environmental contaminants,
which have low pathogenic potential in themselves but can colonize
and infect tissue with impaired local host defenses.

Susceptibility of Soft Tissues to Infection

Subcutaneous and soft tissue infections most often arise from
breaks in local host defenses. Soft tissue infections, however,
are not the natural consequence of simple microbial innoculation

into tissue. Large numbers of bacteria are necessary to produce suppuration in intact tissue. Roettinger et al (1) found that 3×10^6 S. aureus was noninfective when injected into the soft tissues of guinea pigs; 2×10^9 S. aureus were required to produce infections consistently. With E. coli, 3×10^6 organisms were required to infect more than half the sites. The site of innoculation (tongue, subcutaneous fat, skin or skeletal muscle) did not influence the rate of infection.

Differences in the infection rates at different sites is most likely related to the inherent pathogenicity of the local bacteria, the susceptibility of the tissue to trauma, and the size of the inoculum rather than to different degrees of local immunity. In men performing manual labor, the hands and arms are the most frequently infected sites, presumably owing to the high incidence of trauma. In women, the axillae and submammary regions are frequently infected - minor trauma in both areas results in exposure to a relatively large bacterial inoculum growing in moist intertriginous areas.

Differences in blood supply or tissue pO_2 are additional factors in regional differences in infection (2). Ischemic limbs and areas affected by radiation vasculitis and fibrosis are prone to infection. The local injection of epinephrine increases the experimental infection rates for a given bacterial inoculum (1).

Role of Trauma and Foreign Bodies in Soft Tissue Infection

Trauma not only inoculates the bacteria into the soft tissue, but also impairs host defenses. The degree of tissue damage is probably the most important factor in the pathogenesis of soft tissue infections. For this reason, the nature and velocity of the wounding agent is a critical factor in the development of infection after soft tissue trauma.

Foreign bodies have long been recognized as one of the most important adjuvant factors increasing the infectivity of small bacterial inocula. Cotton dust (3) and suture material are classic adjuvants. Environmental contaminants (e.g. soil) have also been implicated (4). Devitalized endogenous tissue may play such a role. Fibrin is known to trap large bacterial inocula within its strands. Furthermore fibrin tends to isolate the trapped bacteria from invading phagocytes. Hemolyzed blood fosters the growth of iron-dependent bacteria and the red cell stroma impairs phagocytosis. For these reasons debridement of devitalized tissues and implanted exogenous foreign bodies is necessary to eliminate infection after trauma.

Not all foreign bodies potentiate infection. Injection of a liquid silicone or a local anesthetic does not stimulate the development of experimental staphylococcal infections. Different suture materials enhance the development of infection to varying degrees.

GANGRENOUS INFECTIONS OF SUBCUTANEOUS TISSUE

Meleney (5) coined the term "infectious gangrene" to describe infections that cause extensive necrosis of the subcutaneous tissues (superficial fascia) and may cause gangrene of the overlying skin. A number of these infections have been described as separate clinical entities. Attempts to discriminate one from the other on clinical grounds alone are difficult (Table I) since the pattern of infection is basically similar in all. The manifestations depend on the etiologic agents, predisposing conditions, and anatomic location of the infection. Almost all forms of infectious gangrene involve a greater or lesser degree of necrosis of the subcutaneous tissues, with hemorrhage, vasculitis, and thrombosis of small arteries and veins and infiltration by polymorphonuclear leukocytes. In clostridial cellulitis and gangrene, leukocytes are notably absent and gas is abundant. The presence of gas in tissue, long considered pathognomonic of clostridial infections, simply means that anaerobic bacterial metabolism has produced insoluble gases such as hydrogen, nitrogen, and methane. Both facultative and obligate anaerobes are capable of such a metabolic activity. Trapped air disseminated by muscular activity can also lead to a similar picture.

In most clinical situations, infectious gangrene results after inoculation of the infecting organisms into the tissues. The precipitating event is usually obvious - an area of crush injury, an operative incision, enterotomy stoma, or a secondarily infected cutaneous ulcer. Perineal fistulas are less visible but common sources of infection. More rarely, rupture of a viscus into the subcutaneous tissues of the abdomen, perineum or thigh can occur, or infectious gangrene can begin at a site of metastatic hematogenous infection in immunodepressed patients.

The extent of skin gangrene is variable. Necrotizing faciitis due to mixed aerobes and anaerobes typically spreads in the fascial cleft between the subcutaneous tissue and deep fascia, sparing the vascular plexus within the subcutaneous tissue and preserving extensive areas of skin. Debridement can frequently be carried out without removing all the skin. In contrast, streptococcal gangrene leads to relatively early necrosis of the overlying skin.

STREPTOCOCCAL GANGRENE

Etiology

Acute streptococcal gangrene is a classic but rare form of necrotizing faciitis caused by S. pyogenes, Lancefield group A (beta-hemolytic streptococci). Although Meleney first described

TABLE I. DIFFERENTIAL DIAGNOSES OF GANGRENOUS INFECTIONS OF SUBCUTANEOUS TISSUES AND SKIN

	Bacterial Synergistic Gangrene	Necrotizing Fasciitis	Streptococcal Gangrene	Gas Gangrene	Necrotizing Cutaneous Mucormycosis	Bacteremia Gangrenous Cellulitis	Pyoderma Gangrenosum
Predisposing conditions	Wound infection; draining sinus	Wound infection; perineal infections; diabetes; drug addiction	Occasionally diabetes or myxedema; after abdominal surgery	Local trauma to deep soft tissues	Diabetes; corticosteroid therapy	Burns; immunosuppression; cancer chemotherapy	Ulcerative colitis, rheumatoid arthritis
Pain	Severe	Variable	Severe	Severe	Minimal	Minimal	Moderate
Toxicity	Minimal	Marked	Marked	Very Marked	Variable	Marked	Minimal
Fever	Minimal	Moderate	High	Moderate or high	Low	High	Low
Crepitus	Absent	Frequent	Absent	Frequent	Absent	Absent	Absent
Appearance	Central shaggy necrotic ulcer surrounded by dusky margin and erythematous periphery	Drainage from single or multiple areas of skin necrosis; extensive undermining of skin along fascial	Extensive undermining of subcutaneous tissue; bullae and necrotic "burned" appearance of overlying skin	Marked swelling; yellow-bronzed discoloration of skin; brown bullae green-black	A central black necrotic area with purple raised margin	A sharply demarcated necrotic area with black eschar and surrounding erythema, resembling a decubitus ulcer	Begin as bullae, pustules, or erythematous nodules that ulcerate deeply; often multiple;

TABLE I.   DIFFERENTIAL DIAGNOSES OF GANGRENOUS INFECTIONS OF SUBCUTANEOUS TISSUES AND SKIN

	Bacterial Synergistic Gangrene	Necrotizing Fasciitis	Streptococcal Gangrene	Gas Gangrene	Necrotizing Cutaneous Mucormycosis	Bacteremia Gangrenous Cellulitis	Pyoderma Gangrenosum
		plane		patches of necrosis; serosanguinous discharge		evolve from initial hemorrhagic bullae	large and coalesce; usually on lower extremities or abdomen
Etiology	Microaerophilic streptococcus plus S. aureus (or Proteus)	Usually a mixture of aerobic and anaerobic organisms	Primarily group A streptococci	C. perfringens (occasionally) other clostridia	Rhizopus, Mucor, Absidia	P. aeruginosa S. aureus	Not a primary infection; secondary by polymicrobial flora

Modified from Wilson, C.B., Siber, G.R., O'Brien, T.F., Morgan, A.P.:   Phycomycotic gangrenous cellulitis. Arch. Surg. 111:532, 1976.

the condition and its treatment in 1924 (5), this disease was probably the "hospital gangrene" of the Civil War, and is also known as "necrotizing erysipelas".

Basically, streptococcal gangrene is a fulminant type of necrotizing fasciitis with extensive skin necrosis. The gangrene results from thrombosis of the blood vessels that supply the skin within the superficial fascia. Destruction of cutaneous nerves may produce late anesthesia. Meleney first believed this disease was an allergic or schwartzman type of reaction, but it is more likely that the gangrene is due to a tendency of the streptococcus organism to affect vascular structures of all types.

Clinical Manifestations

The clinical course is fulminating. The affected skin is hot, red, swollen, and extremely painful at first. Fever, chills, tachycardia, and prostration are also present. Within 2 to 4 days, the skin overlying the infection develops dusky, irregular patches and large bullae containing bacteria and a dark exudate. Without treatment, these areas progress to frank cutaneous gangrene and a burnlike eschar. Muscle and bone are generally spared. If the untreated patient survives, the slough separates from the underlying tissue in 2 to 3 weeks. The essential undermining nature of the infection is best recognized by passing a probe through a skin incision along the fascial cleft overlying the deep fasciitis without resistance.

The differential diagnosis must include gas gangrene caused by C. perfringens, erysipelas, and cellulitis. The blister fluid will frequently show gram-positive streptococci on smear. Gas and odor are notably absent. Lymphangitis is uncommon.

Treatment

High-dose parenteral penicillin G is the treatment of choice, but always in conjunction with surgical debridement within a few hours. An incision along the entire length of the undermined area should be carried down to the muscles. All the necrotic tissue is excised, but viable skin is not removed even though undermined. Some authors spare patient blood vessels to minimize more extensive gangrene. Sometimes muscular edema will be extensive and require fasciotomy.

After incision and debridement through the superficial fascia, the wound is treated by rest, elevation, and frequent dressing changes, which aid in the mechanical debridement. If gangrene progresses, repeated debridement may be necessary. Skin grafting can be carried out in denuded areas when a granulating base has been established.

NECROTIZING FASCIITIS

Definition

Although the term necrotizing fasciitis originally described streptococcal gangrene, currently it more commonly refers to mixed bacterial infections. Necrotizing fasciitis, clostridial cellulitis, nonclostridial anaerobic cellulitis, anaerobic cutaneous gangrene, Fournier's gangrene, and synergistic necrotizing cellulitis all have a similar pathogenesis, treatment, and prognosis. Each is essentially an infection of the subcutaneous tissues (i.e., the superficial fascia), which spreads in the fascial clefts overlying deep fascia and spares the skin. Skin gangrene results only after the vessels to the skin thrombose. Each of these syndromes was originally described separately, and new terminology is constantly appearing in the literature (Table I).

Etiology

A variety of organisms have been reported as predominant in these infections, including beta-hemolytic streptococcus, the hemolytic staphylococcus, and gram-negative organisms, in addition to gram-positive cocci. Rea and Wyrick (6) confirmed that mixtures of bacteria were typical and claimed that inadequate collection or laboratory bacteriology techniques were responsible for failure to document the mixed etiology of this infection.

Most available data now suggest that necrotizing fasciitis is most often a synergistic bacterial surgical infection, produced by the combination of gram-positive cocci and gram-negative bacilli. Both aerobes and anaerobes are typically found. Modern bacteriologic techniques have clarified the etiology to some degree. Giuliano et al found a total of 75 bacterial species were in 16 patients. At least one facultative Streptococcus was recovered from 15 patients, a Bacteroides species was recovered from 10, and a Peptostreptococcus from eight. Giuliano et al concluded that there are two types of necrotizing fasciitis, most commonly anaerobic bacteria and facultative anaerobic bacteria (Enterobacteriaceae and streptococci other than group A) that act in combination; anaerobes were never cultured alone. In the second group, group A streptococcus was isolated alone or in combination with S. aureus or S. epidermidis representing classical streptococcal gangrene.

The organisms cultured by Stone and Martin (7) were different in many regards. Giuliano's patients (8) were primarily drug addicts with infections of the upper extremities, trunk, and shoulders, whereas the patients of Stone and Martin were debilitated bedridden patients, frequently with diabetes, with

infections of the lower extremities, trunk, and perineal regions.
No beta-hemolytic streptococci were found, but there was a higher
incidence of facultative (aerobic) gram-negative bacilli (62
percent) and enterococcus (19 percent) in combination with
anaerobic Streptococcus (51 percent) and Bacteroides species (24
percent)(7). Both sets of investigators speculate that synergism
between aerobic and anaerobic organisms is taking place (7,8).

Pathogenesis and Pathology

The infection is almost always introduced through a break in
the skin or gut-the injection of illicit drugs, an incised
wound, an enterostomy, a decubitus ulcer, perineal fistula, or
diabetic foot. Of the 63 patients studied by Stone and Martin
(7), 47 had diabetes, 33 cardiovascular and renal disease, and 54
were either starved or obese. In drug addicts, extremity
infections are most common; in other patients, infections of the
trunk, perineum, buttocks, and thighs represent spread of
infection from previously infected sites that had been overlooked
or ignored. Phycomycotic gangrene must be considered in all such
infections.

Little is known about synergistic infections of the soft
tissues. It is assumed that facultative bacteria assist the
growth of anaerobes by utilizing oxygen, diminishing the redox
potential, or supplying catalase which detoxifies H_2O_2. Proof
of bacterial synergism in these infections is lacking. S.
pyogenes, group A, is capable of producing a necrotizing fasciitis
either alone or in the presence of staphylococcus.

Clinical Manifestations

Usually the portal of entry is obvious-the site of trauma,
postoperative wound infection, or extension from a previous site
of primary infection, i.e., perirectal abscess, infected
decubitus ulcer, infected diabetic ulcer. It may remain an
indolent undermining infection or may become suddenly fulminant
and rapidly progress to gangrene and death, in a manner similar to
acute streptococcal gangrene.

In the chronic progressive type, cellulitis, rather than
gangrene, predominates. Multiple skin ulcers drain a thin,
reddish-brown foul-smelling fluid characterized by Stone and
Martin (7) as "dishwater pust". The telltale signs are multiple
ulcers, which communicate beneath superficially normal, but
extensively undermined, intervening skin. Superficial gangrene
is limited. Crepitance in the soft tissues is frequent, and
sensation may range from exquisite local tenderness to anesthesia.

The diagnosis is easily made by passing a probing instrument
through the area of necrosis and determining that undermining

exists between the subcutaneous tissue and deep fascia. In
simple cellulitis or abscess, such a probing instrument cannot be
passed laterally into the fascial cleft parallel to the skin
surface.

Frank pus is an unusual finding despite widespread necrosis.
Thus, the extent of the necrosis is frequently overlooked until
suddent systemic toxicity supervenes. In fact, most patients are
admitted with symptoms and signs of septicemia. At that time,
blood cultures are freuqently positive, and hypercalcemia may
occur when necrosis of the subcutaneous tissues is extensive.
Only then are the rather insignificant ulcerating lesions
recognized as the septic source. In short, the classic clinical
picture is a manifestation of neglect. Without question, the
undermining infection takes a long time to develop. The factors
which foster a septicemic rather than indolent outcome are un-
known-but diabetes, anemia, and renal failure are commonly
found (7).

At the other clinical extreme, a picture identical with
acute streptococcal gangrene can be seen in which clinical
attention is immediately focused on extensive areas of cutaneous
gangrene involving the skin, with patchy areas of dusky necrosis
progressing to frank eschar formation or bullae. These patients
also demonstrate fever, chills, and shock, but the local process
is obvious.

Numerous terms have been applied to these subcutaneous
necrotizing infections (Table I). Some deserve special comment:

1. Clostridial anaerobic cellulitis is a necrotizing
clostridial infection of devitalized subcutaneous tissues without
involvement of deep fascia or muscle. Gas formation is often
extensive. Clostridial species, usually C. perfringens or C.
septicum, can be seen on Gram stain and culture. The infection
is usually found at the sites of dirty or inadequately debrided
traumatic wounds, especially around the perineum, abdominal wall,
buttocks, and lower extremities, i.e., areas contaminated with
fecal flora. The clinical picture is similar to necrotizing
fasciitis but has few of the features of gas gangrene. A dark
foul-smelling drainage, often containing fat globules, has been
described; frank crepitus seems to extend widely beyond the
areas of active infection. Roentgenograms of soft tissue show
abundant gas. Sometimes, the clostridia are present in mixed
culture with facultative organisms.

2. Nonclostridial anaerobic cellulitis presents a picture
similar to that of clostridial anaerobic cellulitis. The syndrome
is essentially identical to necrotizing fasciitis, but mixed
anaerobic flora predominate.

3. Synergistic necrotizing cellulitis refers to a variant of
necrotizing fasciitis with systemic toxicity and bacteremia ocur-
ring in patients with diabetes mellitus, obesity, advanced age,
and cardiorenal disease (7). Most infections are located on the
lower extremities or near the perineum. Bacteremia and death are

common.

4. <u>Fornier's gangrene</u> (9) occurs about the male genitals. It may involve the scrotum and surrounding perineum, penis and abdominal wall in patients with diabetes, local trauma, paraphismosis, periurethral extravasation of urine, perirectal or perineal infections, and may follow operation in the area. The extensive gangrene of the skin is due to the blood supply to the skin is readily involved by spreading perineal necrotizing fasciitis. The organisms are those seen in necrotizing fasciitis in this region, including facultative enteric organisms (<u>E.coli</u>, <u>Klebsiella</u>, enterococci) and anaerobes (<u>Bacteroides</u>, <u>Fusobacterium</u>, <u>Clostridia</u>, anaerobic peptostreptococci).

Treatment

Infections of the trunk, perineum, perirectal area, periurethral, buttock, and thigh frequently involve four types of organisms: Enterobacteriaceae, enterococci, anaerobic streptococci, and <u>Bacteroides</u>. It would seem appropriate in these potentially fatal infections to begin triple drug therapy, including ampicillin (for enterococci and anaerobic peptostreptococci), and aminoglycoside for the <u>Enterobacteriaceae</u>, and clindamycin for <u>B. fragilis</u> and peptostreptococci. The new broad-spectrum cephalosporin antibiotics, such as cefoxitin or moxalactam, have not yet been evaluated for these mixed infections. Other antibiotic combinations, such as carbenicillin and tobramycin, may be effective but remain second choices. Cloramphenicol with its broad spectrum and efficacy in vitro against <u>B. fragilis</u> is a useful alternative, but because it is bacteriostatic, potentially toxic, and occasionally ineffective against <u>B. fragilis</u>, it is not recommended as a first choice. Penicillin G is effective for clostridial or beta-hemolytic streptococcal necrotizing fasciitis.

Blood culture results are frequently positive in patients with necrotizing fasciitis, and one might choose an antibiotic based on these results. Stone and Martin (7) found the blood cultures were positive for gram-negative rods in more than one-third of the cases, and an anaerobe could be isolated from the blood in 20 percent. Mixed bacteria were only isolated from the blood cultures in six of 63 patients, but mixed infections were always present in the wounds. Antibiotic therapy should not be based only on blood cultures but on the presumptive bacteria in the wound. Frequently, clinical laboratories fail to culture the anaerobic organisms in mixed infections, so that the clinician is tempted to prematurely discontinue those agents directed at presumptive anaerobes.

The primary therapy of necrotizing fasciitis is radical debridement. The incision should extend beyond the outermost extent of the fascial involvement in all planes. The dead material is resected, although the skin can frequently be preserved after removal of the necrotic underlying fat. The wounds are packed loosely open with fine mesh gauze, and several small catheters are placed in the wound for constant delivery of local antibiotics. Baxter (10) recommends a solution containing 100 mg of neomycin and 100 mg of polymixin B per liter of normal saline. Other workers would prefer less toxic antibiotics (e.g. carbenicillin).

The fine mesh gauze should be changed frequently during the first days after the operation. These dressing changes aid in superficial debridement of the wound and permit examination to determine whether additional surgical debridement is necessary.

Repeated culturing of the wound is necessary as secondary inoculation with <u>Pseudomonas</u>, <u>Serratia</u>, and <u>Candida</u> occurs. Fascial porcine heterografts can be used to cover the wound, as in burns. The porcine heterografts can be left in place until there is complete adherence of the biologic dressing. When the wound is ready (less than 10^5 organisms per gram of tissue) under the biologic cover, the large skin flaps may be replaced, and any remaining open areas grafted with split thickness skin grafts. A meshed graft is advantageous for covering these large wounds. Sulfamylon or silver sulfadiazine can be applied to the open wounds, as in treatment for burns, to prevent secondary infection.

Prognosis

The prognosis is grave and depends in part on the underlying disease, the physiologic condition of the patient, delay in treatment, the site of infection, and the bacteriology of the wound. In young drug addicts with mixed gram-positive aerobic and anaerobic infections, amputation is occasionally necessary for infections of the distal extremity. In the series of Giuliano et al (8) only two of 16 patients died. In the more chronically debilitated patients treated by Stone and Martin (7), the overall mortality was 76 percent and almost 50 percent of the patients died within a week after admission. All surviving patients have considerable residual morbidity and a prolonged hospital course.

Patients with severe renal disease almost never survive, and diabetes mellitus significantly worsens the prognosis (85 percent mortality). One of the most decisive influences on survival was the area of involvement. When the infection developed within an extremity, radical debridement by either amputation or disarticulation was usually practical. All patients with deep infections of the pelvis and neck died, and there were only two survivors of the 24 patients with extension from a perirectal origin, whereas infections of the buttock and distal extremities had a lower mortlaity. If these progressive lesions had been recognized before the onset of septemic toxicity, survival results certainly would have been better.

BACTERIAL SYNERGISTIC GANGRENE

Bacterial synergistic gangrene (progressive synergistic gangrene, Meleney synergistic gangrene) is an infection primarily of the subcutaneous tissue, which rarely spreads in the fascial planes, although it is caused by the same organisms found in aerobic and anaerobic cellulitis, subcutaneous abscesses, and necrotizing fasciitis.

Etiology

The classic etiology is the combination of a microaerophilic nonhemolytic streptococcus that is found primarily in the spreading periphery of the lesion, and S. aureus in the zone of gangrene. The microaerophilic streptococcus has been found to be S. evolutus (11). The Streptococcus can be an obligate anaerobe, and a wide variety of other organisms can be seen instead of or in addition to the Staphylococcus; Proteus, Enterobacter, Pseudomonas, and Clostridium species have been isolated. The microaerophilic streptococcus may be difficult to isolate in culture.

Clinical Manifestations

Bacterial synergistic gangrene develops most often following abdominal or thoracic surgery or drainage of a peritoneal abscess or thoracic empyema. Sometimes, it develops around a colostomy or ileostomy site or following a trivial accidental wound. The major symptom is severe pain and tenderness. The lesion first appears about 2 weeks after wounding, in an area around the foreign body suture or wound closure. A purple central area of induration becomes surrounded by a zone of erythema. Tenderness is pronounced. As the lesion progresses, three zones become demarcated: 1) the outer zone is fiery red, 2) the middle zone is purple and tender, and 3) the central portion of the purplish area becomes frankly gangrenous, the color changing to a dirty gray-brown or a yellow-green with a typical suede leather appearance. As the lesion spreads outward, the inner margin of the gangrenous zone becomes undermined and melts away. Eventually, the center of the lesion becomes a granulating ulcer, and epithelium may be seen to generate here. The progression is slow but unremitting. The depth is usually limited to the upper third of the subcutaneous fat and rarely extends deep to fascia. Satellite lesions may surface as the infection tunnels through the fat. Fever is minimal, but anemia and malnutrition are common.

Chronic undermining ulcer or Meleney ulcer is probably the same disease. In this form, the satellite lesions attract attention, and multiple ulcers and sinuses may develop at a distance from the original ulcer with undermining of the intervening skin.

Treatment

Initially, wide excision alone with zinc peroxide ointment was considered necessary for cure. However, antimicrobial therapy alone may suffice to prevent spread, and debridement will then effect cure. The progress of this disease is slow, and zealous excision is no longer required. The fact that two cases of antibiotic control followed by local steroid treatment have resulted in cure suggests that part of the process may be delayed hypersensitivity response (11).

GANGRENOUS INFECTIONS OF MUSCLE

Gas Gangrene (Clostridial Myonecrosis)

Gas gangrene is a rapidly progressive, life-threatening, toxemic infection of skeletal muscles due to Clostridia species. It usually follows the contamination by animal or human feces of severe crushing muscle injury. It may be part of clostridial cellulitis, but in its classical form, muscle is principally involved.

Etiology

C. perfringens is isolated from 80 to 95 percent of the cases. C. novyi is found in 10 to 40 percent, C. septicum in 5 to 20 percent, and C. bifermentans, C. histolyticum, and C. phallax have all been implicated. Other aerobes and facultative organisms are also usually isolated. The clinical syndromes produced are all similar. C. novyi is supposed to produce toxemia and massive gelatinous edema with little gas. C. septicum is most often associated with colon carcinoma (11). All Clostridium species sporulate, producing potentially lethal organisms resistant to almost all physical and many chemical agents.

Epidemiology and Pathogenesis

C. perfringens and other histotoxic clostridial species are
essential for true gas gangrene. They can be inoculated by
accidental traumatic or high-velocity wounds, which severly impair
muscle viability. Compound fractures are said to be particularly
susceptible because of local calcium salts which favor clostridial
growth. In addition, they are sometimes seen in wounds after
large bowel or biliary tract surgery, or in the presence of
ischemic impairment of a muscular region, especially after
amputations of the lower extremity for ischemic gangrene. Cases
have followed contaminated injections, especially of vasopastic
agents, such as epinephrine in oil. Three factors are usually
present: 1) contamination of wounds with clostridia (e.g. fecal
contamination), 2) devitalized tissue creating an anaerobic
environment, and 3) foreign bodies. Debridement and delayed
primary closure of war wounds substantially reduces the incidence.
Primary carcinomas of the colon with or without penetration of
perforation, have been associated with gas gangrene. Immunocompromised patients have a high risk even in the presence of minor
trauma.

CLINICAL MANIFESTATIONS

The incubation period of clostridial myonecrosis is much
shorter than for most pyogenic infections; the full-blown picture
may be present within 1 to 3 days of wounding. Only group A
streptococci or clostridial infections are normally so fulminant.
The onset is usually acute–a pain so severe that a vascular
catastrophe must be suspected. No other soft tissue infection
produces a comparable degree of pain.

The local lesion becomes rapidly edematous, cool, and
exquisitely tender. Swollen muscle may herniate through an open
wound, and a serosanguinous dirty appearing discharge, which
contains numerous organisms but few leukocytes, escapes. The
wound has a peculiar sweet but foul odor; gas bubbles may be
visible in the discharge. Crepitus, if present, is not as
prominent as in other anaerobic soft tissue infections. The skin
adjacent to the wound is initially swollen and pale, but rapidly
takes on a yellowish or bronze discoloration. Tense blebs containing thick, dark fluid develop in the overlying skin, and
areas of green-black cutaneous necrosis appear.

Toxemia is usually severe long before cutaneous gangrene
appears. Although the systemic signs are nonspecific, they are a
prominent part of the clinical picture. The patient is severely
ill, pale, sweaty, and apprehensive. Delirium may follow. Tachycardia, hypotension, shock, and renal failure follow in rapid
succession. Fever is generally not too high, and hypothermia is
associated with terminal shock, as is jaundice.

Diagnosis

Operative exploration must be carried out on suspicion. Bacteremia with C̲. perfringens occurs in only 15 percent of the patients with gas gangrene, but hemolysis, presumably associated with bacteremia, is a common complication, especially after intra-uterine infections.

Gram-stained smears of the wound exudate or an aspirate from one of the blebs reveals large gram-positive bacilli with blunt ends but few polymorphonuclear leukocytes. Spores are usually not evident. Other gram-positive and gram-negative bacteria may be present, particularly in grossly contaminated wounds, so that the diagnosis can be overlooked if only bacteriologic diagnosis is sought.

Roentgenograms of the involved areas shown extensive and pro-gressive gaseous dissection of muscle and fascial planes.

The differential diagnosis is outlined in Table I. The degree of toxemia, the rather limited crepitance usually masked by edema, the severe degree of local pain, and the characteristic skin lesions with bronzing, dark blebs, and gross ischemic necrosis differentiate this disease from nonclostridial crepitant myositis and cellulitis. The absence of leukocytes and the presence of Clostridia on smear are helpful diagnostic signs, although Clostridia can be part of mixed bacterial crepitant and noncrepitant infections such as necrotizing fasciitis.

At exploration, the infected muscle itself may be unimpres-sive; it may exhibit only pallid edema and elasticity, fail to contract on stimulation, and not bleed from a cut surface. Later, it becomes discolored to a reddish purple before becoming black and friable.

Treatment

Treatment includes emergency operation to define the nature and extent of the gangrenous process, directly examine the muscles at the site of infection, and widely excise the infected tissue. Gram stains of the infected muscle should be carried out during debridement. Only when resected muscle is free of bacteria should debridement be stopped. Some surgeons irrigate the wound in the postoperative period with H_2O_2; others pack the wound with zinc peroxide. All infected or possibly infected muscles should be excised, and fasciiotomies performed to decompress and drain the swollen or potentially swollen fascial compartments of adjacent uninfected muscle groups. Amputation is a highly effective treatment of distal infections and should be carried out promptly in any patient with clostridial myonecrosis who manifests systemic toxicity. For this reason, the mortality is much higher for truncal and perineal gas gangrene than for limb infections. All wounds should be left to close by secondary intention.

Repeated inspection of the wound in the operating room is necessary at frequent intervals after primary debridement to determine if further excision is required.

Antibiotic Therapy. Antibiotic therapy is essential. Penicillin G is administered intravenously in a dosage of 1 to 2 million units every 2 to 3 hours. Most authorities advocate a second antibiotic (chloramphenicol for mixed infections or an aminoglycoside)(12). Chloramphenicol is a good alternative drug in the penicillin-allergic patient. A few strains of Clostridia are resistant to tetracycline and clindamycin.

Ancillary Surgical Therapy. If autogenous fecal contamination is responsible for the infection, diversion of the fecal stream will be required. Skin grafting and other reconstructive procedures are almost always required in survivors.

Hyperbaric Oxygen Therapy. Hyperbaric oxygen therapy has been advocated as an additive treatment, particularly for patients with diffuse spreading infections (13). Until controlled clinical trials are completed, it may be useful in the management of patients with extensive involvement of the trunk or perineum where adequate surgical debridement is impossible. It is not a substitute for debridement or antibiotics.

General Maintenance. Attention to fluid and electrolyte balance and nutrition is essential in the management of these patients. Renal failure and secondary organ failure syndromes are common.

Antitoxin. A polyvalent gas gangrene antitoxin is no longer available, and its usefulness was controversial. Before the ready availability of penicillin, military surgeons were convinced of its value (11), though the mechanism of action was unclear. Finegold strongly advocates its use when there is evidence of hemolysis (11).

Prevention

The disease in wartime is more rare than in civilian practice. The military medical policy of wide debridement of all fresh wounds with delayed (4 day) primary closure has effectively reduced the incidence. Prophylactic antibiotics for wounded patients may be useful adjuncts, but excision of all devitalized tissue is the principal prophylactic maneuver. Only 22 cases occurred in 139,000 casualties in Vietnam, where this policy was generally followed. There were 27 cases in Miami in a recent 10 year period, suggesting that the policy is not followed in civilian practice (14).

NONCLOSTRIDIAL INFECTIOUS MYONECROSIS

Myonecrosis can be caused by organisms other than Clostridia—most prominent among them is the anaerobic Streptococcus.

Anaerobic Streptococcal Myonecrosis

Anaerobic streptococcal myonecrosis is a rare disease even in wartime. The anaerobic streptococci are usually accompanied by S. aureus or group A streptococci. The predisposing causes are the same as for clostridial myonecrosis, but the incubation period is longer (3 to 4 days) and the course less fulminating. The wounded area is edematous, and seropurulent drainage is seen. Pain is not the initial symptom but can become severe. Gas is present but not extensive. The odor may be sour. Toxemia is a later and preterminal sign. When S. pyogenes or S. aureus are present, the wound takes on some of the clinical characteristics of infections with these organisms. Treatment with wide debridement and penicillin is appropriate. Penicillinase-resistant penicillins or cephalosporins should be added for S. aureus.

Synergistic Nonclostridial Anaerobic Myonecrosis

The disease is similar to necrotizing cellulitis or necrotizing cutaneous myositis (10), in which the skin, subcutaneous tissue, fascia, and muscle are all involved. As in necrotizing fasciitis, many patients have diabetes or other debilitating conditions. B. fragilis is the key pathogen, in combination with aerobic or anaerobic streptococci and facultative gram-negative enteric organisms. Basically, this disease is necrotizing fasciitis with muscular involvement. Combination antibiotics (aminoglycoside plus clindamycin) are required as adjuncts to wide debridement.

Infected Vascular Gangrene

Infected vascular gangrene is simply secondary infection of a dead extremity in which amputation has been delayed. A variety of organisms have been reported, and true gas gangrene also occurs.

REFERENCES

1. Roettinger, W., Edgerton, M.T., Kurtz, L.D., Prusak, M., Edlich, R.F.: Role of inoculation site as a determinant of infection in soft tissue wounds. Am. J. Surg. 126:354, 1973.
2. Duncan, W.C., McBride, M.E., Knox, J.M.: Experimental production of infections in humans. J. Invest. Dermatol. 54:319,1970.

3. Agarwal, D.S.: Subcutaneous staphylococcal infection in mice. I. The role of cotton-dust in enhancing infection. Br. J. Exp. Pathol. 48:436, 1967.

4. Haury, B.B., Rodeheaver, G.T., Pettry, D., Edgerton, M.T., Edlich, R.F.: Inhibition of nonspecific defenses by soil infection potentiating factors. Surg. Gynecol. Obstet. 144: 19, 1977.

5. Meleney, F.L.: Hemolytic streptococcus gangrene. Arch. Surg. 9:317, 1924.

6. Rea, W.J., Wyrick, W.J., Jr.: Necrotizing fasciitis. Ann. Surg. 172:957, 1970.

7. Stone, H.H., Martin, J.D., Jr.: Synergistic necrotizing cellulitis. Ann. Surg. 175:702, 1972.

8. Giuliano, A., Lewis, F., Jr., Hadley, K., Blaisdell, F.W., Bacteriology of necrotizing fasciitis. Am. J. Surg. 134:52, 1977.

9. Rudolph, R., Soloway, M., DePalms, R.G., Persky, L.: Fournier's syndrome: synergistic gangrene of the scrotum. Am. J. Surg. 129:591, 1975.

10. Baxter, C.R.: Surgical management of soft tissue infections. Surg. Clin. North Am. 52:1483, 1972.

11. Finegold, S.M. (ed): Infections of the skin, soft tissue and muscle. In Anaerobic Bacteria in Human Disease. New York, Academic, 1977, p. 386.

12. Burbrick, M.P., Hitchcock, C.R.: Necrotizing anorectal and perineal infections. Surgery 86:655, 1979.

13. Roding, B., Groenveld, P.H.A., Borema, I.: Ten years of experience in the treatment of gas gangrene with hyperbaric oxygen. Surg. Gynecol. Obstet. 134:579, 1972.

14. Brown, P.W., Kinman, P.B.: Gas gangrene in a metropolitan community. Bone Joint Surg. 56A:1445, 1974.

PART VII
BACTERIAL INFECTIONS OF SPECIAL IMPORTANCE

GROUP A STREPTOCOCCAL INFECTIONS
AND THEIR NON-SUPPURATIVE COMPLICATIONS,
RHEUMATIC FEVER AND NEPHRITIS

Lewis W. Wannamaker

Departments of Pediatrics and of Microbiology
University of Minnesota
Minneapolis, Minn., U.S.A.

I. INTRODUCTION

Throughout the world, group A streptococcal infections are one of the most commonly encountered problems of bacterial infection. In vast areas of the globe (e.g. Central and South America, Africa, India), non-suppurative complications of group A streptococcal infections are among the leading causes of diseases of the heart and of the kidney (Strasser, 1978). In the developing countries, including tropical countries, where it was formerly considered to be rare, rheumatic fever is the major cause of heart disease in the 5 to 30 year age group and may be increasing due to urbanization (Markowitz, 1981).

In the past several decades, useful approaches to the control of streptococcal diseases with antimicrobial agents have been developed. However, these methods require continuous vigilance and/or persistent compliance and have not succeeded in eliminating the problem (Wannamaker, 1981). Indeed, despite their exquisite sensitivity to penicillin, group A streptococci are still commonly found in throat cultures and may be a cause of confusion and concern on the part of the parent or the physician.

II. RELATIONSHIP OF STREPTOCOCCAL INFECTIONS TO RHEUMATIC FEVER AND NEPHRITIS

Evidence for the relationship of streptococcal infections to rheumatic fever and acute nephritis comes from a variety of sources: epidemiological, clinical and laboratory sources and finally from successful intervention by antimicrobial agents

(Stollerman, 1975). An understanding of this relationship is essential for a rational approach to the management and control of these diseases.

A. *Rheumatic Fever*

   1. Requisites and Risks. The only known agent clearly associated with the development of acute rheumatic fever is the group A streptococcus. There also seems to be an absolute requirement that the infection take place in the upper respiratory tract and for the streptococcus to persist in the throat for 1-2 weeks and to produce an antibody response (Wannamaker, 1973). These last two requisites may serve to separate true infection from transitory and chronic carrier states.

   The risk of developing acute rheumatic fever varies from less than 1% to 3%, depending on the strictness of the criteria for defining streptococcal infection and perhaps on the epidemiological circumstances or the serotype of the infecting strain (Siegel et al., 1961; Bisno, 1980). In the absence of a clear laboratory marker for "rheumatogenicity", it has been difficult to establish definite differences in the capacity of strains to produce this complication, and it seems likely that most strains causing clinical infection of the throat possess this potentiality, at least to some degree.

   The failure of rheumatic fever to occur after cutaneous infections with group A streptococci is not understood. Possibilities include biologic differences between throat and skin strains, differences in the immune response related to the site of infection, inhibition of the cytotoxic (e.g. cardiotoxic) properties of streptolysin O by non-esterified cholesterol in the skin, and direct lymphatic connections between the tonsils and the heart (Wannamaker, 1973).

   2. Immunologic Studies. Most current theories on the pathogenesis of rheumatic fever propose an immunologic basis. The numerous immunologic cross reactions and, at least in several instances, biochemical similarities between different components of the streptococcal cell and various mammalian tissues suggest an autoimmune possibility (Ayoub, 1972; Husby et al., 1976; Manjula and Fischetti, 1980). A hyperresponsiveness in the production of antibodies to streptococcal antigens (Stetson, 1954) and an enhanced cellular immune response to streptococcal cell membranes (Read et al., 1974) have been reported in patients with acute rheumatic fever, whereas a suppressed cellular immune response to streptococcal extracellular antigens has been documented in patients with rheumatic heart disease (Gray et al., 1981).

3. Genetic Studies. The recent association of a B cell alloantigen with susceptibility to rheumatic fever reopens the question of genetic differences in rheumatic patients (Patarroya et al., 1979). Variations in the frequency of rheumatic fever and rheumatic heart disease in population groups has generally been attributed to differences in frequency of streptococcal infections, but some studies, notably those comparing the Maori and Caucasian populations of New Zealand (Frankish et al., 1978) have suggested an ethnic or possibly genetic basis.

B. *Acute Glomerulonephritis*

Acute glomerulonephritis has been associated with a variety of different infectious agents, but clearly one of the most common is the group A streptococcus. Certain serotypes (e.g. types 1, 4 and 12) have been associated with streptococcal infections of the throat leading to this complication (Rammelkamp and Weaver, 1953) whereas other serotypes (e.g. 2, 49, 55, 57) have been related to the development of nephritis after skin infections (Dillon, 1972). Recent studies have suggested that these "nephritogenic" strains produce an extracellular antigen not present in the mixture of extracellular components produced by "non-nephritogenic" strains (Villarreal et al., 1980).

Although a direct toxic effect of some streptococcal substance is possibly responsible for the development of acute post-streptococcal glomerulonephritis, the most popular current theory would incriminate antigen-antibody complexes. The low complement levels in the acute stage of the human disease and the production of similar pathologic lesions in experimental animals by injection of non-streptococcal immune complexes have supported this view, but the recognition of immune complexes in patients with rheumatic fever as well as in patients with acute nephritis (van de Rijn et al., 1978) has clouded their specificity for renal complications.

C. *Epidemiology and Latent Periods of Non-Suppurative Complications*

Many of the epidemiologic features (e.g. season, age) of acute nephritis and acute rheumatic fever can be related to the epidemiology of the preceding streptococcal infection, skin or throat in the case of acute nephritis and throat only in the case of rheumatic fever (Wannamaker, 1970). The average latent period of pharyngitis-related nephritis is

short (10 days) as compared with that of impetigo- or
pyoderma-related nephritis which, oddly enough, is similar to
that of rheumatic fever (3 weeks). Long latent periods (2 to
6 months) are characteristic of Sydenham's chorea (Taranta,
1956). The apparent geographic shift in the frequency of
rheumatic fever and rheumatic heart disease from temperate to
tropical and semi-tropical countries (Markowitz, 1981) is a
puzzling phenomenon which suggests there may be other
unidentified factors in the pathogenesis of this disease
complex.

III. PREVENTION OF NON-SUPPURATIVE COMPLICATIONS BY CONTROL OF
STREPTOCOCCAL INFECTIONS

A. *Antimicrobial Agents in the Control of Rheumatic Fever*

1. *Prevention of Recurrences.* The most impressive inroad
in the control of rheumatic fever has been the prevention of
recurrent attacks by the continuous use of antimicrobial
agents in patients with well-documented rheumatic fever or
rheumatic heart disease (American Heart Association Committee
Report, 1977). A monthly intramuscular injection of
benzathine penicillin G (1,200,000 units) has proved to be
more effective than oral penicillin (200,000 - 250,000 units
twice daily) or oral sulfadiazine (1 gram once a day for
adults and children over 60 pounds, 0.5 gram in smaller
children) and is especially recommended for high risk and
non-compliant patients (e.g. those with severe carditis or
multiple attacks). Injections of benzathine penicillin at 3-
week rather than monthly intervals have been tried in some
high risk populations, but without definitive advantages.
Oral erythromycin (250 mg. twice daily) has been recommended
for those rare patients who are sensitive to both penicillin
and sulfadiazine. Since patients with pure Sydenham's chorea
may develop cardiac damage with future rheumatic attacks, they
should also be put on continuous prophylaxis. Any decision to
discontinue prophylaxis in older adults should be carefully
weighed in view of the chance of home and occupational
exposure to streptococcal infection and the peril of
additional cardiac disability resulting from a recurrence.

2. *Prevention of First Attacks.* Although it has been well
documented that adequate penicillin treatment of acute
streptococcal infections will reduce the risk of rheumatic
fever by 10 fold (Denny et al., 1951), there are some

difficulties in applying this to non-epidemic situations. The recognition of acute streptococcal infections and their differentiation from non-streptococcal infections of the upper respiratory tract and from streptococcal carrier states pose a number of problems (Wannamaker, 1972).

   a. *Throat cultures for beta-hemolytic streptococci.* Ideally patients with clinical findings suggestive of streptococcal infection (acute onset with fever plus pharyngeal inflammation, tender anterior cervical nodes or diffuse erythematous rash) should be cultured by thorough swabbing of the posterior pharynx and tonsillar areas. If the clinical indications of streptococcal infection are strong or the patient is unlikely to return, treatment can be instituted at once, although there is no significant increase in the risk of rheumatic fever by delaying treatment for 1 or 2 days until the results of the throat culture are available.
   Most strains of group A streptococci show clear hemolysis on aerobic surface cultures. An additional few will be detected only by anaerobic conditions, e.g. by stabs into the medium. Strains of group A streptococci that are non-hemolytic even on anaerobic cultures appear to be very rare but have been reported in association with an outbreak of rheumatic fever (James and McFarland, 1971). Sensitivity to bacitracin, as tested by specially prepared discs, is a simple though presumptive indicator that the strain is group A (Maxted, 1953).

   b. *The problem of carriers.* The prevalence of strep- tococcal carriers raises many questions about interpretation of culture results and about appropriate management (Kaplan, 1980). The differentiation of streptococcal carriers from clinical or subclinical cases of acute streptococcal infection may be impossible, except in retrospect by serial antibody determinations. Although most cases of true infection have more than a few colonies of beta hemolytic streptococci on throat culture, quantitation of cultures does not satis- factorily separate carriers from cases. Streptococcal carriers presenting with viral infections may be misdiagnosed as acute streptococcal infection. Routine throat culture surveys in schools often turn up chronic carriers who are not personally at risk of developing complications or likely to spread infection; no benefit is likely to result from treatment of such carriers. In the absence of evidence of epidemic streptococcal disease or an unusually high risk situation, these surveys are probably not indicated.

c. *Treatment regimens.* In order to prevent rheumatic fever, the infecting strain of streptococcus must be eradicated (Cantanzaro, 1958). A single intramuscular injection of benzathine penicillin G (1,200,000 in adults and older children, 600,000 units in children under 60 pounds) has been recommended (American Heart Association Committee Report, 1977). If oral treatment is used, it must be taken for 10 days, which is difficult to enforce in an illness that lasts only a few days. The recommended oral drugs are penicillin G (200,000 or 250,000 units 3 or 4 times daily) and for penicillin-sensitive individuals erythromycin (250 mg. 4 times a day in adults and older children, 40 mg per kg. per day in younger children).

d. *Treatment Failures.* Bacteriologic treatment failures may occur even with "adequate" treatment as recommended above. In orally treated patients, failures may be due to non-compliance or to reinfection with the same strain. However, recent studies have shown bacteriologic failures in 20% of patients treated with intramuscular benzathine penicillin G and even higher rates with further courses of antibiotics (Gastanaduy et al., 1980). Except in high risk situations (e.g. rheumatic patients, rheumatic families or harborers of nephritogenic strains), it does not seem worthwhile to persist in attempts to eradicate residual streptococci after two "adequate" trials at least one of which is with intramuscular benzathine penicillin G. Some of the treatment failures that have been reported may be in carriers who may be hard to distinguish from acutely infected patients and in whom the relatively quiescent streptococci may be more difficult to kill with penicillin.

e. *Subclinical infections.* Some patients develop rheumatic fever in the absence of a recognized streptococcal illness, pointing up the problem of subclinical infections. As many as one half of the streptococcal infections may be asymptomatic or may produce such minimal symptomatology that they are not brought to the attention of a physician. They are difficult to identify and to separate from carriers except by changes in streptococcal antibody titers.

f. *Contacts.* Close contacts of patients with streptococcal pharyngitis should be watched for clinical symptoms of streptococcal infection. Whether they should be cultured routinely is debatable, except in high risk situations.

Spread within the family may have occurred before identification and treatment of the index case of streptococcal
pharyngitis.

B. *Antimicrobial Agents in the Control of Acute Nephritis*

Unlike rheumatic fever, repeated attacks of acute
nephritis are rare, and, therefore, continuous antimicrobial
prophylaxis is not recommended. Infections of various kinds
(viral, streptococcal or other bacterial) may result in a
transitory enhancement in the number of red blood cells seen
on Addis count for a period of 6 to 12 months after subsidence
of the acute disease. Short term penicillin prophylaxis for
this period of time has been used but its value has not been
established.

Prevention of acute nephritis by treatment of the
preceding streptococcal infection is uncertain. One report
indicates a 50% reduction in risk of nephritis by penicillin
treatment of patients with pharyngitis due to a nephritogenic
strain (Stetson et al., 1955). There are no studies
documenting the prevention of acute nephritis by treatment of
preceding streptococcal infection of the skin. Because of the
long latent period, spread has usually occurred within the
family and among other close contacts before the index case of
impetigo- or pyoderma-related nephritis is identified.

Most cases of streptococcal impetigo are not brought to the
attention of a physician during the early transient vesicular
stage, at which time with careful culturing the group A
streptococcus can be isolated in pure culture. During the
typical honey colored, thick crusted stage, the secondarily
invading staphlococci often overgrow the streptococci unless
inhibitory media are used (Dajani et al., 1973). Primary
staphylococcal impetigo presents in a different manner, as
bullous lesions with paper thin crusts on rupture.

Intramuscular benzathine penicillin G has been found to be
effective in streptococcal skin infections (Derrick, and
Dillon, 1970) though it may not be the preferred method of
treatment, especially in the absence of evidence of a
nephritogenic strain. Oral treatment with penicillin or
erythromycin has also been successful and even local treatment
alone may be satisfactory for less extensive infections. One
difficult problem is repeated infection in patients who remain
in a high risk environment. Continuous penicillin prophylaxis
is generally effective in controlling repeated infections
(Ferrieri et al., 1974) and may be especially indicated when
nephritogenic strains are prevalent.

C. *Other Approaches to Control of Streptococcal Diseases*

1. Tonsillectomy. The value of tonsillectomy in
controlling streptococcal infections is moot. The removal of
tonsils may result in fewer clinically recognizable
streptococcal illnesses, converting them to less obvious
infections which may go untreated (Chamovitz et al., 1960).
One report indicates that large tonsils in established
rheumatics are associated with an increased incidence of
recurrences (Feinstein and Levitt, 1970), perhaps justifying
their removal in non-compliant rheumatics with a history of
repeated attacks.

2. Streptococcal Vaccines. The more than 60 recognized
serological types of group A streptococci (based on their
type-specific antiphagocytic M proteins) present a formidable
barrier to the development of a vaccine. It is possible that
a vaccine could be developed for the most prevalent types with
the hope that its use would not result in a shift of types.
There is also the nagging possibility of toxicity to a
vaccine, not only immediate reactions but also the inducement
of rheumatic fever-like findings. Recently progress has been
made in methods of extracting and purifying the M proteins
(Beachey et al., 1974). Preparations produced by these
methods may be free of toxic elements and may ultimately lead
to vaccines suitable for testing in man.

IV. STREPTOCOCCAL ANTIBODY TESTS AS AIDS IN THE DIAGNOSIS OF
     NON-SUPPURATIVE SEQUELAE

    Streptococcal antibody tests do not differentiate between
patients who do and those who do not develop complications.
Therefore, in diagnosing acute rheumatic fever or acute
nephritis, they should be used only in conjunction with
careful documentation and analysis of the clinical indicators
of these complications. Local data on the distribution of
titers in normal individuals of different ages and from
different population groups are necessary for interpretation
of the significance of a streptococcal antibody titer on a
single serum specimen. Except in Sydenham's chorea, the
antibody titers may still be rising in patients presenting
with complications of streptococcal infection, providing the
possibility of obtaining more definitive serological evidence
of streptococcal infection. Since the latent period in chorea
is so long, several antibody tests may be needed to find one
that is still elevated (Ayoub and Wannamaker, 1966).

Of the several commercially available antibody tests, the antistreptolysin O assay has been most widely used. The anti-DNase B test is a very reproducible assay which has the added advantage that it is usually markedly elevated in patients with streptococcal pyoderma and pyoderma-associated nephritis whereas the antistreptolysin O response is often feeble in cutaneous infections (Wannamaker, 1970). The "streptozyme" test has the attraction of simplicity and of reflecting antibodies to a mixture of streptococcal antigens, but problems of variation in reagent lots and in interpretation of results have detracted from its usefulness (Kaplan and Huwe, 1980).

ACKNOWLEDGMENTS

Lewis W. Wannamaker is a Career Investigator of the American Heart Association.

REFERENCES

American Heart Association Committee Report (1977). *Circulation* 55,1.

Ayoub, E.M. (1972). *In* "Streptococci and Streptococcal Diseases" (L.W. Wannamaker and J.M. Matsen, eds.) p. 451. Academic Press, New York.

Beachey, E.H., Campbell, G.L., and Ofek, I. (1974). *Infect. Immun.* 9, 891.

Bisno, A.L. (1980). *In* "Streptococcal Diseases and the Immune Response" (S.E. Read and J.B. Zabriskie, eds.) p. 789. Academic Press, New York.

Cantanzaro, F.J., Rammelkamp, C.H., Jr., and Chamovitz, R. (1958). *N. Engl. J. Med.* 259, 51.

Chamovitz, R., Rammelkamp, C.H., Jr., Wannamaker, L.W., and Denny, F.W., Jr. (1960). *Pediatrics* 26, 1960.

Dajani, A.S., Ferrieri, P., and Wannamaker, L.W. (1973). *Arch. Dermatol.* 108, 517.

Denny, F.W., Wannamaker, L.W., Brink, W.R., Rammelkamp, C.H., Jr., and Custer, E.A. (1950). *J.A.M.A.* 143, 151.

Derrick, C.W., and Dillon, H.C., Jr. (1970). *J. Pediatr.* 77, 696.

Dillon, H.C. (1972). *In* "Streptococci and Streptococcal Diseases" (L.W. Wannamaker and J.M. Matsen, eds.) p. 571. Academic Press, New York.

Feinstein, A., and Levitt, M. (1970). *N. Engl. J. Med.* 282, 285.
Ferrieri, P., Dajani, A.S., and Wannamaker, L.W. (1974).
     J. Infect. Dis. 129, 429.
Frankish, J.D., Stanhope, J.M., Martin, D.R., Clarkson, P.M.,
     Leslie, P.N., and Langley, R.B. (1978). *New Zealand J.
     Med.* 87, 33.
Gastanaduy, A.S., Kaplan, E.L., Huwe, B.B., McKay, C., and
     Wannamaker, L.W. (1980). *Lancet ii*, 498.
Gray, E.D., Wannamaker, L.W., Ayoub, E.M., El Kholy, A., and
     Abdin, Z.H. (1981). *J. Clin. Invest.* 68, 665.
Husby, G., van de Rijn, I., Zabriskie, J.B., Abdin, Z.H., and
     Williams, R.C. (1976). *J. Exp. Med.* 144, 1094.
James, L., and McFarland, R.B. (1971). *N. Engl. J. Med.* 284, 750.
Kaplan, E.L. (1980). *J. Pediatr.* 97, 337.
Kaplan, E.L. and Huwe, B. (1980). *J. Pediatr.* 96, 367.
Manjkula, B.N., and Fischetti, V.A. (1980). *J. Exp. Med.*
     151, 695.
Markowitz, M. (1981). *Clinical Therapeutics.* In press.
Maxted, W.R. (1953). *J. Clin. Pathol.* 6, 224.
Patarroyo, M.E., Winchester, R.J., Vejerano, A., Gibofsky, A.,
     Chalem, F., Zabriskie, J.B., and Kunkel, H.G. (1979).
     Nature 278, 173.
Rammelkamp, C.H., Jr., and Weaver, R.S. (1953). *J. Clin. Invest.*
     32, 345.
Read, S.E., Fischetti, V.A., Utermohlen, V., Valk, R.E., and
     Zabriskie, J.B. (1974). *J. Clin. Invest.* 54, 439.
Siegel, A.C., Johnson, E.E., and Stollerman, G.H. (1961).
     N. Engl. J. Med. 265, 559.
Stetson, C.A. (1954). *In* "Streptococcal Infections" (M. McCarty,
     ed.) p. 208. Columbia Univ. Press, New York.
Stetson, C.A., Rammelkamp, C.H., Jr., Krause, R.M., Kohen, R.J.,
     and Perry, W.D. (1955). *Medicine* (Balt.) 34, 431.
Stollerman, G.H. (1975). "Rheumatic Fever and Streptococcal
     Infection," Grune and Stratton, New York.
Strasser, T. (1978). *WHO Chronicle* 32, 18.
Taranta, A., and Stollerman, G.H. (1956). *Am. J. Med.* 20, 170.
van de Rijn, I., Fillit, H., Brandeis, W.E., Ried, H., Poon-King
     T., McCarty, M., Day, N.K., and Zabriskie, J.B. (1978).
     Clin. Exp. Immunol. 34, 318.
Villarreal, H., Jr., Fischetti, V., van de Rijn, I., and
     Zabriskie, J.B. (1980). *In* "Streptococcal Diseases and the
     Immune Response" (S.E. Read and J.B. Zabriskie, eds.)
     p. 185. Academic Press, New York.
Wannamaker, L.W. (1970). *N. Engl. J. Med.* 282, 23.
Wannamaker, L.W. (1972). *Am. J. Dis. Child.* 124, 352.
Wannamaker, L.W. (1973). *Circulation* 48, 9.
Wannamaker, L.W. (1981). *Robert Koch Foundation Bulletin and
     Communications* 3, 23.

GRAM-NEGATIVE BACTEREMIA AND SEPTIC SHOCK

Michael Dan
George Goldsand

Division of Infectious Diseases
Department of Medicine
University of Alberta
Edmonton, Alberta, Canada

Introduction

In contrast to the preantibiotic era, gram-negative bacilli are now the most frequent microbial causes of bacteremia in the United States (1) and other developed countries (2). The frequency of gram-negative bacteremia (GNB) is greater in secondary and tertiary care hospitals than in smaller community hospitals because patient populations in the former are more likely to have underlying diseases and will undergo more diagnostic and treatment procedures which may predispose to bacteremia. Categorization into hospital-acquired (nosocomial) or community-acquired infections is convenient. Community-acquired bacteremia usually originates from the genitourinary or gastrointestinal tracts. Hospital-acquired infections, which account for three-fourths of cases, often originate from bladder or intravenous catheters and are caused by a variety of gram-negative bacilli which tend to be more antibiotic-resistant than community-acquired infections (3). Two-thirds of endemic nosocomial bacteremias and 80 percent of hospital epidemics are caused by aerobic gram-negative bacilli (4). Gram-negative organisms are unique among bacteria in their ability to produce shock almost immediately following bloodstream invasion. Only cardiac disease exceeds GNB as a cause of shock among hospitalized patients. Fatality rates of 47% among patients with GNB complicated by the development of shock contrast to a 7% rate among bacteremic patients without this complication (5).

I. THE DISEASE ENTITY

A. Predisposing Factors

GNB occurs most commonly in patients with deficient host defenses. The severity of underlying disease, old age and degree of
granulocytopenia are all important predisposing factors. Both the
frequency and the severity of bacteremia are markedly increased in
patients with a granulocyte count below 1000/mm^3 (6). Although
the risk of acquiring an infection and its severity are increased
in patients with neoplastic disease (7,8), there is no evidence
this is due to malignancy per se rather than to the associated
granulocytopenia, more frequent use of procedures capable of inducing infection, and more frequent and prolonged hospitalization.
    When associated with diabetes, congestive heart failure and
uremia or when acquired in hospital, GNB has a less favorable
outcome, independent of the severity of the underlying disease
(9). Irradiation and therapy with drugs such as cortical
steriods and cytotoxic agents have contributed significantly to
the increasing frequency and severity of GNB (5) probably as a
result of the immunosuppression (mainly granulocytopenia) which
they induce.
    Gram-negative bacilli are relatively resistant to drying,
moisture and chemical agents. In fact, Pseudomonas aeruginosa
has been shown to proliferate in the disinfectant, benzalkonium
chloride. The ability of pseudomonas and others to persist in
certain fluids has led to the identification of many hospital
materials, including intravascular catheters (10), urethral
catheters (11), and ventilatory equipment (12) as frequent
sources of GNB. Outbreaks of infection have also resulted from
contaminated intravenous fluids, blood, incubators for infants,
and hand lotions. Some diagnostic procedures like cystoscopy,
proctosigmoidoscopy and bronchoscopy may also be associated with
bacteremia, but this tends to be transient and of little clinical
significance in otherwise healthy patients.
    Factors predisposing to shock are less clearly defined than
those leading to bacteremia alone. Shock is more frequent in
patients with rapidly fatal or ultimately fatal underlying
disease, those over age 50, and in association with diabetes,
congestive heart failure, azotemia, antibiotic or immunosuppressive drug therapy. On the other hand, no difference has been
detected in the frequency of shock in bacteremia caused by various species of bacilli or magnitude of bacteremia as determined
by colony counts of blood cultures (13).

B. Microbiology

Although almost all species of aerobic and anaerobic gram-negative bacilli have caused bacteremia, the vast majority of cases are associated with Escherichia coli, Klebsiella pneumoniae, Enterobacter aerogenes, Pseudomonas aeruginosa, and various species of Proteus and Bacteroides. Bacteremic episodes caused by more than one species of bacteria have been reported in up to 16% of cases. No significant differences in fatality rates could be demonstrated for bacteremias caused by individual species of gram-negative bacilli when comparisons were made between patients with underlying disease of similar severity (14).

C. Pathophysiology

Lipopolysaccharides incorporated in the cell wall of gram-negative bacteria are called endotoxins. Whether free or associated with intact bacteria these lipopolysaccharides, together with still incompletely understood other factors, are able to initiate a series of events characterized by fever, hypotension and shock. Eventual activation of Hageman factor (Factor XII) results in sequential stimulation of the coagulation system leading to the changes of disseminated intravascular coagulation (DIC). These details of pathophysiology of bacteremic shock are the subject of a recent extensive review by McCabe et al (15).

The evolution of bacteremic shock is characterized by two successive phases (16): the earliest hemodynamic alterations are those of a hyperdynamic state ("warm shock") with a fall in vascular resistance and a disproportionate increase in cardiac output resulting in inadequate tissue and organ perfusion. Hyperventilation with subsequent respiratory alkalosis is a relatively consistent early finding and often a valuable clue to the development of septic shock. If shock proceeds uncorrected, modest early increases in serum lactate levels progress with development of frank metabolic acidosis. The second phase ("cold shock") is characterized by the classical pattern of shock with cyanosis and cold clammy extremities. Pathophysiologic alterations consist of increased peripheral resistance, decreased cardiac output, decreased venous pressure, hyperventilation, and metabolic acidosis. The factors responsible for the transition from one phase to the other have yet to be defined; recent studies have suggested that a fall in tissue oxygen consumption, resulting from failure of extraction rather than failure of oxygen delivery (17), and/or myocardial depression by circulating cardiodepressant substances (17, 18) may lead to these changes.

D. Clinical Features

The onset of bacteremia may vary from an insidious to a
rapidly fulminant presentation (5,13,14). The specific microorganism producing bacteremia does not influence the mode of
presentation, nor can it be predicted on the basis of clinical
findings. In its classical form, bacteremia presents with rigors,
high fever, hypotension, prostration, and occasionally nausea,
vomiting and/or diarrhea a few hours following a manipulative
procedure. Shock usually occurs during the first few hours after
appearance of the initial signs of bacteremia. However, only
about one-third of patients present with this typical pattern.
In the remainder, onset of bacteremia is less apparent; almost all
patients are febrile, but the degree of fever may be minimal in
the elderly and in patients with uremia or receiving corticosteroids (5). Bacteremia may also present as initially unexplained hypotension, oliguria, or metabolic acidosis. Confusion or
agitation may be the first sign in the elderly. Features of
local infections, such as urinary or respiratory tract infections,
may predominate in some patients and mask features of bacteremia.
Ecthyma gangrenosum, (tender, indurated skin lesions with black
necrotic centers, or bullous or vesicular lesions surrounded by
an erythematous margin) is considered to be specific for bacteremia caused by P. aeruginosa or Aeromonas spp., although it is
also described with other gram-negative bacilli, or candida (19),
and identical lesions may even appear in the absence of infection
(20). The spectrum of cutaneous and soft tissue manifestations
of sepsis due to gram-negative enteric bacilli has been reviewed
recently by Musher (20).
Some degree of shock occurs in about 40% of the patients with
GNB (15). It may be the first sign of gram-negative bacteremia
or develop more insidiously during the course of the illness.
Early clues include an unexplained increase in respiratory rate,
often associated with respiratory alkalosis, or otherwise unexplained mental changes in the elderly. During the early phase
"warm shock", the patient is often alert with plethoric skin.
Hyperventilation, warm dry skin, and a bounding pulse with hypotension are typically present. In the second "cold shock" phase,
the patient is obtunded, cyanotic, has cold, clammy skin, and a
rapid but weak pulse. In some instances shock may be unrecognized until oliguria or coagulation abnormalities appear.
DIC associated with bacteremia is almost always associated
with shock. Though GNB appears to be the most frequent cause of
DIC, relatively few patients with GNB suffer from this
complication (21). Thrombocytopenia is found in approximately
60%, laboratory evidence of DIC in about 12%, but DIC-associated
bleeding occurs in less than 3% (5). Clinically, DIC presents as
bleeding from skin (particularly venipuncture sites), subcutaneous tissues, or from mucous membranes of the mouth, nose, or

gastrointestinal tract. Laboratory findings consist of thrombocytopenia, increased circulating fibrin-split products and
decreased levels of coagulation factors II, V, and VII. Abnormalities of clotting function are associated with a greater frequency of shock and fatal outcome in each category of underlying
host disease (5).

Bacteremic shock is a common cause of adult respiratory distress syndrome (ARDS). ARDS increases the fatality rate of GNB.
When caused by bacteremia,ARDS carries a higher fatality rate
than that due to other causes (22). Pulmonary abnormalities may
occur after recovery from bacteremic shock, and present with
tachypnea after a latent period of 12-24 hours. Chest roentgenograms typically show bilateral alveolar infiltrates, and blood
gases reveal marked hypoxia, hypocapnia and often respiratory
alkalosis. Supportive management requires assisted mechanical
ventilation using distending airway pressures.

Total leukocyte count increases with onset of bacteremia.
Although failure to develop a leukocytosis was considered to be a
poor prognostic sign (23), these findings have not been confirmed
in a recent study (24).

The overall fatality rate in patients with GNB is about 25%
(14). Though representing a decrease in comparison to mortality
rates during the 1950's, the fatality rate of GNB has remained
relatively stable in the last decade. Increased fatality rates
were found to be associated with inappropriate antibiotic therapy
(5), delayed admission to an intensive care unit, significant
lactate accumulation, and decreased cardiac output which is
resistant to therapy (25). The decrease in frequency of fatal
outcome observed in recent studies seems more reflective of
earlier diagnosis and therapy than to the effect of introducing
new antimicrobial agents.

II. DIAGNOSIS

The diagnosis of bacteremia can be definitively established
only by blood cultures. Since prompt recognition and diagnosis
of GNB are crucial for early optimal therapy, more rapid diagnostic methods are required. Non-specific tests to indicate a
bacterial cause of a febrile episode, such as the nitroblue
tetrazolium (NBT), and limulus assay have failed to fulfill their
early promise. More specific immunologic assays, such as counter-
immunoelectrophoresis (CIE), enzyme-linked immunosorbent assay
(ELISA), etc., are of value for diagnosis of a limited number of
infections, but not useful as yet in the early diagnosis of GNB
(15). This lack of rapid and specific diagnostic tests for
bacteremia means that meticulous patient evaluation and sound
clinical judgment remain the major bases for early diagnosis and
treatment. Leukocyte counts showing a "shift to the left" and

toxic granulation, strongly suggest bacterial infection.
Bacteriologic diagnosis and determination of the antimicrobial
susceptibility of infecting organisms is essential though therapy
should not be delayed while awaiting this laboratory data. In
addition to the obvious need for blood cultures, valuable information can be obtained by careful collection of specimens from
suspect primary sites of infection in the urinary or respiratory
tracts, infected wounds, abscesses or cannulae sites. Immediate
gram smears may reveal the suspect gram-negative bacilli, indicate
gram-positive organisms or a "mixed" bacterial population, all of
which would influence the details of initial antimicrobial therapy.
Proper culture by appropriate aerobic and anaerobic techniques
should be ensured.

The differential diagnosis of GNB and shock may be especially
difficult in older patients referred from chronic care facilities.
These patients may be hypovolemic, often have only low-grade
fever, and have a higher than normal incidence of decubiti and
urinary tract infections caused by gram-negative bacilli. In
patients with severe cardiac disease the frequent use of intravenous and bladder catheters may serve as a source for bacteremia
and lead to confusion regarding the etiology of shock. T waves
and ST segment abnormalities on EKG's and elevations of SGOT and
LDH may develop in bacteremic shock and be misconstrued as myocardial infarction. On the other hand, some patients with suspected bacteremic shock may have adrenal insufficiency, which can
also present with fever and hypotension, but would usually show
the typical electrolyte changes and eosinophilia. Also potentially confusing is pulmonary embolism where tachypnea and hyper-
pnea may be attributed to bacteremia and pulmonary infiltrates to
bacterial pneumonia. Wherever doubt remains after careful clinical assessment and bacteremia cannot be excluded, antibiotics
should be administered until results of blood and other cultures
are available.

III. TREATMENT AND PREVENTION

The management of GNB demands attention to treatment of the
infection with appropriate antibiotics; surgical intervention
where necessary to drain abscesses, debride necrotic tissue or
remove foreign bodies (including intravenous cannulae); and
prompt control of life-threatening hematologic, ventilatory and
hemodynamic complications, the latter best carried out within an
intensive care unit.

The importance of early antibiotic therapy has been unequiv-
ocally established in a series of investigations which demonstrated enhanced survival in bacteremia treated with appropriate
antibacterial agents (9,13,14). Early appropriate treatment
affords a two-fold reduction in the frequency of shock among

patients with GNB whatever the severity of underlying disease.
Even when initiated after onset of shock, appropriate antibiotic
therapy significantly improved survival rates over those of
patients who received inappropriate agents. Selection of an
effective antibiotic is guided by culture and antibiotic susceptibility results. When these results are unavailable or pending,
initial antibiotic therapy is selected by the process of identifying the site of origin of bacteremia, knowledge of those
bacteria which produce infections most often at these sites, and
where available, gram smear findings. Also to be considered are
the usual nosocomial pathogens in a specific hospital and their
antimicrobial susceptibility. The urinary tract is the most frequent source of GNB, E. coli being the predominant organism.
Bacteria of the Klebsiella-Enterobacter-Serratia and Proteus
families, and P. aeruginosa are less frequently involved, and
occur more often in patients who have had prolonged hospitalization and previous antibiotic therapy. E. coli is also the most
common etiologic agent of bacteremias originating from the gastrointestinal and female genital tract; but anaerobic bacilli, especially B. fragilis, must also be considered in bacteremias originating from these sites. The biliary tract is a relatively frequent site of origin of bacteremia, particularly in the elderly
and tends to occur with organisms similar to those producing
bacteremia from a urinary tract source. Bacteremias originating
from decubitus ulcers and the respiratory tract are often secondary to nosocomial infections of these sites and occur with organisms that tend to be more antibiotic resistant. In 30% of
patients, predominantly those with more severe underlying disease,
the original source might not be identified (14).
     The need to include antibiotics with the broadest spectra
against gram-negative bacilli has led to extensive use of aminoglycosides for empiric initial therapy of suspected bacteremia.
The aminoglycosides most frequently used are gentamicin (1.5 mg/
kg IV q8h) or tobramycin (1.5 mg/kg IV q8h), but amikacin (5.0 -
7.5 mg/kg q8-12h) should be considered in those hospital environments where gentamicin and tobramycin resistance is documented
among gram-negative isolates. In studies comparing the efficacy
of single antibiotics with combinations in the treatment of GNB
(26-28), enhanced survival rates could be demonstrated for combinations subsequently shown to be synergistic. The nature of
second or third drugs varies depending on assessment of origin
site and probability of certain micro-organisms being responsible.
Many regimes include one of the first generation cephalosporins
such as cephalothin (2g IV q4-6h) or cefazolin (2g IM or IV q8h),
however, the inefficacy of this combination against enterococci
should be considered and where bacteremia with this organism is
suspected, either penicillin (2.5-5.0 million units IV q4-6h) or
ampicillin (2g IV q4-6h) should be given in addition to the
aminoglycoside. Ampicillin may be preferrable because of its
extended spectrum against some gram-negative bacilli, particularly

if they are not hospital-acquired. Enterococci produce bacteremia most frequently from a urinary tract source and can be easily
seen in gram smear of urine. If pseudomonas is suspected, either
carbenicillin (4-6g IV q4-6h) or ticarcillin (3-6g IV q6h) should
be given in addition to the aminoglycoside and/or cephalosporin.
Suspected bacteremia from a colonic or vaginal source should be
treated by adding to the aminoglycoside, either clindamycin (450-
600 mg IV q6h), chloramphenicol (0.5-1 g IV q6h), metronidazole
(250-750 mg IV q8h) or cefoxitin (2g IV q4h), all agents with
proven efficacy against B. fragilis. Carbenicillin and ticarcillin in large doses are also inhibitory to B. fragilis but are
not conventionally used as principal agents in treatment of anaerobic infections.

Though initial antimicrobial therapy should include multiple
drug coverage for all probable bacteremic microbial agents, it is
important to alter antibiotic therapy once organisms are identified in the laboratory and sensitivities determined. Depending
on the total clinical picture and the patients' initial response,
one should strive towards using the narrowest spectrum antibio-
tic(s) which will predictably reach the site of infection and
eradicate the responsible micro-organisms. There is an unfortunate tendency by many physicians to maintain patients on the wide-
spectrum antibiotics given at onset of bacteremia for fear that
the initial favorable response will not be sustained. This is a
potentially dangerous habit because it increases the risk of antibiotic toxicity in the patient and contributes to the development
of a more antibiotic-resistant flora within the hospital environment.

The frequently changing hemodynamic and hematologic picture
in patients with shock requires close monitoring of antibiotic
dosages. The degree of renal failure should be reviewed daily
and antibiotic dosages altered in accordance with published
guidelines (29). Use of serum levels as guides to aminoglycoside
dosage is particularly important in view of the narrow therapeutic
index of these agents and their high toxic potential. Inhibition
of platelet function by carbenicillin and ticarcillin should be
considered and lead to cautious use of these drugs, particularly
in the presence of renal failure and DIC.

The problems of antibiotic therapy relating to the need for
use of multiple drugs with toxic potential will hopefully be reduced by introduction of safer drugs with a sufficiently wide
spectrum to cover not only the conventional aerobic gram-negative
bacilli, but also pseudomonas and B. fragilis.

The newly introduced second generation cephalosporins, cefamandole and cefoxitin, do not appear likely to replace aminoglycosides as agents of choice for initial therapy of bacteremia
because of significant gaps in their spectrum against gram-
negative bacilli (30), but several newer cephalosporins, still
currently under investigation appear to have a wider spectrum of
activity including pseudomonas and B. fragilis and may eventually
replace aminoglycosides as the agents of choice for empiric therapy.

Duration of antibiotic therapy is determined primarily by the nature of the original local infection and patient response. They should be continued for a minimum of 5 afebrile days or even longer if local infection or granulocytopenia persists.

Treatment of GNB in granulocytopenic patients presents special problems. In these, the results of surveillance cultures (especially gingival and rectal cultures obtained once or twice weekly) can be used to guide initial empiric therapy. One should also be cautious about changing to a single antibiotic (if and when a causative organism is isolated from the blood) in patients with persistent neutropenia because recovery rate in these special patients appears to be increased if antimicrobial therapy includes 2 agents to which the pathogen is susceptible (31). Granulocyte transfusions, though not useful prophylactically, are indicated if prolonged marrow aplasia is predicted and the patient is not responding to appropriate antibiotic therapy (32).

Ventilation, removal or replacement of foreign bodies (intravascular and urinary catheters, etc.) drainage of purulent accumulations, and correction of hemodynamic abnormalities are essential components in the management of bacteremia and shock. The need for drainage of abscesses and debridement of necrotic tissue (particularly in anaerobic infections) is of particular importance. Volume expansion by fluid administration is an important initial step in correcting the hemodynamic defect, and will also improve the cardiac output. If volume expansion does not produce prompt improvement, vasoactive agents such as dopamine may be considered to increase cardiac output further. The effectiveness and hazards of corticosteroids in the therapy of septic shock continue to be controversial. Some studies suggest improved survival (33-35), while others indicate no benefit (36,37) and even significant increase in fatality rates (5). An answer to the riddle of steroids in bacteremic shock continues to await further clarification.

The major thrust in reducing GNB should be better control of hospital infection and antibiotic usage. This would hopefully reduce the frequency of nosocomially acquired GNB, particularly with resistant organisms. Control should be directed toward the three most frequent sources of infection: indwelling intravenous and bladder catheters and ventilatory therapy equipment. They should be used only when absolutely necessary and withdrawn as soon as possible. Bladder catheterization should be done under sterile conditions and only closed drainage systems used. Intravenous catheters should be inspected regularly with a view to their removal at the earliest sign of sepsis at entry sites, and changed every 48-72 hours (38). Ventilatory equipment should be disposable and fluid reservoirs regularly changed and cleaned. Routine care of tracheostomies, wounds, tube drainage, and catheters should be done with sterile technique. The importance of preventing decubitus ulcers is self-evident.

Control and audit of antibiotic use by appropriate hospital specialists can help reduce the overuse of wide-spectrum antibiotics in situations where they are unnecessary or narrower spectrum drugs will suffice. Though possibly creating some political controversy in certain hospitals, this procedure may help reduce the proliferation of resistant organisms in the hospital environment and help control at least some of the factors contributing to development of GNB and its potentially lethal complications.

IV. FUTURE DEVELOPMENTS

Major research efforts aimed at preventing the lethal sequelae of GNB have been mainly directed to granulocytopenic patients in whom mortality from GNB is highest. Gurwith, Ronald and co-workers in Winnipeg, showed a decreased occurrence of bacteremia among granulocytopenic patients with acute leukemia and other malignancies by the administration of cotrimoxazole (2 tablets b.i.d.) at onset of granulocytopenia below $1000/mm^3$ (39). Zeigler, McCutchan and Braude, using passive immunization with an antiserum prepared from the lipopolysaccharide of the J5 mutant of E. coli 0111, succeeded in protecting animals from the lethal effects of endotoxin from unrelated gram-negative organisms. In a subsequent study in humans, they were able to significantly reduce mortality from both GNB and septic shock following administration of human antiserum (40). Prevention by means of active immunization awaits better definition of an antigenic factor common to most species of gram-negative bacilli which produce lethal bacteremia. To date some preliminary studies using a polyvalent pseudomonas vaccine in burn patients have been encouraging (41), but the potential for ongoing research in this area remains massive.

REFERENCES

1. McCabe WR. Gram-negative bacteremia. Disease-a-Month. Chicago: Year Book Medical Publishers; February: 1975.
2. Svanbom M. Septicemia I. A prospective study on etiology, underlying factors and source of infection. Scan J Infect Dis. 1978;10:187.
3. Craven DE, Kreger BE, McCabe WR. Adult bacteremia caused by gram-negative bacilli. Clin Obstet Gynecol. 1979;22:361.
4. Maki DG. Nosocomial bacteremia. An epidemiologic overview. Am J Med. 1981;70:719.

5. Kreger BE, Craven DE, McCabe WR. Gram-negative bacteremia IV. Re-evaluation of clinical features and treatment in 612 patients. Am J Med. 1980;68:344.
6. Bodey GP, Buckley M, Sathe YS, et al. Quantitative relationships between circulating leukocytes and infections in patients with acute leukemia. Ann Intern Med. 1966;64:328.
7. Levine AJ, Graw RH, Young RC. Management of infections in patients with leukemia and lymphoma. Current concepts and experimental approaches. Semin Hematol. 1972;9:141.
8. Singer C, Kaplan MH, Armstrong D. Bacteremia and fungemia complicating neoplastic disease. Am J Med. 1977;62:731.
9. Bryant RE, Hood AF, Hood CF, Koenig MG. Factors affecting gram-negative rod bacteremia. Arch Intern Med. 1971;127:120.
10. Collins RN, Braun PA, Zinner SH, Kass EH. Risk of local and systemic infection with polyethylene catheters. N Eng J Med. 1968;279:340.
11. Martin CM, Vaquer F, Meyers M, El-Dadah A. Preventions of gram-negative rod bacteremia associated with indwelling urinary catheterization. In: Antimicrob Agents Chemother. Washington, American Society of Microbiol. 1964:617.
12. Pierce AK, Sanford JP, Thomas GD, Leonard JS. Long-term evaluation of decontamination of inhalation therapy equipment and the occurrence of necrotizing pneumonia. N Eng J Med. 1970;282:528.
13. DuPont HC, Spink WW. Infections due to gram-negative organisms. An analysis of 860 patients with bacteremia at the University of Minnesota Medical Center 1958-1966. Medicine. 1969;48:307.
14. Kreger BE, Craven DE, Carling PC, McCabe WB. Gram-negative bacteremia III. Reassessment of etiology, epidemiology and ecology in 612 patients. Am J Med. 1980;68:332.
15. McCabe WR, Olans RN. Shock in gram-negative bacteremia: Prediagnosing factors, pathophysiology and treatment. In: Remington JS, et al. eds. Current clinical topics in infectious diseases. New York: McGraw-Hill Book Company; 1981:121.
16. Gunnar RM, Loeb HS, Winslow EJ, Blain C, Robinson J. Hemodynamic measurements in bacteremia and septic shock. J Infect Dis. 1973;128:295.
17. Lefer AM. Mechanisms of cardiosuppression in endotoxin shock. Circ Shock (Suppl.). 1979;1:1.
18. Goldfarb RD. Characteristics of shock-induced circulating cardiodepressant substances. A brief review. Circ Shock (Suppl.). 1979;1:23.
19. Fine DJ, Miller JA, Harrist TJ, Haynes HA. Cutaneous lesions in disseminated candidiasis mimicking ecthyma gangrenosum. Am J Med. 1981;70:1133.
20. Musher DM. Cutaneous and soft tissue manifestations of sepsis due to gram-negative enteric bacilli. Rev Infect Dis. 1980;2:854.

21. Yoshikawa T, Tanaka KR, Guze LB. Infection and disseminated intravascular coagulation. Medicine. 1971;50:237.
22. Kaplan RL, Sahn SA, Petty TL. Outcome of the respiratory distress syndrome in gram-negative sepsis. Arch Intern Med. 1979;139:867.
23. Hanninen P, Tarho P, Toivanen A. Septicemia in a pediatric unit. A 20 year study. Scand J Infect Dis. 1971;3:201.
24. Svanbom M. A prospective study on septicemia. II. Clinical manifestations and complications, results of antimicrobial treatment and report on a follow-up study. Scand J Infect Dis. 1980;12:189.
25. MacLean LD, Mulligan WG, McLean AP, et al. Pattern of septic shock in man. A detailed study of 56 patients. Ann Surg. 1967;166:543.
26. Anderson ET, Young LS, Hewitt WL. Antimicrobial synergism in the therapy of gram-negative rod bacteremia. Chemother. 1978; 24:45.
27. Klastersky J, Meunier-Carpentier F, Prevost JM. Significance of antimicrobial synergism in the outcome of gram-negative sepsis. Am J Med Sci. 1977; 273:157.
28. Young LS, Martin WJ, Mayer RD, Weinstein MD, Anderson ET. Gram-negative rod bacteremia: microbiologic, immunologic and therapeutic considerations. Ann Intern Med. 1977;86:456.
29. Bennett WM, Muther RS, Parker RA, Feig P, Morrison G, Golper TA. Drug therapy in renal failure: dosing guidelines for adults. Part I: antimicrobial agents, analgesics. Ann Intern Med. 1980;93:62.
30. Eickoff TC, Ehret JM. "In vitro" comparison of cefoxitin, cefamandole, cephalexin and cephalothin. Antimicrob Agents Chemother. 1976;9:994.
31. Love LJ, Schimpff SC, Schiffer CA, Wernick PH. Improved prognosis for granulocytopenic patients with gram-negative bacteremia. Am J Med. 1980;68:643.
32. Winston DJ, Ho WG, Gale RP. Prophylactic granulocyte transfusions during chemotherapy of acute nonlymphocytic leukemia. Ann Intern Med. 1981;94:616.
33. Christy JH. Treatment of gram-negative shock. Am J Med. 1971; 50:77.
34. Schumer W. Steroids in the treatment of clinical septic shock. Ann Surg. 1976;184:333.
35. Hinshow LB, Archer LT, Beller-Todd BK, Coalson JJ, Flournoy DJ, Passey R, Benjamin B, White GL. Survival of primates in LD$_{100}$ septic shock following steroid/antibiotic therapy. J Surg Research. 1980;28:151.
36. Bennett IL, Finland M, Hamburger M, et al. A double-blind study of the effectiveness of cortisol in the management of severe infections. Trans Assoc Am Physicians. 1962;75:198.
37. Klastersky J, Cappel R, Debusscher LE. Effectiveness of betamethasone in the management of severe infections. N Eng J Med. 1971;284:1248.

38. Corso JA. Maintenance of venous polyethylene catheters to reduce risk of infection. JAMA. 1969;210:2075.
39. Gurwith MJ, Brunton JL, Lank BA, Harding GKM, Ronald AR. A prospective controlled investigation of prophylactic trimethoprim/sulfamethoxazole in hospitalized granulocyto-penic patients. Am J Med. 1979;66:248.
40. Zeigler EJ, McCutchan JA, Braude AI. Successful treatment of human gram-negative bacteremia with antiserum against endotoxin core. Clin Research. 1981;29:576A (Abstract).
41. Jones RJ, Roe EA, Gupta JL. Controlled trials of a polyvalent pseudomonas vaccine in burns. Lancet. 1979;2:977.

TOXIC SHOCK SYNDROME AND KAWASAKI SYNDROME

Walter R. Wilson

Department of Infectious Diseases
Mayo Clinic
Rochester, Minnesota

I. TOXIC SHOCK SYNDROME

The toxic shock syndrome (TSS) was first described in 1978
by Todd et al who reported seven cases in children 8-17 years
old (1). The illness was characterized by high fever, headache, confusion, conjunctival injection, scarlatiniform rash,
subcutaneous edema, oliguria, and hypotension. These symptoms
were usually accompanied by sore throat, vomiting, watery
diarrhea, and shock. During recovery, all patients had fine
desquamation of affected skin, particularly of the palms and
soles. Toxin-producing strains of Staphylococcus aureus were
recovered from various body sites in each of five children.
Since this initial report several hundred additional cases
have been reported to the Center for Disease Control in
Atlanta, Georgia. Because of the age group involved and the
alleged association with the use of tampons, the TSS has been
a subject of widespread interest among the lay population and
press and has resulted in withdrawl from the market of one
brand of tampon which has been incriminated as a cause of TSS.
The widespread publicity attached to this disease and to the
tampon withdrawn from the market has resulted in a large
number of legal claims against the manufacturer of the tampon
amounting to hundreds of millions of dollars.
    Our criteria for TSS are all five of the following:
1) hypotension with sustained blood pressure of less than 90 mm
of mercury, 2) fever greater than 38.9° C, 3) erythematous
rash followed by desquamation, 4) involvement of at least four
organ systems, and 5) reasonable evidence for absence of other
causes.

The incidence of TSS per 100,000 menstruating females depends upon the age group. An incidence of 7.5 was calculated for females aged 10-19. For women aged 10-29, the incidence decreased to 3.8 and for women aged 10-49, the incidence was 2.4 per 100,000 (2).

The majority of women affected with TSS are young. The mean age of patients reported by McKenna et al (2) was 20.6 years with a range of 13-43 years. Most of the cases of TSS have the onset of symptoms from day 2 through day 5 of the menstrual cycle with the peak number of cases occurring on day 4.

Table 1 shows the most common clinical features of TSS observed in 19 episodes (11 patients) seen at Mayo Clinic. These data are remarkably similar to those published elsewhere (3,4).

Table 2 shows the frequency of abnormal laboratory findings in patients with TSS.

Multiple episodes of TSS in the same patient occur frequently. Sixty-four percent of the patients reported by McKenna and associates and 27% of the patients reported by Davis et al (3) and Shands and colleagues (4) had more than one episode of TSS. In the majority of instances, subsequent episodes are less severe than the first, suggesting that some degree of immunity may develop.

TABLE 1.   Clinical Findings of TSS[a]

Finding	% of episodes with finding
Fever	100
Menstruating	100
Myalgias	100
Rash: diffuse erythematous	100
desquamation	94
Mental status change	89
Sore throat	84
Hypotension (< 90 mm of Hg)	83
Diarrhea	79
Abdominal pain	79
Vomiting	74
Conjunctivitis	63
Headache	58
Prolonged refractory shock	37
Adult respiratory distress syndrome	21

[a]From McKenna N. G., et al, Mayo Clinic Proceedings. 55:663, 1980.

TABLE 2. Abnormal Laboratory Findings in TSS[a]

Finding	%
Abnormal urinary sediment	100
Increased urea	92
Hypocalcemia	92
Hypoproteinemia	90
Leukoytosis	85
Anemia	77
Hyperglycemia	77
Hypokalemia	75
Increased hepatic enzymes	69
Increased creatine kinase	64
Hypophosphatemia	60
Hyperbilirubinemia	54
Increased LDH	50
Thrombocytopenia	50

[a]From McKenna N. G. et al, Mayo Clinic Proceedings. 55:663, 1980.

Treatment of patients with TSS with a beta-lactamase resistant antibiotic during the first or subsequent episodes reduces the frequency of recurrence of TSS. Among patients treated during the initial episode, none of 19 patients during the first month, one of 19 during the second month, and one of 16 during the third month experienced recurrence of TSS (3). Among patients who have not been treated with a beta-lactamase resistant antibiotic during the first episode, eight of 13 experienced recurrence during the first month, nine of 13 during the second month, and nine of 13 during the third month. These differences between antibiotic treated patients and those receiving no antibiotics were statistically significant (P value of < 0.001). The recurrence rate of TSS was lower following treatment with a beta-lactamase antibiotic during any episode of TSS but the reduced frequency was not as great as that observed among patients treated during the first episode (P $= \leq 0.02$).

The mortality of patients with TSS is approximately 2%. Early recognition of TSS and agressive management of complications reduce the mortality.

The major factors which are thought to be associated with TSS are menstruation, infection or colonization with S. aureus, and the use of tampons. Among the patients reported in the three major studies, 95%-100% of patients were menstruating at the time of onset of TSS. The isolation of S. aureus from vaginal cultures has been shown to be associated with the development of TSS.

The frequency of isolation of S. aureus from vaginal cultures in patients with TSS has been reported to range from 66-100% (2-4). Only 10% of normal patients has S. aureus isolated from vaginal cultures (P = < 0.001) (4).

One hundred percent of patients with TSS reported using tampons compared with 85% of normal controls (P = < 0.02) (4). The continuous use of tampons is more likely to be associated with TSS than intermittent use. Among patients with TSS, 33 reported continuous use and one intermittent use. Among controls 9 patients reported continuous use and one intermittent use (P = < 0.05).

A number of factors have been reported to be unassociated with the development of TSS. Despite the widespread publicity concerning the brand of tampon which was withdrawn from the market, three major reported studies did not link the brand of tampon used, the degree of absorbency of tampons, or the frequency of tampon change with the development of TSS (2-4). Other factors which have been found to be unrelated to TSS are infection with Herpes simplex, frequency of sexual intercourse, sexual intercourse during menstruation, and use or brand of oral contraceptives.

A number of mechanisms have been proposed for the pathogenesis of TSS. The most prominent theory is that one or more toxins produced by S. aureus may be responsible for the TSS. Staphylococci are capable of producing exotoxins and enterotoxins. An exotoxin has been incriminated in the scaled skin syndrome in children and this, or a similar toxin, may be responsible for the development of the clinical syndrome of TSS in adults.

Several theories concerning the role of tampons have been proposed. Tampons may serve as a culture medium for staphylococci, especially when endometrial blood is pooled on the surface of the tampon. Tampons may serve as a substrate for the production of some as yet identified toxin or may facilitate the production of staphylococcal toxins. It has been speculated that tampons, especially when used continuously, may cause a partial obstruction of the vagina or cervix which could result in rapid growth of staphylococci or other bacteria which may result in TSS. Tampon use has also been associated with ulcerations of the vagina. These ulcerations may permit entrance of toxins or bacteria which could produce the syndrome.

Based on our experience and the published reports we make the following recommendations: 1) Menstruating females who have not had previous episodes of TSS need not discontinue use of tampons, however, if tampons are used, we suggest that they be used intermittently instead of continuously during the menstrual cycle. 2) If patients have a history of TSS, then the use of tampons should be avoided. 3) Patients with TSS should be treated with a beta-lactamase resistant antibiotic during the first and any subsequent episodes of TSS. 4) Patients who develop symptoms suggestive of TSS should immediately remove the tampon from the vagina and should consult their local physician promptly.

II. KAWASAKI SYNDROME

Kawasaki syndrome (KS) is an acute febrile illness of unknown etiology which occurs almost exclusively in children less than five years old (5,6). The criteria for the diagnosis of KS are 1) fever greater than five days in duration together with at least four of the following: bilateral conjuctivitis, oropharyngeal mucous membrane changes, rash, lymphadenopathy, pharyngitis, erythema or fissuring of the lips, and peripheral extremity abnormalities including edema and erythema. 2) no other identifiable cause.

KS is endemic in Japan where the majority of cases have been reported. At least 20,000 cases have been identified in Japan since surveillance began in 1967. In the United States more than 650 cases have been reported to the Center for Disease Control since 1976. The majority of cases in Japan and in the United States have occurred sporadically, although clustering of cases may occur. A cluster of 57 cases of KS occurred recently in Massachusetts (7).

Rash is the most prominent physical finding in patients with KS. The rash is macular or finely papular and involves the trunk and the extremities including the palms and soles. Frequently the rash progresses to desquamation of the skin, similar to that which occurs in the toxic shock syndrome.

There are no specific laboratory abnormalities which occur in patients with KS. Among the most commonly observed abnormalities are thrombocytosis and an elevated erythrocyte sedimentation rate.

Cardiac involvement in children with KS is relatively common. Among the 57 children with KS reported in the cluster of cases in Massachusetts, 30% had evidence of cardiac abnormalities. Seventeen percent had pericardial effusions which resolved spontaneously; 10.5% had transient electrocardiographic changes consistent with diffuse ischemia or myocarditis; 8.5% had transient cardiomegaly and decreased left ventricular function; 8.5% had coronary artery aneurysm demonstrated by echocardiography; and 3.5% had evidence of myocardial infarction.

Extensive epidemiologic and laboratory investigation has failed to identify the cause of KS. Evaluation of the cluster of cases of KS has revealed no common source of exposure for patients with KS or for family members of patients. Person to person transmission of KS has not been demonstrated.

Children with KS should receive supportive care and physicians should be alert to the possibility of cardiac involvement. The use of salicylates in patients with KS may reduce the frequency of coronary artery aneurysm formation. The use of corticosteroids has not proven to be efficacious and may increase the frequency of coronary artery aneurysm. The mortality of KS is approximately 2%. Virtually all fatal cases occur among patients with cardiac involvement. The leading causes of death among these patients are rupture of coronary artery aneurysm or myocardial infarction.

Physicians should be alert to the possibility of KS and should report suspected cases to the Center for Disease Control through the local and state health departments. Further epidemiologic, laboratory, and clinical studies are underway at the Center for Disease Control and elsewhere.

REFERENCES

(1) Todd, J., Fishaut, M., Kapral F., Welch, T.:   Toxic-shock syndrome associated with phage-group-I staphylococci. Lancet, 2:1116-1118, 1978.

(2) McKenna, U. G., Meadows, J. A., Brewer, N. S., Wilson, W. R., Perrault, J.: Toxic shock syndrome, a newly recognized disease entity. Mayo Clinic Proceedings, 55:663, 1980.

(3) Davis, J. P., Chesney, P. J., Wand, P. J., LaVenture, M. and the Investigation and Laboratory Team: Toxic-shock syndrome: epidemiologic features, recurrence, risk factors, and prevention. N Engl J Med, 303:1429, 1980.

(4) Shands, K. N., Schmid, G. P., Dan, B. B., Blum, D., Guidotti, R. J., Hargrett, N. T., Anderson, R. L., Hill, D.L., Broome, C. B., Band, J. D., Fraser, D. W.:   Toxic-shock syndrome in menstruating women: its association with tampon use and Staphylococcus aureus and the clinical features in 52 cases. N Engl J Med, 303:1436, 1980.

(5) Todd, J., Fishaut, M., Dapral, F., Welch, T.:   Toxic-shock syndrome associated with phage-group-I staphylococci. Lancet, 2:116-1118, 1978.

(6) Follow-up on toxic-shock syndrome. MMWR, 29:441-5, 1980.

(7) Kawasaki syndrome--Massachusetts. MMWR, 29:369, 1980.

PART VIII
VIRAL INFECTIONS OF SPECIAL IMPORTANCE

CLINICAL MANAGEMENT OF HERPESVIRUS INFECTIONS, 1982

A. Martin Lerner

Department of Medicine
Wayne State University School of Medicine
Detroit, Michigan

Here, the current treatment of herpesvirus infections will
be reviewed. Therapy of herpes simplex viruses and varicella-
zoster virus infections has progressed beyond the investigational
phase to the benefit of our patients. We, as general physicians,
need to be cognizant of these advances. The human herpesviruses
and their diseases, and, in my judgment, the likely availability
of efficacious treatment within the next several years are listed
in Table 1. There certainly is promising experimental work underway with cytomegalovirus (CMV) and infectious mononucleosis
virus (EBV), but fundamental developmental work is still needed.
Treatment of herpes simplex virus, type 1 (HSV-1), herpes simplex
virus, type 2 (HSV-2) and varicella-zoster virus (VZV) infections
will be discussed.

The clinical syndromes produced by these viruses are shown
in Table 2. Each of these viruses has the unique property of
initial (primary) infection, the maintenance of latent virus in
sensory ganglia for long periods of time, and recurrent infection, the latter occurring with great frequency (HSV-1, HSV-2),
or usually appearing only once many years after primary infection
(VZV).

Effective therapy of herpesvirus diseases can significantly
alter morbidity and mortality. Estimates suggest that 500,000
new patients with genital herpes are recruited each year and 10
million persons suffer from recurrent disease annually. Table 2
indicates the current methods for laboratory diagnosis of HSV and
VZV infections.

THERAPY

Although research efforts continue, vaccine prophylaxis for
HSV or VZV infections are not available in the United States.
Effective antiviral drug treatments for HSV encephalitis, herpe-

TABLE I. Herpesviruses of Humans and the Availability of Antiviral Chemotherapy

Virus	Antiviral Chemotherapy
Herpes simplex virus, type 1 (HSV-1)	Present
Herpes simplex virus, type 2 (HSV-2)	Present
Varicella-zoster virus (VZV)	Present
Cytomegalovirus (CMV)	Absent
Epstein-Barr Virus (EBV)	Absent

TABLE II. Clinical Syndromes of HSV-1, HSV-2 and VZV

Virus	Clinical Syndromes	Laboratory Diagnosis
HSV-1	Primary infection[a] (orofacial or genital)[b] Herpetic whitlow Encephalitis[a] (Eczema herpeticum)[b] Recurrent herpes labialis	1) Isolation of virus from vesicular fluid or base of active ulcer or infected tissue (e.g. brain) 2) Tzanck smear from base of ulcer, intranuclear inclusion bodies plus giant cells 3) Four-fold rise in antibodies from acute to convalescent phase sera by immuno-fluorescent methods, ELISA, radio-immunoassay, or immune adherence hema-gglutination assays 4) Simultaneous assay of antibodies in serum and CSF (S/CSF $\leqq$20, encephalitis)
HSV-2	Herpetic keratitis[a] (Kaposi's varicelliform eruption)[b] Primary genital herpes[a] Herpetic whitlow Disseminated neonatal infection[a], including hepatitis and encephalitis Specific infections of the immunocom-promised patient, esophagitis (pneumonia)[b]	1, 2, 3 and 4 as above
VZV	Chickenpox (Chickenpox pneumonia)[b] Herpes zoster Disseminated herpes zoster[a] Congenital infection with malformation	

[a]Effective therapy has been reported by "double-blind" randomized controlled clinical trials.
[b]Effective therapy "probably" available, but controlled trials have not been reported.

tic keratitis, disseminated neonatal HSV disease and disseminated herpes zoster are available now. "Probably" effective therapy is also present for eczema herpeticum, Kaposi's varicelliform eruption, HSV pneumonia and chickenpox. The drugs for these conditions, which have reached or soon seem likely to enter the marketplace, are trifluorothymidine (TFT); acycloguanosine (ACV, Zovirax); idoxuridine (IDU); adenine arabinoside (ara-A, vidarabine) and adenine arabionoside monophosphate (ara-AMP) (Table 3). Each agent is either a specific inhibitor of viral polymerase and/or is incorporated into the developing viral DNA, and is chain-terminating. Additionally, acyclovir requires HSV specific thymidine kinase for intracellular uptake which appears to add an additional welcome margin of safety. With each antiviral agent, after intracellular uptake, the antiviral nucleoside is progressively phosphorylated to its triphosphate which inhibits viral polymerase.

The antiviral agents mode of administration and herpesvirus disease appropriately treated with each compound, are shown (Table 3). The current agent of choice is listed. Dosages, routes of administration and side effects for each preparation are listed (Table 4).

PERSPECTIVE

The safety and efficacy of acycloguanosine raise the possibility, for the first time, that sufferers with herpes labialis or herpes genitalis, as well as others with disseminated neonatal infection may be treated.

TABLE III. Antiherpesvirus Drug, Mode of Administration
and Clinical Condition Appropriately Treated

Antiviral Agent	Mode of Administration	Disease
Triflurothymidine (TFT)[c]	Local (eye only)	Herpetic keratitis[a] (drug of choice)
Idoxuridine (IDU)	Local (eye only)	Herpetic keratitis
Adenine arabinoside (ara-A)	a) Local (eye)	a) Herpetic keratitis
	b) Intravenous	b) HSV encephalitis[c]:
		Disseminated neonatal[c] infection
		Disseminated varicella-zoster in immunocompromised host
		(Eczema herpeticum)[b]
		(Kaposi's varicelliform eruption)[b]
Adenine arabinoside monophosphate (ara-AMP) - currently being studied		
Acycloguanosine (ACV)	a) Local (eye plus genital)	Herpetic keratitis
		Primary and recurrent herpes genitalis[c]
	b) Oral	Primary and recurrent herpes genitalis

TABLE III. Antiherpesvirus Drug, Mode of Administration and Clinical Condition Appropriately Treated (continued)

Antiviral Agent	Mode of Administration	Disease
	c) Intravenous	Prophylaxis of HSV infection in recipients of Bone Marrow Transplants[a]
		Varicella pneumonia in immunocom‑promised patients[a]

[a]No present agent is effective versus HSV geographic ulcers or deep stromal disease.
[b]Case reports only – no controlled trial has been reported.
[c]Preparation of choice.

TABLE IV. Preparation, Dosage, Frequency and Adverse Effects of Current Antiviral Drugs

Antiviral Agent	Mode of Administration	Disease
1) Trifluorothymidine (Viroptic ophthalmic solution, 1% Burroughs Wellcome)	One drop q2h (x9) for 7 days; then one drop q4h (x5) for an additional 7 days	Mild local reactions
2) Idoxuridine	Not recommended	
3) Adenine arabinoside (Vira-A ophthalmic ointment, 3% Parke-Davis)	Give one half inch into lower conjunctival sac q3h (x5) for 14 days	Mild local reactions
4) Acycloguanosine (eye) (Acyclovir, Burroughs Wellcome)	Not firm at present, but clearly will be effective	Mild local reactions
5) Adenine arabinoside (Vira-A, vidarabine)	10-15 mg/Kg/day I.V. over an eight hour infusion for 7-10 days	Decrease in Hb / Occasional CNS signs / Occasional fall in wbc or platelets
6) Acycloguanosine	Tablet, oral, 200mg q4h (x5)	None
7) Acycloguanosine	5mg/Kg over 1 hr. infusion q8h (x3)/day for 7-10 days	Renal crystalization / Increased creatinine / ? CNS

HEPATITIS

A. Martin Lerner

Department of Medicine
Wayne State University School of Medicine
Detroit, Michigan

Although hepatitis can occur during the course of several systemic virus infections (Table 1), there are three major hepatitis syndromes caused by the viruses, hepatitis A, hepatitis B and hepatitis, non-A, non-B (perhaps 2 or more separate organisms). The characteristics of the viruses and their illnesses are shown in Table 2. Hepatitis A is transmitted by the fecal-oral route and can be recognized by immune electron microscopy as an enterovirus-like agent in feces of patients. Hepatitis B and non-A, non-B viruses are transmitted from blood and secretions such as saliva, urine, semen, breast milk, synovial fluid, CSF bile and vaginal secretions through intimate mucosal contact. Thus, hepatitis B and non-A, non-B are sexually transmissible diseases.

Recovery from acute hepatitis A produces firm long-lasting immunity, while hepatitis B and non-A, non-B may be followed by either a) acute disease with permanent immunity or b) continuing chronic hepatitis with little continuing injury (chronic persistent hepatitis), or progressive hepatic destruction and fibrosis (chronic active hepatitis) leading, ultimately, to hepatic failure. Several essential features of these diseases are listed in Table 2.

The major antigens and their relationships of the hepatitis B virion are shown in Table 3, along with immunochemical characterizations of the acute illness, recovery and chronic carrier states (Table 4). Antibody to HB_S seems necessary for immunity to HBB. Large amounts of HB_S ($\sim 10^8$/ml) are found in carrier plasma and a vaccine is being prepared from this human source. Neither hepatitis B, nor hepatitis, non-A, non-B viruses have been grown in cell culture. Hepatitis A, HBB and non-A, non-B viruses produce hepatitis in chimpanzees. In some populations, a coincident relationship between the HB_S carrier state and hepatoma has been established (e.g. South Africa).

When acquired in the third trimester of pregnancy, hepatitis B may be transmitted from infected vaginal secretions to the neonate.

Steroids increase titers of HB_s and HB_c in plasma and are of dubious value in chronic hepatitis. Interferon and adenine arabinoside given over a protracted period have been shown to decrease or end the carrier state of chronic hepatitis B, but this work remains investigational.

The diagnosis of acute hepatitis A is made by finding IgM antibodies to HBA. Immunity is long-lasting and is defined by IgG antibodies to HBA. These tests can be done by radioimmunoassays or ELISA methods. The diagnosis of HBB is made by defining the presence of HB_s, HB_e, anti-HB_c and DNA polymerase activities along with their antibodies. There are not yet serologic tests to diagnose H (non-A, non-B).

TABLE I. Virus Infections Associated with Hepatitis

Hepatitis virus, type A {HBA}

Hepatitis virus, type B {HBB}

Hepatitis virus(es), non-A, non-B {H, non-A, non-B}

Hepatitis associated with systemic viral infections

       Cytomegalovirus

       Epstein-Barr virus

       Yellow Fever virus

       Coxsackieviruses, group B

       Mumps virus

       Influenza virus

       Rubella virus

TABLE II. Characteristics of Hepatitis Viruses

	Virus		
	A	B	Non-A, Non-B
Transmission	Fecal-oral	Blood, secretions	Blood, secretions
	Epidemic plus endemic (Water and food-borne outbreaks)	Endemic	Endemic
Incubation period	2 to 7 weeks	4 weeks to 6 months	2 to 8 weeks
Disease	Acute only	Acute and chronic	Acute and chronic
Size of virus	27nm	42nm (27nm core)	?
Nucleic acid	RNA	DNA	?
DNA polymerase	—	+	?
Vaccine	—	? (purified coat protein)	—
Passive immunity with immuneglobulin	+	+	?+

TABLE III. Antigens of Hepatitis B Virus

Surface; HB$_s$	Particulate; viral coat protein; found in cytoplasm of infected liver cell
Core ; HB$_c$	Particulate; found in nucleus of infected liver cell
E ; HB$_e$	Soluble; present in viral core
DNA polymerase activity	– indicates presence of whole virion (Dane particle)

TABLE IV. Antigens and Antibodies of Acute and Chronic Hepatitis B

HB	Antigen	Antibody
"Recovery"	s	
Acute Hepatitis	e	
	c	
"Carrier"	s	
Chronic Active Hepatitis	e	
	c	
"Carrier"	s	
Chronic Persistent Hepatitis	e	
	c	

ANIMAL BITES AND RABIES

L.D. Sabath

Department of Medicine
University of Minnesota
Minneapolis, Minnesota

INTRODUCTION

Although animal bites are extremely common, more than 1
million per year being reported in the United States, the disease
rabies in man is exceedingly rare, averaging a bit more than one
case per year over the last several decades. Thus, American
physicians are constantly encountering patients who have
suffered animal bites whereas it is only infrequently they
actually encounter a clinical case of rabies in a human being.

Rabies is a severe, usually fatal, illness of man caused by
a virus known as the rabies virus, which belongs to the rabdovirus
group of RNA viruses. Its shape, as revealed by electronmicro-
scopy, suggests a bullet; no antigenic variation in the virus
has been noted, and therefore, there is only one kind of antiserum.

ANIMAL BITES

Although the fear that animal bites may transmit rabies is
a justified one, the major problem in animal bites is a specific
damage to tissue and possible initiation of an infectious process.
The general care of the wound following an animal bite is basically
that for any other wound, that is, thorough cleaning of the wound,
initiation of a tetanus immunization series if the patient has
not received the complete primary series of immunizations or the
provision of a tetanus booster should the patient have received
the original series of three or four immunizations but not had
a booster within the last ten years. In addition, antibiotic

treatment should be given since all animal mouths and teeth contain numerous organisms. The major special organisms of note
causing infection in animal bites are *Pasteurella multocida*,
especially common following cat bites but also bites of other
animals. Also problems are *Streptobacillus moniliformis* and
Spirillum minus. *Streptobacillus moniliformis* is the cause of
"rat-bite fever". All of these organisms are exquisitely sensitive to Penicillin G. Therefore, following a bite, treatment
with penicillin immediately would be in order. Penicillin V,
2 g daily, (0.5 g approximately q 6 h) would be appropriate.
Erythromycin or tetracycline in identical doses would be appropriate for penicillin allergic patients. For those in whom there
is evidence of infection as well as the physical trauma to the
wound, treatment would obviously be continued longer than a
simple prophylactic single dose or a several day treatment.

NEWER DEVELOPMENTS IN RABIES

There have been more new developments concerning rabies in
the last twelve years than at any other time since Pasteur's
classic work on rabies, in the middle third of the last century.
These specific developments of considerable practical importance
are:

1. New vaccine

A safe, effective, efficient vaccine already licensed in
Europe and available on a limited scale in the United States has
been developed, using human diploid cells for production of the
vaccine. Its advantage is very likely due to the greater
efficiency of producing antigenic material when compared to
older methods. Therefore, a series of five immunization injections
provide much higher and more dependable antibody levels than can
be achieved with a series of 23 injections of duck embryo vaccine.
It has been suggested by one author that if supplies become
adequate, immunization with the human diploid cell vaccine may
be used routinely for individuals who have frequent contact with
rabid animals or are likely to (such as hunters and campers in
areas where rabid wild animals are common).

2. Survival after clinical rabies

Whereas in the past rabies in man was considered an invariably
fatal infection once the clinical disease began, it is now
documented that survival is possible, at least in a few instances.
Since 1970 there have been three documented cases of humans surviving clinical rabies. The first case was a young boy in Ohio,

the second was reported from Argentina, and a third was a laboratory worker in New York State who acquired the disease, apparently
by inhalation of aerosolized rabies virus with which he was
working. In the latter case, although there was survival, there
is considerable neurologic sequelae.

3. Diagnosis of rabies by fluorescent antibody microscopy

In the past, rabies has been diagnosed mainly on the basis
of the clinical picture and subsequently verified by demonstrating
the Negri bodies in postmortem sections of the brain and/or
isolation of virus from patient tissues. It is now possible to
diagnose rabies by demonstration of virus (viral antigen) by
fluorescent antibody tests on either corneal scrapings or hair
follicle biopsies. The latter is considered the most efficient
means of demonstrating rabies antigen in human hosts during
clinical disease; the fluorescent antibody (FA) test material
is often taken from biopsy at the nuchal hairline. The basis for
taking this tissue is that the nerve fibers supplying the
arector pili muscles (which cause erection of hairs) are easy
to locate in this tissue.

4. Spread of the disease in wild animal reservoirs

In the United States the identification of rabies in domestic
animals exceeded the identification of rabies in wild animals
prior to 1960, but since that time there has been a continued
decrease in rabies in domestic animals but an increase in wild
animals. In Europe there has been a continuous spread of rabies
in animals westward towards the English channel, but the major
reservoir there is in red foxes.

5. Conclusive proof of airborne transmission of rabies

There was evidence of airborne transmission of rabies secondary to exposure of humans in bat caves in the southwest of the
United States and more recently, in the case of the New York
State health department worker who developed rabies (and survived)
following an airborne exposure.

6. Use of attenuated virus to influence spread of rabies in wild
   animal populations

In Europe there has been discussion and more recently exper-
imentation on using attenuated virus (distributed in chopped meat)
as a means of immunizing wild animals against rabies, and thus,

hopefully, preventing spread of the disease in this important
reservoir.

7. Non-bite transmission of rabies

In addition to airborne transmission of rabies, there have
been an increasing number of reports of human to human spread
of rabies by organ transplantation. Of the 19 cases of human
rabies reported in the United States since 1966, in nine of those
instances there was no evidence at all of animal bite or animal
exposure. Thus, almost half of the human cases of rabies diagnosed in the United States since 1966 have not been secondary to
animal bites. In September of 1981 the third and fourth cases of
human rabies secondary to corneal transplants were reported
from Thailand. The first and second cases were reported in 1979
(USA) and 1980 (France).

8. Neurological complications of duck embryo vaccine

Although it has been widely accepted that neurological
complications following active immunization with duck embryo
vaccine (DEV) are less frequent than after spinal cord vaccine
(Semple vaccine), it was within the last decade recognized that
neurologic complications to the DEV also occur. This may be
a major problem when large numbers of humans are immunized with
this preparation.

RESERVOIRS

The major reservoirs of rabies in the United States and Canada
are in wild animals, whereas in Mexico the major reservoir is in
dogs. The number of isolates of rabies in animals has continued
to increase in the United States. In the year 1978 there were
3,298 reported cases of rabies in the United States, four of those
in man. The most common species from which rabies was isolated
in that year was the skunk (1,657 animals), the next most common
being bats (567), farm animals (254), foxes (148), dogs (119),
and cats (96). In that same year in Mexico there were 15,029
reports of rabies in animals, of which 14,109 were in dogs,
305 in cats, 206 in rats, 49 in bats, 36 in horses, 16 in swine,
8 in sheep, 19 in squirrels, and only 3 in foxes. The largest
number of animal isolates were from the Distrito Federal (2,122).
In that same year there were 1,641 reports of rabies in animals in
Canada with the largest number being in foxes (809), followed by
isolates in skunks (345), cattle (237), dogs (77), cats (63),
horses (35), bats (24), and sheep (16). Of the 1,641 reports

of animal rabies in Canada in 1978, 1,361 of those were from
Ontario and 122 from Saskatchewan, with 85 in Quebec and 60 in
Manitoba. Within the United States the largest numbers of cases
of animal rabies in 1978 were in Texas (556), California (335),
Georgia (288) and Minnesota (204). There is evidence of a marked
increase in the reporting of animal rabies in the United States
since 1978 whereas the cumulative number of reports in the United
States during the first 37 weeks for the years 1976-1980 was 2,261,
the reports for that 37 week period in 1980 was 4,770 cases and
for the first 37 weeks of 1981 it was 5,255 reports of animal
rabies. Thus, the reports of animal rabies in the United States
is increasing dramatically, the current rate in 1981 being more
than double the median for the 1976-1980 period. Within the
United States the most common animal in which rabies is reported
is the skunk; this is especially true for most of the country.
But the most common animal in which rabies has been identified
in the Southeast is the raccoon; almost all of the reports come
from Georgia and the flanking states of South Carolina, Alabama
and Florida.

CLINICAL PRESENTATION

    Whereas the literature of the past has emphasized the relation-
ship between animal bites and the appearance of rabies indicating
an incubation period of ten days to one year (with a mean of 1 to
2 months) it is extremely important to recognize the fact that
about half of the cases in the last 15 years in the United States
are not associated with animal bites and the recognition of rabies
following corneal transplantation raises the possibility that
some cases of rabies may go unrecognized.
    When the clinical symptoms of rabies appear, the course
tends to be relatively rapid with a prodrome of one to four days,
with a course of survival of about four days and a maximum of
up to 20 days with the exception of those instances of prolonged
survival with use of artifical life support means.
    The presentation may be that of an acute encephalitis with
excitation, confusion, hallucination, sometimes combativeness,
spasms, meningismus, opisthtonos, mental aberration, vocal
paresis and twitching leading to coma and death. Earlier symptoms
may be that of fever, headache, malaise, myalgia, increased
fatiguability, anorexia and nausea and vomiting. Thus there
is very little specific about the presentation of a patient with
rabies and the differential diagnosis is a very long one. The
differential diagnosis should include rabies, pseudo-rabies,
Landry-Guillain-Barré syndrome, poliomyelitis, tetanus, allergic
encephalitis, and basal artery syndromes.

The physical examination is one in which there is often low grade fever and there may be evidence of sympathetic overactivity (demonstrated by pupil dilatation and/or irregularity, increased lacrimation, salivation, perspiration and/or postural hypotension). There may be motor weakness, there may be tingling or paresthesias around the site of the bite, if there is a bite. Increased deep tendon reflexes is common, as are cranial nerve palsies. There may be difficulty swallowing but the classic picture of foaming at the mouth is extraordinarily rare.

Laboratory findings, with the exception of those noted below are very nonspecific. The white count is often slightly elevated.

Specific diagnosis of rabies is by one of four means: 1) isolation of virus, 2) serologic evidence (four-fold rise in antibody titer if there has been no immunization), 3) demonstration of viral antigen in affected tissue such as brain biopsy, corneal scrapings or hair follicle biopsy, 4) presence of antibody in the cerebrospinal fluid (CSF). This presence of antibody in the CSF is thought to be rare, if ever, in immunized patients and when it occurs it probably is <1:64 titer, whereas with the disease, antibody levels of 1:200 to 1:160,000 have been demonstrated. Treatment consists of use of active and passive immunization (see below) and general supportive measures. The official recommendation is for isolation of patients with rabies or suspected rabies (because of possible transmission by infected secretions) but documented evidence of human to human spread other than by organ transplantation (e.g. corneal transplant) are not known to this author.

USE OF ACTIVE AND PASSIVE IMMUNIZATION; CLEANSING OF BITE WOUNDS

All bite wounds should be promptly and vigorously cleaned and disinfected, as detailed in footnote of the Table.

Active immunization is advised pre-exposure for all veterinarians and would wisely also be appropriate as pre-exposure immunization for others whose occupation or activities would indicate a likelihood of bite or other exposure to rabies virus. Active immunization is also recommended for individuals known to be bitten by rabid animals or bitten by possibly rabid animals that escaped. The criteria for deciding whether active immunization after possible exposure should be initiated is suggested in the accompanying table.

There are basically two approaches to active immunization post-exposure. One is the use of duck embryo vaccine (DEV), which is widely available in the United States. Usual immunization with DEV, for post-exposure immunization, would be given as two (different sites) injections daily for one week followed by one injection per day for a second week and then two booster doses at ten and twenty days after the 21st dose.

The second type of active immunization recommended is with the diploid cell vaccine which is only available on a limited basis and may be obtained through either the state health departments in the United States or the Center for Disease Control in Atlanta. As noted above, it is a much more effective vaccine in eliciting antibody and is accompanied by fewer side effects. Clearly, if available, it appears to be a more desirable agent for active immunization.

Passive immunization is recommended for previously unimmunized individuals who have had unequivocal or very likely exposure to rabies virus as suggested in the accompanying table. The usual dose is 20 U/kg of human immunoglobulin (RIG) when available or if none is available, double that dose of equine immunoglobulin. In either case one-half of the total dose is infiltrated around the site of the bite (if there is a bite and this is anatomically possible) and the remainder injected intramuscularly at the same time.

If the duck embryo vaccine is used for active immunization it is desirable to draw serum from the patient after immunization to be sure an adequate level of antibody has been achived (>1-5 if no passive immunization has also been given); if necessary, additional injections are advised until the desired titer is reached.

PROSPECTS FOR THE FUTURE

Obviously future work in the management and control of rabies is required: 1) some means of reducing or eliminating the animal reservoir, 2) development and availability of safe and effective means of producing immunity, 3) a means of maintaining patients who have developed the disease or treating it (possibly by use of interferon or other antiviral materials) and 4) a simpler means of making the diagnosis of rabies in patients with encephalitis or coma of unknown etiology which might have been rabies that was not suspected but which may be rabies (this latter category is rarely screened by laboratory means for the possibility of rabies).

TABLE 1. Recommendations of Expert Committee on Rabies of the World Health Organization

Nature of exposure	Status of Biting Animal Irrespective of Previous Vaccination		Recommended treatment[b]
	At time of exposure	During 10 days[a]	
I. Contact, but no lesions; Indirect contact; no contact	Rabid	–	None
II. Licks of the skin; scratches or abrasions; minor bites (covered areas of arms, trunk, and legs)	(a) Suspected as rabid[c]	Healthy	Start vaccine; stop treatment if animal remains healthy for five days[a,d,f]
		Rabid	Start vaccine; administer serum upon positive diagnosis and complete the course of vaccine[f]
	(b) Rabid; wild animal[e] or animal unavailable for observation		Serum + vaccine[f]
III. Licks of mucosa; major bites (multiple or on face, head, finger or neck)	Suspect[c] or rabid domestic or wild animal[e], or animal unavailable for observation		Serum + vaccine; stop treatment if animal remains healthy for five days[a,d,f]

Table 1 continued next page

TABLE I. Recommendations of Expert Committee on Rabies of the World Health Organization (cont.)

a *Observation period in this chart applies only to dogs and cats.*

b *See explanatory notes in this chart.*

c *All unprovoked bites in endemic areas should be considered suspect unless proved negative by laboratory examination (brain FA). Consult with local or state health department regarding likelihood of rabies in species that caused bite.*

d *Or if its brain is found negative by FA examination.*

e *In general, exposure to rodents and rabbits seldom if ever requires antirabies treatment.*

f *All animal bite wounds should be properly cleaned as soon as possible after bite, by: 1) thoroughly washing with soap and water, 2) thoroughly rinsing away soap with water or ethyl alcohol, and 3) scrubbing with 1 or 2% benzalkonium chloride or 1% cetrimonium bromide.*

REFERENCES

Baer, G.-M. (1975). The Natural History of Rabies. New York, Academic Press.
Centers for Disease Control. (1981). Rabies Surveillance. (Annual Summary 1978). U.S. Department of Health and Human Services, Public Health Service, Atlanta, GA.
Expert Committee on Rabies: Sixth Report. (1973). W140 Techn. Rep. Ser. No. 523.
Houff, S.A., Burton, R.C., Wilson, R.W., *et al.* (1979). Human to human transmission of rabies virus by corneal transplant. *N. Engl. J. Med. 300*:603-604.
Knutson, N., Ward, J., and Roberts, M.A. (1981). Human rabies - Oklahoma. *Morbidity and Mortality Weekly Report 30*:343-349.
Plotkin, S.A., and Wiktor, T.J. (1978). Rabies vaccination. *Ann. Rev. Med. 29*:583.
Rubin, R.H., *et al.* (1973). Adverse reactions to duck embryo vaccine. *Ann. Intern. Med. 78*:643.

PART IX
PARASITIC INFECTIONS OF SPECIAL IMPORTANCE

MALARIA - THE OFTEN NEGLECTED DISEASE

Murray Wittner

Professor of Parasitology and Tropical Medicine
Albert Einstein College of Medicine
Bronx, New York

INTRODUCTION

Malaria is a disease of man and other vertebrates caused by
Sporozoa of the genus *Plasmodium*. The disease has been known
since antiquity. Hippocrates, who studied in Egypt, unmistakably
described the various forms of malaria. Long before the etiology
of malaria was discovered by Laveran at the end of the nineteenth
century it was clear that malaria was related to the emanations
of the swamps; thus the name "malaria". At present there are
four species of *Plasmodium* recognized as the usual etiologic
agents of human malaria: *P. falciparum, P. vivax, P. malariae,*
and *P. ovale*. These species cause, respectively, malignant
tertian or falciparum malaria, benign tertian or vivax malaria,
quartan malaria and ovale malaria. The latter two species are
least commonly encountered. Although some cases of naturally
acquired simian malaria have been reported, it is not clear
how widespread this situation may be.

Malaria infects an estimated 100-150 million individuals
throughout the world and accounts for about 10 million deaths
annually. It is found, with few exceptions, throughout the
tropical and subtropical zones and parts of the temperate
zones, wherever a suitable species of anopheline mosquito exists.
Extensive malaria eradication programs have eliminated or reduced
malaria in many parts of the world. Recently, however, in many
of these underdeveloped nations there has been a marked resur-
gence of this disease, especially as the cost of mosquito control
and prophylaxis became prohibitive and these programs were largely
abandoned. In addition, widespread resistance of mosquitos to
insecticides reduced effectiveness of residual spray programs
and the emergence of drug resistant strains of malaria -
especially chloroquine resistant *P. falciparum* - has changed the

lofty goals of malarial eradication to that of control. These
adverse events have engendered renewed interest in understanding
malaria immunity with the aim of developing an effective vaccine.
Towards this end the recent work of Trager and Jensen in developing continuous *in vitro* culture methods for the propagation of
P. falciparum makes the possibility of obtaining large quantities
of parasite material for development of a vaccine an attainable
achievement for the near future. Moreover, with widespread
low-priced travel becoming commonplace, it is essential to con--
sider malaria in those individuals who have returned from malarious regions.

LIFE HISTORY

Malaria is transmitted through the bite of female anopheline
mosquitos that inoculate sporozoites into the bite wound and
enter the blood stream. Within 1 hour they invade hepatic
parenchymal cells where they undergo successive nuclear divisions,
producing as the end product of schizogony many thousands of merozoites. The parasitized host cell ruptures, releasing these merozoites, many of which are phagocytized; others invade red blood
cells of the host. During the pre-erythrocytic cycle the
patient's blood is free of parasites and he cannot transmit the
disease (this is the prepatent period). As this period ends,
(a minimum of 5.5 days in falciparum malaria) merozoites leave
the liver and invade red blood cells, initiating the erythrocyte
cycle. Within parasitized erythrocytes, schizogony is repeated
regularly, releasing new groups of merozoites into the bloodstream. This event is often associated with the clinical symptoms
of malaria. Moreover, it is not unusual for parasites to develop
synchronously so that the clinical features of the disease may
exhibit a 48 hour (falciparum, vivax, ovale) or 72 hour (malariae)
periodicity. After a week to 10 days some of the merozoites
within the erythrocytes develop into macrogametocytes or micro-
gametocytes. These subsequently must be ingested by a suitable
female mosquito in order to undergo further development. Sporo-
zoite-induced vivax and ovale infections are often characterized
by relapses believed to be caused by retained tissue forms. These
forms have recently been identified and termed "hypnozoites".
It has been suggested that hypnozoite polymorphism may account
for this feature by genetically different populations of hypnozoites maturing periodically and subsequently undergoing schizogony. This, however, does not appear to be the case in sporo-
zoite-induced falciparum infections and is of utmost importance
with regard to therapy. It remains unclear whether residual
tissue forms are present in *P. malariae* infections despite the
well recognized extended chronicity that may characterize this
form of malaria. Moreover, tissue forms are not found in blood
induced malaria, i.e. transfusion malaria.

Shortly after a suitable anopheline mosquito ingests gametocytes together with her blood meal, gametocyte maturation and
fertilization takes place. The resulting zygote (ookinete)
develops into an oocyst and sporozoites soon develop within the
oocyst. The sporozoites next invade the mosquito's salivary
glands. When the mosquito next feeds, infective sporozoites are
inoculated into the human host; depending on climatic conditions
and other host factors the mosquito cycle takes 7 to 20 days or
longer.

PATHOLOGY AND PATHOGENESIS

Other than destruction of a few liver cells no pathologic
damage occurs in the preerythrocytic or exoerythrocytic stages.
Moreover, invasion and cyclical destruction of erythrocytes
and progressive increase of peripheral parasitemia only partly
account for the developing anemia which is of varying severity
and usually depends on the species of *Plasmodium* involved. Thus,
observations of Kitchen suggest that *P. vivax* invades reticulo-
cytes, *P. malariae* prefers mature erythrocytes and *P. falciparum*
invades all ages of erythrocytes. This may in part account for
the greater parasitemia often encountered in falciparum malaria.
Erythrocyte destruction is also enhanced by erythrophagocytosis
of non-parasitized cells. It is unusual to detect red cell
sensitization by either direct or indirect Coombs test. During
acute episodes there may be moderate leukocytosis, although
leukopenia and thrombocytopenia are also frequently encountered.
With increased destruction of erythrocytes, malarial pigment
(hemozoin), as well as hemosiderin, cell debris, and merozoites,
may stimulate reticuloendothelial activity. The viscera, including the brain, may take on a slate gray to black appearance as a
result of sequestered malarial pigment.
The spleen may enlarge during an acute attack. At this time
the capsule is thin and easily torn and the pulp is diffluent.
After many years of chronic disease however the capsule becomes
thickened and the pulp fibrous. Splenomegaly is then irreversible. Liver function usually is not seriously impaired, although
there may be increases in conjugated bilirubin, SGOT/SGPT, and
alkaline phosphatase. Serum albumin may decrease and there is
almost always an absolute increase in serum globulins. A
false positive serological test for syphilis is often encountered.
For many years it has been recognized that erythrocytes
infected with *P. falciparum* become sequestered in visceral capillaries where schizogony takes place. Recent experimental evidence
has shown electron dense changes of the cell membrane of erythrocytes parasitized by late-stage trophozoites and schzonts. It is
believed that these "knobs" are responsible for the tendency of
red cells to clump and adhere to capillary endothelium.

The development of immunity to malaria involves both humoral and cellular mechanisms. Increased phagocytic activity, hyperplasia of reticuloendothelial components and the appearance of high titers of strain-specific protective antibodies in serum are important features of the immune response. Humoral immunity is developed against the erythrocytic phase of the infection with the production of high levels of IgM, and followed shortly by IgG and IgA. In endemic or hyperendemic regions infants are born with passive immunity to malaria as a result of placental transfer of protective IgG antibodies. During the first few years of life repeated infection and active disease may result in acquired active immunity which may decrease clinical attacks even in the presence of significant parasitemia. Serum IgG levels are markedly elevated with the development of immunity although much of the IgG is non protective and probably represents polyclonal B-cell activation. Inoculation of hyperimmune globulin however has been shown to prevent or diminish an acute malaria attack. During an acute episode levels of circulating complement decline and immune complexes have been localized by immunofluorescence to the renal glomerular basement membrane. Whether these findings can be implicated in the nephrotic syndrome of *P. malariae* is not entirely clear, although species specific immune complexes have been eluted from renal biopsy material.

The role of fixed macrophages in malaria as an expression of cell-mediated immunity is highly suggestive. A number of studies have shown that a large portion of the normal circulating erythrocyte population, as well as platelets, may be engulfed by activated macrophages in the spleen, liver, and marrow, significantly contributing to the anemia. Whether this represents macrophage activation by lymphocyte products or a nonspecific host hyperphagocytic state is not settled. It seems likely, however, that the enhanced host phagocytic activity is responsible at least in part, for the frequent pathologic findings in malaria of hepatosplenomegaly, anemia and thrombocytopenia.

CLINICAL ASPECTS

Older children and adults may exhibit the typical clinical picture of malaria characterized by intermittent febrile episodes, anemia and splenomegaly. The incubation period in the nonimmune subject varies widely from a week to many weeks depending on the species and strain of *Plasmodium*. Certain strains of *P. vivax* may have incubation periods of 6 to 12 months or more, and following the discontinuance of suppressant drugs, delayed primary attacks of many months can be seen.

The initial or primary attack in the nonimmune often is
heralded by a short prodromal period of several days to a week
and consists of irregular fevers, anorexia, chilliness, arthralgias, abdominal discomfort and mild diarrhea. This is followed
by the primary attack that lasts several weeks, during which there
are recurring intermittent paroxysms classically consisting of
four more or less distinct stages: shaking chills, high fever,
drenching sweats, and an apyretic period. Paroxysms recur at
approximately 48 hour intervals with *P. vivax, P. ovale* and
P. falciparum (tertian fevers); *P. malariae* recurs every 72 hours
(quartan fever); initially, the attacks may be non-periodic with
daily remitting fever episodes.

   P. falciparum accounts for most of the severe or pernicious
complications and nearly all the deaths. A wide range of
symptoms referable to central nervous system involvement may be
seen, presumably related to those areas of the brain in which
capillary occlusion and/or hypoxemia have occurred. The onset
of cerebral malaria may appear unheralded and may occur when the
parasitemia is low or high. Nevertheless, it should be emphasized
that the degree of parasitemia is most often correlated with a
fatal outcome in falciparum malaria. Disseminated intravascular
coagulation is sometimes reported, but is uncommon. Blackwater
fever, which is characterized by massive intravascular hemolysis,
jaundice, acute renal failure and hemoglobinuria is believed
to be related to red cell injury by antibody. Previously many
authors have suggested that it was caused by quinine acting as a
haptene in those cases of incompletely treated falciparum malaria.
However, blackwater fever is occasionally seen in untreated
falciparum as well as other forms of malaria. Acute renal failure
can occur without warning with or without massive hemolysis.
Vascular collapse (algid malaria) may suddenly intervene and is
particularly difficult to treat even with vasopressors. Meningeal signs are especially common in children, but examination of
the cerebrospinal fluid usually is normal. Alternatively, severe
gastrointestinal, cardiovascular, respiratory, or urogenital
symptoms can dominate the picture and may have a fatal termination.
Glomerulonephritis in children associated with *P. malariae*
usually has a poor prognosis and does not respond to steroid
therapy.

   The natural history of untreated malaria is such that clinical
attacks or relapses become less frequent and after a variable
period clinical disease disappears. *P. falciparum* infection lasts
about 9 months to 1 year and *P. vivax* 1 to 8 years, but *P. malariae* can persist for decades as a latent infection, and relapses
have occurred after 30 years. While congenital malaria undoubtedly occurs in endemic areas, it is a rare event. In most instances a nonimmune mother acquired the disease during pregnancy,
or the child may develop malaria early in the perinatal period.

Considerable evidence has accumulated indicating that individuals, with abnormal hemoglobins, especially sickle cell trait,
have fewer parasites and milder disease than those with normal
hemoglobin. Recent experimental evidence has shown that *P. falciparum* invades HbS-trait cells as readily as normal hemoglobin-
containing cells. Similarly, they appear to grow just as well in
both types of red cells. However, under low oxygen tensions, such
as would be present in visceral capillaries, they do not grow and
the trophozoites subsequently succomb. Individuals with erythrocyte glucose-6-phosphate dehydrogenase deficiency are said to be
similarly disposed. Epidemiologic studies from Africa seem to
implicate malaria as an important factor in the etiology of
Burkitt's lymphoma. It has been suggested that the profound
immuno-suppression that occurs in chronic malaria lowers the
immune surveillance mechanism of the host increasing susceptibility
to neoplastic transformation by Epstein-Barr virus. In recent
studies it has been shown that infectivity of merozoites for red
blood cells depends upon an appropriate red cell receptor in order
for the parasite to attach and subsequently invade the erythrocyte.
The almost universal absence of the Duffy blood group determinants
in West African and American blacks has been convincingly correlated with their innate resistance to *P. vivax* in contrast with
their marked susceptibility to the other three species of human
malaria. Experimental studies have strongly suggested that
P. vivax merozoites require the Duffy site or one very closely
linked to it as the receptor site.

DIAGNOSIS

The definitive diagnosis of malaria is made by microscopic
identification of the organisms on stained thin and thick blood
smears. It is important to examine thick films, since they provide a higher concentration of parasites, which is indispensable
when parasitemia is low or thin films are negative. Preferably,
the blood smear should be stained with Giemsa's stain, although
Wright's stain can be used. Since parasites are continuously
present in peripheral red blood cells during schizogony, blood
can be taken and examined at any time with *P. vivax, P. ovale,*
and *P. malariae* infections. In *P. falciparum* infections, however,
only ring forms may be present immediately after the fever peaks
and no parasites may be evident a few hours later, since infected
erythrocytes are sequestered in visceral capillaries. If symptoms
have been present for 7 to 9 days, gametocytes will usually be
present in the peripheral blood, and species identification can
readily be made. The correct species diagnosis is important in
order to establish proper therapy and prognosis. Moreover, it
should be remembered that mixed infections (more than one
 pecies) occur in about 1 to 2% of cases and could explain why

a diagnosed case of *P. vivax* has failed to respond to chloroquine therapy when, in fact, a chloroquine-resistant strain of *P. falciparum* is also present.

TREATMENT

The management of malaria demands prompt chemotherapy, but the patient must also be given supportive care while being kept under careful observation. It is essential, especially in *P. falciparum* malaria, to assess the parasitemia frequently by examination of blood smears three to four times daily. Fatalities rise dramatically when the parasitemia exceed $100,000/mm^3$; patient management must be guided by this criterion.

Antimalarial chemotherapy is outlined in Table 1. Treatment of the acute attack is aimed at destroying erythrocytic stages of the parasite as rapidly as possible. For this purpose chloroquine is the drug of choice; it is a powerful schizonticidal 4-amino-quinoline that may be administered by the oral route or, if necessary, by the intramuscular route. Clinical and parasitic response can usually be detected for several weeks thereafter.

Certain strains of *P. falciparum* from Southeast Asia, the Indian subcontinent, part of Central and South America and East Africa have been found resistant to therapeutic doses of chloroquine. Quinine should be employed when resistance is encountered. It is preferable to use oral quinine, but in serious situations, or if vomiting intervenes, it may be given by the intravenous route. Toxicity to quinine can develop rapidly if renal function is impaired. The use of quinine alone is often associated with a significant recrudescence rate, which can be reduced appreciably by also giving an absorbable sulfa drug such such as sulfadiazine, 100 mg/kg/day in four divided doses for 5 days (2 g maximum), and pyrimethamine, 1 mg/kg in two divided doses daily for 3 days (maximum 25 mg twice a day for 3 days).

Primaquine should be given for the eradication of persisting hepatic (exoerythrocytic) stages of *P. vivax* and *P. ovale*. It is unnecessary, however, for *P. falciparum* malaria, since tissue forms apparently are not present. Similarly, it is unnecessary in the treatment of transfusion malaria, since erythrocytic forms do not establish an exoerythrocytic cycle. Primaquine may cause hemolysis in individuals with glucose-6-phosphate dehydrogenase deficiency. In high doses it may cause hemolytic anemia, methemoglobinemia, and leukopenia. It should not be used concurrently with quinacrine (Atabrine), quinine, or sulfonamides. In order to avoid primaquine-induced hemolysis, which may occur in patients with glucose-6-phosphate dehydrogenase (G-6-PD) deficiency a G-6-PD determination should be obtained on each patient prior to initiating therapy with primaquine. It should be

Table 1.   Summary of Chemotherapy and Chemoprophylaxis in Malaria

Clinical Situation	Drug and Usual Preparation	Route of Administration	Dose as Active Base or Salt	Dosage and Schedule of Administration
Clinical attack	Chloroquine phosphate, UPS XVIII*	Oral	Base	0 hours, 10 mg/kg; 6 hours, 5 mg/kg; 24 hours 5 mg/kg; 48 hours
	Quinine sulfate, USP XV +	Oral	Salt	20-30 mg/kg/day divided into 3 doses for 7-10 days
	Pyrimethamine +	Oral	Base	1 mg/kg daily for 3 days in 2 divided doses (see text)
	Sulfadiazine	Oral		100 mg/kg day divided in 4 doses for 3 days (see text)
Emergency requirement for parenteral route	Chloroquine dihydrochloride	Intramuscular	Base	5 mg/kg may be repeated once in 24-hour period
	Quinine hydrochloride, USP XV	Intravenous	Salt	10 mg/kg well diluted in saline over 1-hour period, may be repeated twice in 24-hour period
Eradication, exoerythrocytic stage	Primaquine phosphate	Oral	Base	0.3 mg/kg once a day for 14 days

Table 1. Summary of Chemotherapy and Chemoprophylaxis in Malaria - CONTINUED

Clinical Situation	Drug and Usual Preparation	Route of Administration	Dose as Active Base or Salt	Dosage and Schedule of Administration
Personal prophylactic suppression				
Chloroquine sensitive	Chloroquine phosphate USP XVII#	Oral	Base	5 mg/kg once a week
Chloroquine resistant	Pyrimethamine** Sulfadoxine	Oral Oral	Base Base	6-11 mos. 1/8 tab/wk 1-3 yrs. 1/4 tab/wk 4-8 yrs. 1/2 tab/wk 9-14 yrs. 3/4 tab/wk 14 yrs. 1 tab/wk

* Drug of choice; maximal initial dose 600 mg of the base.
For use only in case of resistance to chloroquine and other antimalarials; maximal total daily dose 2 g.
Use oral route as soon as possible; maximal single dose 300 mg of the base.
Use oral route as soon as possible; maximal single dose 650 mg.
Do not use concurrently with quinacrine or sulfonamides; discontinue if evidence of hemolysis; maximal single dose 15 mg of the base. (see text)

Start 1 week before and continue 1 month after being in malarious area; maximal single dose 300 mg of the base/

** Pyrimethamine and Sulfadoxine comes in a fixed-dose combination: Fansidar-Roche

remembered that primaquine therapy does not always prevent relapses especially with vivax malaria. If a relapse should occur after appropriate chloroquine-primaquine therapy then the complete course of therapy should be given again.

Chemoprophylaxis with chloroquine is highly effective and will suppress all clinical activity of the disease except for resistant strains of *P. falciparum*. However, it is important to realize that prophylaxis with chloroquine does not prevent infection; it only destroys erythrocytic stages. Hepatic or exoerythrocytic stages remain unaffected, and clinical disease may become evident once prophylaxis is discontinued. Therefore, on leaving a malarious area, it is essential to initiate primaquine therapy before suppression with chloroquine is discontinued (Table 1). Prophylaxis for chloroquine-resistant *P. falciparum* can be achieved with pyrimethamine and sulfadoxine taken weekly (see Table 1). Unfortunately sulfadoxine or the fixed-dose combination (Fansidar-Roche) is not available in the United States, nor is it readily available in many areas overseas where chloroquine resistance is encountered. Following a *P. falciparum* infection a patient may develop a fever several weeks after discharge. Recrudescence of the infection should be entertained and blood smears examined without delay and at regular intervals since the smears may be negative initially.

The transfusion of whole blood or plasma has increasingly become recognized as a means of acquiring malaria. Similarly, drug addiction or the use of unclean hypodermic needles have been implicated as a means of transmitting the disease. With this means of infection the incubation period is usually short, generally depending on the number of parasites transmitted with the donor's blood. Malaria acquired as a result of blood transfusion can be an especially hazardous complication in view of the perilous condition of the patient requiring a blood transfusion and the difficulty in making the diagnosis of malaria for an unsuspecting physician, especially in nonmalarious areas.

REFERENCES

Brooks, M.H., Kiel, F.W., Sheehy, T.W., Barry, K.G. (1968). Acute pulmonary edema in falciparum malaria. *New Engl. J. Med. 279*, 732.

Coatney, G.R. (1976). Relapse in malaria - An enigma. *J. Parasit. 62*, 3.

Cohen, S. (1979). Immunity to malaria. *Proc. Roy. Soc. (Ser B) 203*, 323.

Hendricksen, R. (1972). Quartan malarial nephrotic syndrome. *Lancet 1*, 143.

Maegraith, B., and Fletcher, R. (1972). The pathogenesis of mammalian malaria. *Adv. Parasit. 10*, 49.

Miller, L.H., and Carter, R. (1976).   Innate resistance in
    malaria. *Exper. Parasit. 40,* 132.
Miller, L.H., Mason, S.J., Clyde, D.F., McGinniss, M.H. (1976).
    The resistance factor to Plasmodium vivax in Blacks.
    New Engl. J. Med. 295, 302.
Najem, G.R., and Sulzer, A.J. (1976). Transfusion - induced
    malaria from an asymptomatic carrier. *Transfusion 16,* 473.
Russell, P.F., West L.S., Manwell, R.D., MacDonald, G. (1963).
    Practical Malariology. 2nd Ed. London, Oxford Univ. Press.
World Health Organization. (1973). Chemotherapy of Malaria and
    Resistance to Antimalarials. WHO Tech. Rep. Series No. 529.
World Health Organization. (1975). Developments in Malaria
    Immunology. WHO Tech. Rep. Series No. 579.

SCHISTOSOMIASIS

Murray Wittner

Professor of Parasitology and Tropical Medicine
Albert Einstein College of Medicine
Bronx, New York

DEFINITION

Schistosomiasis, a chronic disease afflicting over 200 million people, is caused by several trematode species of the genus, *Schistosoma*. There are three medically important schistosomes: *S. mansoni, S. japonicum,* and *S. haematobium* causing either hepatosplenic or urinary tract disease. A fourth species infecting man has recently been described.

EPIDEMIOLOGY

The three common species are widely distributed in the tropical and subtropical world. *S. mansoni* is found in Africa, Puerto Rico, Vieques, portions of Santo Domingo, Surinam, Venezuela, Brazil, Guadeloupe, Martinique, St. Lucia and Arabia including Yemen. It has not been found in the Central American countries. *S. haematobium* is widespread in Africa and the Middle East. *S. japonicum* is a disease of the orient including China, Japan, Laos, Thailand, Celebes and the Philippines.

Of particular importance to American physicians is the influx of individuals from Puerto Rico, Santo Domingo and South America into urban areas. Currently it is estimated that perhaps 10-12 percent of the 1.5 million Puerto Ricans in mainland United States have chronic *Schistosoma mansoni* infection.

Among other ethnic groups the Yemeni population of the San Joaquin Valley in California has recently been surveyed and 56 percent of those studied had positive stool examination for *S. mansoni*. The lack of an appropriate snail intermediate host in continental United States, however, makes transmission of the disease here unlikely. Finally, as a result of agricultural irrigation development projects there has been a marked increase in schistosomiasis in Egypt and Rhodesia due to the spread of snail vectors into previously arid areas.

ETIOLOGY AND LIFE CYCLE

Adult worms of *S. mansoni* reside in mesenteric venules of the large intestine; those of *S. japonicum* in the small intestine and *S. haematobium* are found in the vesicle plexus of the urinary bladder. After pairing in the liver the slender female worm lies in a fold of the male body known as the gynecophoric canal. The ova are fully mature when passed in the feces and are readily distinguishable by their morphologic characteristics. The ovum of *S. mansoni* is ovoid 114 to 175 μM by 45 to 68 μM and possesses a characteristic lateral spine; *S. haematobium* has a terminal spine and measures 112 to 170 μM by 40 to 70 μM; and the *S. japonicum* ovum is ovoid 70 to 100 by 50 to 65 μM with an inconspicuous lateral spine. The average life span of a gravid female worm is probably about 5-10 years although they may live for much longer periods, i.e. 20 to 40 years. Ova are able to pass from blood vessels into the lumen of neighboring viscera, in part, by means of lytic enzyme secretions of the enclosed larva.

When excreta is diluted with fresh water the eggs hatch and a free-swimming ciliated larva, the miracidium, emerges, which has a life span of approximately six hours. If the miracidium penetrates an appropriate snail host, it rapidly undergoes development into a first generation sporocyst which subsequently produces hundreds of second generation sporocysts. Each sporocyst, in turn, may produce many fork-tailed cercariae. The end result is that one miracidium ultimately can produce thousands of cercariae.

Each of the schistosome species requires a specific snail host such as *Biomphalaria sp.* for *S. mansoni*, *Bulinus sp.* for *S. haematobium* and *Onchomelania sp.* for *S. japonicum*. The emerging cercariae rapidly penetrate the skin by mechanical as well as enzymatic means, shed their tails and enter the venous circulation as schistosomiles.

After about four days in the pulmonary circulation the schistosomules migrate to the liver, mature, pair and mate in the intrahepatic portal vessels. The adult worm pairs next, migrate out of the liver against the portal blood flow, and reach their destination in either mesenteric or vesicle venules where ovi-

position is initiated. Eggs may be found in the stool in 4-6
weeks for *S. japonicum*; 6-8 weeks for *S. mansoni* and in the urine
in 10-14 weeks for *S. haematobium*.

PATHOLOGY AND PATHOGENESIS

Ova may have one of three fates: 1) they may be excreted with
the feces or urine; 2) trapped in the intestinal or bladder wall
or 3) carried in the portal or systemic circulation only to be
filtered out in various organs. Eggs deposited in tissues provoke
granulomatous inflammation and eventually fibroblastic proliferation. An affected intestinal wall may become thickened, fibrotic,
rigid and lead to pseudopolyp formation.

In the liver ova evoke the formation of granulomata or "pseudo-
tubercules". Typically, these granuloma are composed of mononuclear cells, giant cells and eosinophiles. Recent studies
suggest that granuloma formation is a manifestation of cell
mediated immunity stimulated by the secretion from the ova of
"soluble egg antigen".

Pseudotubercule formation eventually leads to periportal
fibrosis (Symmer's "pipe stem fibrosis"). However, despite these
pathologic changes the hepatic parenchyma generally remains
functionally normal. Over many years, there is the gradual
development of presinusoidal hypertension and fibrocongestive
splenomegaly. As collateral venous circulation becomes prominent,
esophogeal varices, hemorrhoids, "caput medusae" or other manifestations of collateral venous varices may be seen. Ova embo-
lizing to the lung may cause endarteriolitis, periarteriolitis
with formation of angiomatoid bodies, as well as pulmonary
fibrosis.

S. haematobium infection often causes mucosal inflammation,
hyperplasia, pipillomata, fibrosis and calcification of the
urinary bladder. Hydronephrosis and pyelonephritis are common
complications. Squamous metaplasia, papillary carcinoma and
squamous cell carcinoma are found in heavily infected individuals.
Most authorities believe *S. haematobium* infection is responsible
for these neoplastic changes.

IMMUNOLOGIC ASPECTS

The terms "premunition" or "concomitant immunity" are used to
describe a form of acquired immunity in which the established
parasitic infection persists long after resistance has developed
against a challenge infection, perhaps the best example being
that of schistosomiasis. If adult schistosomes are transferred
to the portal vein of monkeys who have never experienced cercar-

ial invasion, they become resistant to subsequent infection with cercariae but their immune response does not reject the transferred adults. Thus the question is raised as to how it is possible for adult worms to engender an immune response which can prevent further infection by cercariae while remaining unaffected by the immune response they have stimulated. Among many explanations proposed for this phenomenon two have been most widely discussed. The first suggests that the parasite has evolved antigenic determinants similar to the host's by a process of natural selection. However, among the many objections to this hypothesis is that the adult worm can live in a variety of mammalian hosts and it is highly unlikely that it could have evolved major antigens common to all of these hosts. An alternative hypothesis suggested by Smithers and Terry is that schistosomes adapt to the range of hosts in which they live by appropriating host molecules onto their surface and, in effect, "disguise" themselves as being of host origin. Recent experimental evidence has amply demonstrated this phenomenon in *S. mansoni*. Thus, adult worms transferred from mice to monkeys that had been immunized against mouse erythrocytes failed to establish themselves and were killed by the monkey's immune system.

Moreover, in order to adequately explain concomitant immunity, it is further necessary to assume that host antigens are acquired by the adult worms but are not found on immature forms such as cercariae and early schistosomules. Recent studies suggest this to be the case.

In human infection host antigens acquired by schistosomulae and adults are believed to be human blood group antigens. In the mouse model, however, Scher has presented evidence that schistosomulae can acquire mouse histocompatibility antigens. This offers another means by which the parasite may disguise itself. There is, however, no conclusive evidence in human infection which establishes conclusively that such "mimicry" or antigenic disguise is responsible for the failure of rejection of adult worms by the host.

CLINICAL SYNDROMES

Several clinical syndromes are recognized in schistosomiasis. Penetration of the skin by cercariae may be accompanied by intense itching ("Kabure itch"), urticarial rash and occasional vesiculation. Systemic symptoms, however, are usually absent until the parasites have reached maturity.

The acute form of schistosomiasis is rarely seen in the United States. In the experience of the author during the past several years, only one case in over 200 seen in New York City had this syndrome. "Katayama fever", as it is often called, begins several weeks after exposure to cercariae and is most commonly associated with heavy *S. japonicum* infections although it is seen with the other species. The syndrome is characterized by intermittent bouts of fever, chills, abdominal pain, lymphadenopathy, hepatosplenomegaly, arthralgias, urticaria and periorbital edema. "Schistosomal dysentery" is a frequent finding especially in acute *S. mansoni* infection in which bloody diarrhea and mucous strands may be seen. A striking eosinophilia ranging from 20-60 percent is not uncommon and hypergammaglobinemia is often pronounced. The onset of Katayama fever is associated with the early egg laying period of the initial infection and may be so severe as to lead to the patient's demise. Recent studies suggest that acute schistosomiasis may be a form of immune complex disease.

Chronic schistosomiasis is most commonly encountered in practice and is the result of granulomatous inflammation and subsequent fibrosis in liver, bowel and urinary tract. The most severe cases usually result from heavy worm burdens whereas light infections rarely cause clinically important disease.

INTESTINAL SCHISTOSOMIASIS

Few ova trapped in the intestinal wall may be of little consequence. In some patients, however, if large numbers of eggs have been deposited, the large bowel and terminal ileum may be the site of major pathology. During the first few years of *Schistosomiasis mansoni* (or *japonicum*) patients may present with intermittent episodes of bloody diarrhea associated with mucous and tenesmus. Schistosomal granulomas may lead to the formation of papillomata or large polypoid non-neoplastic tumors. These lesions may be found in any portion of the large bowel and in some cases be palpable on abdominal examination. When present in the rectum, polyps may be mistaken for internal hemorrhoids and rectal prolapse has been reported. Polypoid lesions in the cecum may lead to intussusception. Enlarged, palpable abdominal lymph nodes are sometimes found. A rare patient may have schistosomal tumors of the peritoneum that closely resemble carcinomatosis. Barium enema sigmoidoscopy and colonoscopy are useful in confirming these bowel lesions.

HEPATOSPLENIC SCHISTOSOMIASIS

Hepatic involvement in schistosomiasis is the most common consequence of both *S. mansoni* and *japonicum* infections. One often finds hepatomegaly as the earliest sign of hepatic disease.

At this time the liver parenchyma is functionally spared as reflected by normal laboratory values for serum transaminases, albumin and bilirubin. Mild to moderate increases in alkaline phosphatase are seen.

As granulomatous inflammation progresses to portal fibrosis presinusoidal portal hypertension intervenes; often the spleen is enlarged and easily palpable. Because hepatic lesions are presinusoidal, intrasplenic and portal pressures are elevated whereas wedged hepatic vein pressure is normal. Total hepatic blood flow is normal as a result of increased hepatic arterial perfusion. When significant portal hypertension occurs hepatosplenomegaly increases and esophageal and gastric varices may result. Hematemesis from these ruptured vessels is the major life-threatening complication of this syndrome. Anemia and pancytopenia often is the result of hypersplenism. Most other clinical stigmata of chronic liver disease such as palmar erythema, spider angiomata, ascites and edema are not often found in *S. mansoni* infection. In some patients hepatic dysfunction may be progressive leading ultimately to cirrhosis and liver failure. It should be recognized, however, that progression of hepatic-splenic disease may take place over a 15 to 20 year period. Where alcoholism and drug abuse co-exist with schistosomiasis, the natural course of hepatosplenic disease may be accelerated.

SCHISTOSOMIASIS OF THE GENITO-URINARY TRACT

Infection with *S. haematobium* results in fibrosis and calcification of the bladder and ureters. The most characteristic early manifestation of urinary tract disease is terminal hematuria which may be accompanied by dysuria, frequency, urgency and suprapubic pain. Hematuria is often exacerbated by physical exertion. This clinical sign is usually the result of mucosal ulceration of the bladder, especially in those areas in which large collections of eggs have calcified. These areas have a characteristic quality on cystoscopy and are called "sandy patches". As the disease progresses, blood is seen throughout the urinary stream. When reinfection does not occur, the hematuria gradually disappears over months to years although egg excretion continues. *S. haematobium* ova can become the nucleus of stone formation. Eventually the bladder wall becomes fibrotic, irregular and loses its elasticity. Finally, the bladder becomes calcified and contracted with limitation on volume and motility. Frequency and dribbling are seen as a consequence of these findings. Bacterial cystitis associated with hematuria and pyuria may complicate schistosomiasis of the bladder. Obstructive lesions of the ureter lead to dilation and hydronephrosis and are often associated with decreased maximal urine concentration with early antischistosomal therapy. These lesions may be reversible.

Ureteral stenosis and vesicoureteric reflux may lead to frequent urinary tract infections. These repeated bouts of infection may ultimately lead to renal impairment. Patients with urinary tract schistosomiasis may be chronic *Salmonella* excreters.

PULMONARY SCHISTOSOMIASIS

Pulmonary involvement in schistosomiasis can be seen with any of the three schistosome species. In *S. haematobium* infection, ova frequently embolize from the vesicle plexus via the vena cava to the lung. In hepatosplenic disease caused by *S. japonicum* and *S. mansoni*, severe pulmonary involvement is often seen in those patients with portal hypertension. The collateral circulation resulting from portal hypertension enables the ova to bypass the liver only to be trapped in the pulmonary circulation. These ova obstruct the pulmonary arterioles occasionally reaching the capillaries.

Patients with clinically significant pulmonary schistosomiasis present with dyspnea and an accentuated second pulmonic sound. The chest x-ray may reveal mottled lung fields, pulmonary fibrosis, enlargement of the right ventricle and of the pulmonary artery segment in the hilum. As disease progresses hemoptysis, cough, chest pain and cyanosis are seen and pulmonary function tests may confirm arterial desaturation. Abnormalities in diffusion capacity are pronounced at this time. An occasional patient has been reported in whom a "coin lesion" on chest x-ray was found to be a large schistosome granuloma.

SCHISTOSOMIASIS OF THE CENTRAL NERVOUS SYSTEM

Schistosomal involvement of the central nervous system is an uncommon clinical complication. *S. japonicum* may involve the brain, whereas *S. haematobium* and *S. mansoni* are most often reported to affect the spinal cord. *S. japonicum* may present as generalized encephalitis or as a space occupying lesion and may be an important cause of epilepsy in endemic areas.

DIAGNOSIS

The diagnosis of schistosomiasis should be considered in anyone coming from an endemic area who has hepatic disease, abdominal pain, abnormalities in bowel habits, terminal hematuria or dysuria. It should be noted, however, that the only definitive method of diagnosing schistosomiasis is the demonstration of viable ova in stool, urine, bladder or rectal biopsy.

Since eggs are not excreted at regular intervals, at least three separate stool specimens on three consecutive days should be examined. In those cases where there is heavy infection, ova may be seen on direct smear. However, it is routine to employ concentration and/or sedimentation methods in order to increase the chances of finding eggs, moreover because of the direct correlation between fecal egg excretion and intensity of infection, a quantitative egg count such as the one developed by Kato is often used. In patients suspected of having *S. haematobium* infection a midday urine should be centrifuged and the sediment examined for ova. Early in the disease these ova are frequently observed in terminal bloody urine but as the disease progresses, ova are found with equal frequency throughout the urine stream. It should be emphasized that the discovery of eggs alone is not sufficient to initiate therapy since therapy is directed only at active cases, i.e. those in which viable ova can be demonstrated. For this purpose ova are viewed under a microscope in which transmitted light is reduced in order that the miracidium's flame cell flagellum can be seen actively beating, or the finding of free swimming miracidia in distilled water (hatch test). Rectal biopsy specimens should be obtained from the valve area, pressed between two microscope slides and viewed under a microscope for evidence of viability as described above.

There are several immunological methods available for the diagnosis of schistosomiasis. Skin tests may be useful in adults but less so in children. However, the *Schistosoma* skin test may cross react with that of trichinosis. In patients with CNS schistosomiasis and negative stool examination the skin test may provide the only positive indication of schistosomal infection. The complement fixation test becomes positive early in the infection but the titers usually decline with chronicity; the circumoval precipitin test is a research tool which is specific, and can be used as a guide in evaluating therapy; it becomes negative about six months after therapeutic cure. It should be recognized that in evaluating an individual for therapy with possible exception of CNS schistosomiasis; the presence of viable eggs in stool, urine or biopsy must establish the definitive diagnosis.

TREATMENT

Medical treatment of schistosomiasis has changed markedly
in the past several years. New, highly effective, and orally
administered drugs with low toxicity have been introduced.
For *S. mansoni* infections a new FDA approved drug, Oxamniquine,
is the drug of choice. It is administered to patients from the
Caribbean or South America in a single oral dose of 15 mg/kg
of body weight. For those patients from Africa the dose is
60 mg/kg. Side effects include a short period of dizziness,
abdominal pain and discoloration of the urine. A seizure history
is the only contraindication. For *S. haematobium* infection
Metrifonate is the drug of choice. It is given orally as 10 mg/
kg body weight every other week for 3 doses. Red cell levels
of acetylcholine esterase should be monitored and each dose
given only after the esterase has returned to at least 70% of
the base line level.

S. japonicum is treated orally with Niridazole at 25 mg/kg/day
for 10 days. This drug has numerous side effects such as nausea,
vomiting, insomnia and discoloration of urine. Occasionally
severe neuropsychiatric symptoms occur and may require cessation
of therapy. Surgical intervention for portal hypertension
is occasionally required.

A new oral drug which is highly effective against *S. japoni-*
cum, Praziquantel, is not available in the United States at
this time.

PREVENTION

Though mass education programs have been partially successful
in reducing schistosomiasis in some areas, especially Puerto
Rico, in other areas almost 100 percent of the population over
two years of age are infected. The use of molluscicides such as
copper salts, biological methods and mass chemotherapy have all
met with little success.

Currently, research is aimed at developing a vaccine for
prevention as well as new therapeutic agents of low toxicity that
can be administered safely to large populations.

PROGNOSIS

In most cases of schistosomiasis light infection has little
if any sequelae even if untreated. The best prognosis is in early
or light infections treated promptly. In moderate to heavy

infection, severe intestinal or hepatosplenic disease with portal
hypertension, bleeding esophageal varices and hepatic failure
may result. Advanced cases of *S. haematobium* infections may lead
to irreversible renal failure.

REFERENCES

Warren, K.S. (1972). The immunopathogenesis of schistosomiasis.
A multidisciplinary approach. *Trans. Roy. Soc. Trop. Med.
& Hyg. 66*, 217–434.
Cavallo, T., Galvanek, E.G., Ward, R.A. and von Lichtonberg, F.
(1974). The nephropathy of experimental hepatosplenic
schistosomiasis. *Am. J. Path. 76*, 433–446.
Warren, K.S. (1966). The pathogenesis of "clay-pipe stem cirr-
hosis" in mice with chronic schistosomiasis mansoni with a
note on the longevity of schistosomes. *Amer. J. Path. 49*,
477–489.
Cheever, A.W. (1968). A quantitative postmortem study of
Schistosomiasis mansoni in man. *Amer. J. Trop. Med. Hyg.
17*, 38.
Warren, K.S., Mahmound, A.A.F., Cummings, P., Murphy, D.J., and
Houser, H.B. (1974). Schistosomiasis mansoni in Yemeni
in California, duration of infection, presence of disease,
therapeutic management. *Am. J. Trop. Med. Hyg. 23*, 902–909.
Mahmound, A.A.F, and Warren, K.S. (1974). Anti-inflammatory
effect of tartar emetic and niridazole: suppression of
schistosome egg granuloma. *J. Imm. 112*, 222–228.
Smith, J.H., Said, M.N., and Kelada, A.S. (1977). Studies
on schistosomiasis rectal and colonicpolyposis. *Am. J.
Trop. Med. Hyg. 26*, 80–84.

CHAGAS' DISEASE

Publio Toala
Alberto Brown
Carlos Russo

University of Panama Medical School
Complejo Hospitalario Metropolitano del
Seguro Social and Hospital Santo Tomas
Panama City, Panama

Chagas' disease (American trypanosomiasis) is a zoonotic disease caused by *Trypanosoma cruzi* (Chagas 1909). *Trypanosoma rangeli* (Tejera 1920), produces a mild parasitemia in man, but does not invade or destroy tissue cells nor cause other evidence of disease. It was in our hospital, Santo Tomas, that the first three cases of Chagas' disease were diagnosed, early in 1930 in the Republic of Panama. Since then a great deal of research has been done clinically, experimentally and in the epidemiology of the disease.

ETIOLOGY

T. cruzi is a flagellate protozoan that circulates in the blood of man and undergoes intracellular transformation to oval or spherical nonflagellate forms, the leishmanial form. *T. cruzi* can be distinguished by a tendency to assume a "C" or "U" shape when fixed, by the location and size of the kinetoplast at the extreme posterior (aflagellate), by its narrow undulating membrane, and by its length, 16-22 microns (average 20). *T. rangeli* has a broader undulating membrane, a less prominent kinetoplast located between the compact nucleus and the posterior end, and measures 27-32 microns (average 31). Contrary to *T. cruzi*, *T. rangeli* multiplies in the blood of man by binary fusion. Intracellular forms of this parasite haven't been described. In both species the blepharoplast, the parabasal rod from which the flagellum arises, and the nucleus stain red with Giemsa stain;

309

the cytoplasm and undulating membrane stain light blue. *T. cruzi*
grows well in tissue cultures, but the Novy, McNeal and Nicolles
medium, a saline agar with 10 percent defibrinated rabbit blood
in which the parasites develop in the water of condensation
after one to six weeks, is most commonly employed. Although
the most common developmental form of the parasite which is
usually seen in an intracellular location is the leishmanial
form, the leptomonad, crithidial and trypanosome forms also occur.

TRANSMISSION

Several species of triatomid (reduviid) bugs transmit
T. cruzi. A bug may remain infected for life (years). Larvae,
nymphs, and adult bugs ingest trypanosomes when taking blood
meals from infected animals. The parasites then multiply and
differentiate in the alimentary tract of the bug from leishmanial
forms, to crithidial forms, and finally to metacyclic trypomasti-
gotes (trypanosomes). The latter congregate in the rectum of
the bug and are discharged in its feces. Infection of mammals
takes place by ingestion of infected bugs and also by contamination of mucous membranes, conjunctivae, and abraded skin with
fecal material from infected bugs. Reservoir hosts of *T. cruzi*
include marsupials, edentates, bats, rodents, carnivores, pigs,
and primates.
T. cruzi infections of man have been acquired by blood
transfusion, by accidental contamination with infected blood or
cultures in laboratories, and congenitally by transplacental
passage of parasites. There are approximately 25,000 cases of
transfusion-induced Chagas' disease in Brazil annually. This
is due to the fact that many blood donors have an inapparent
parasitemia with *T. cruzi* and are free of clinical manifestations.
Transplacental transmission and congenital infection are well-
recognized causes of abortion and neonatal morbidity in endemic
areas. Less is known about the transmission of *T. rangeli,* but
T. rangeli is transmitted by only a few species of triatomid
bugs, most or all of which belong to the genus Rhodnius.
Infection by blood meal and multiplication and growth of various
forms in the alimentary tract of the bugs proceed as with
T. cruzi, except for the site of the development of metacyclic
trypanosomes. About six weeks post-infection, flagellated
parasites penetrate the gut wall, pass through the hemocoelom
and invade the salivary glands of the bug. Here, metacyclic
trypanosomes develop and multiply. Thus, the actual bites
of infected bugs transmit *T. rangeli*, a more efficient mechanism
than the fecal contamination method of *T. cruzi*.

GEOGRAPHICAL DISTRIBUTION

More than eight million persons living in the region from Argentina to Texas are infected with *T. cruzi*. The major focus of infection is located in the state of Minas Gerais in Brazil. The World Health Organization estimated that over 35 million persons in Latin America are exposed to this infection.

Bugs and mammals infected with *T. cruzi* have been found on the American continents between latitudes of 42N (northern California and Maryland) and 43S (southern Argentina and Chile), and on the islands of Aruba and Trinidad.

Infection by *T. cruzi* is most often acquired by rural and suburban poor people whose homes and ways of life permit close contact with infected bugs. Some species of triatomid are wild and rarely infect man; others, such as *Triatoma infestans*, *T. sordida*, and *T. dimidiata* are domestic or paradomestic and cause thousands or millions of infections in man. Infections of bugs, man, and other reservoir hosts with *T. rangeli* have been found with variable prevalence in most Central and South American countries. This variation depends on distribution and on sampling. *T. rangeli* is common in Panama.

PATHOGENESIS AND PATHOLOGY

Acute Chagas' Disease

The trypanosomes directly invade the cells of the reticulo-endothelial system, myocardium, smooth and skeletal muscles, and the central and autonomic nervous systems. The extent of actual destruction in the acute phase of the disease is the most important determinant of the chronic state. In the acute state, leishmanial pseudocysts can be demonstrated in most tissues.

The pathological findings in fatal cases of acute Chagas' disease were described in detail by Chagas (1911), Cronwell (1923) and others. The main macroscopic findings are generalized edema, especially in the face, generalized swelling of the lymph nodes, serous effusions in the body cavities, hyperemia and edema of the brain, spinal cord and meninges, punctiform hemorrhages in the brain, dilatation of the heart with flabby, friable and spotted myocardium, serofibrinous pericarditis, acute swelling of the liver and the spleen. Microscopically, in all organs or tissues are found variable quantities of parasitic pseudocysts and acute inflammatory foci, containing numerous eosinophils. In the heart, collections of parasites are present in the myofibers. Rupture of fibers is associated with microabscesses, phagocytosis and digestion of parasites, and an extensive and severe inflammatory reaction with lymphocytes, macrophages and plasma cells. Fragmentation, vacuolization, hyalinization, destruction of myofibers,

interstitial edema, and obliteration of capillaries and veins
are present. The coronary arteries are spared, but some degree
of endocarditis and pericarditis is usual. Inflammation and
parasitization of the sinus node and atrio-ventricular node
have been found. Parasites invade neurons and glial cells of the
brain and spinal cord, and, less commonly, the perivascular
spaces. Inflammatory reaction includes perivascular cuffing
by lymphocytes, focal infiltrates of lymphocytes in the meninges,
and small nodules comprised of glial cells, lymphocytes, and
plasma cells.

Congenital Chagas' Disease

In some pregnant women with parasitemia, the placenta and
fetus are infected even without maternal symptoms. This commonly
leads to abortion. Most babies born alive with *T. cruzi* infections die within a few days or weeks of Chagasic encephalitis.
Congenital Chagas' disease should be distinguished from the
common occurrence of a mother with a positive complement fixation (CF) test giving birth to a CF positive baby because of a
transient persistence of maternal antibody in the baby's blood.
It has been stated that the rate of transmission of *T. cruzi*
from infected humans to their offspring is low, and the reason
that *T. cruzi* crosses the placenta in such a small proportion is
unknown. Experimentally it has been shown that the transplacental
transmission of *T. cruzi* in mice is dependent on two factors:
pathogenicity of the strain of *T. cruzi*, and blockade of phagocytic activity, suggesting that transplacental transmission of
T. cruzi is related to interference with the phagocytic activity
of the placenta.

Chronic Chagas' Disease

Chronic Chagas' Disease afflicts millions of Americans. In
most of these, chronic Chagas' disease develops years or decades
after an episode of undetected parasitemia, or, less commonly,
following a recognized episode of acute Chagas' disease. As
the disease becomes chronic, the leishmanial forms are difficult
to locate. Chronic chagasic cardiopathy is present wherever
there is chronic Chagas' disease. The principal gross change
in the heart is generalized enlargement and dilatation with
predominant involvement of the right heart and strikingly of the
right atrium. There is frequently a yellowish mottling of the
myocardium. Thinning of the muscle wall of the ventricles and
principally of the right atrium is very characteristic. Transillumination shows the translucent areas very distinctly. In the
great majority of cases the chagasic heart shows dilatation of

all chambers, again predominantly on the right side and almost
always excessively pronounced in the right atrium, which appears
translucent. The thickness of the wall of the ventricles is
variable according to the degree of the dilatation of the
cavities and to the secondary degenerative lesions of the
myocardium.

More than half of the chagasic hearts disclose a very odd
alteration at the apex. This lesion consists of a thinning and
bulging of the apical region, mainly of the left ventricle,
producing the so-called aneurysm of the heart. Thrombosis of
this aneurysm is common. Even without aneurysm formation, extensive mural thrombosis in the lower part of the left ventricle may
be seen, and in cases with cardiomegaly a massive thrombosis of
the right auricle is almost always present. Thrombosis of the
left auricle is uncommon. The myocardium of the lower part of
the ventricles shows fibrotic scars. Marked atrophy and slight
fibrosis on the tracular carneae of both apical regions, as well
as in the papillary muscles of the left ventricle in cases of
accentuated cardiomegaly, are frequent.

Although coronary arteries are usually normal, capillaries
and small veins are dilated and irregular. Microscopically,
focal areas of chronic myocarditis contain infiltrates of
lymphocytes and plasma cells and streaks and patches of interstitial fibrosis among hypertrophied myofibers. Apical lesions
regularly appear as segments of acellular fibrous tissue
associated with epicardial vessels and adipose tissue. Fibrosis,
inflammation, and atrophy with partial replacement by adipose
tissue may be found in the A-V node or in the major conduction
bundles. Köberle has found decreased numbers of ganglion cells
in the posterior wall of the right atrium. Rarely nests of
leishmania may be found in the center of the circumscribed or
granulomatous inflammatory foci. Parasitic pseudocysts are rarely
seen.

In chronic Chagas' disease alterations of motility of hollow
muscular organs and its final morphological expression, hypertrophy of the muscle wall and dilatation of the organ, are known
as enteromegaly (megaesophagus, megacolon, megaureter, etc.).
In 800 autopsies of chagasic patients Köberle found 172 (34.4%)
cases of megacolon and 158 cases of megaesophagus (31.6%). It
is interesting to emphasize that in our experience and others in
Panama and Central America we have not found such cases of enteromegaly. Gross examination shows the characteristic dilatation
and hypertrophy of the musculature. Microscopically the most
impressive feature is the hypertrophy of the muscularis propia.
The increase in thickness of this muscular mass is always more
evident in the inner layer than in the outer layer. Köberle
has found an absence of 95% of the ganglion cells of the myenteric
plexuses.

CLINICAL MANIFESTATIONS

Acute Chagas' Disease

After an incubation period of one to two weeks the disease begins with tiredness, headache, and fever of variable intensity. Other complaints include irritability, palpitations and diarrhea. Very infrequently the site of the bug bite is evident with local adenopathy. Unilateral periorbital edema with mild conjunctivitis, a darkish discoloration of the skin and satellite lymphadenopathy are characteristic findings (Romaña's sign). The usual patient is a toxic, febrile infant or young adult with nontender generalized lymphadenopathy, tender hepatosplenomegaly, tachycardia with a gallop rhythm, and other signs of congestive heart failure. Acute meningoencephalitis is often fatal. Between 10 and 20 percent of patients die of irreversible cardiac failure or ventricular fibrillation. Survivors recover slowly and are often well six to eight weeks after the onset. Some have persistent electrocardiographic changes, particularly right bundle branch block. Infections acquired by blood transfusions are frequently fatal, probably because of the massive infective dose. Laboratory workers that have been infected accidentally by animal blood or cultures sometimes develop severe myocarditis.

Congenital Chagas' Disease

Abortion is a common feature in pregnant women with parasitemia. As stated previously, most infected babies die within a few days or weeks of contracting Chagas' disease.

Chronic Chagas' Disease

Chronic Chagas' myocardiopathy is manifested as palpitations, syncopal episodes, or recurrent congestive heart failure. Cardiac death may occur from cardiac failure, but the most characteristic death is a sudden and unexpected one. Chagas reported that in Minais Gerais, almost every family lost one or more of its members by this typical sudden cardiac death. A multiplicity of electrocardiographic changes include ventricular extrasystoles, right bundle branch block and atrioventricular blocks. Mural thrombosis is common and results in cerebral, renal, splenic and pulmonary embolism.

Megaesophagus is manifested by dysphagia for solid foods, progressing to difficulty in swallowing liquids and the regurgitation of food. X-ray examination shows dilatation of the esophagus mainly of the lower segment. Advanced cases also show elongation of the esophagus. Functional study reveals retention

of contrast material which passes gradually at long and irregular
intervals through the cardia into the stomach. The main symptom
of megacolon is a difficulty or an impossibility of evacuation.
Patients who do not defecate for two to four months are not unusual
and in some cases this may even last five or six months. It is
remarkable that many of these patients feel no discomfort and
come to the hospital because of some complication, e.g., volvulus
of a dilated sigmoid loop, fecaloma with decubitus ulcer, peritonitis due to perforation of the ulcer, etc.

DIAGNOSIS

The demonstration of *T. cruzi* in the peripheral blood on
microscopic examination or by xenodiagnosis is diagnostic of
acute Chagas' disease. Xenodiagnosis utilizes laboratory bred
triatomes which are allowed to feed on the patients for 15
minutes. They are then examined at 30 and 60 days for trypanosomes in the feces or the gut. Recent research utilizing first
instar *Dipetalogaster maximus* provides a more economic method
for testing patients.
    Agglutination and precipitin tests are immediately positive.
After 30 days the CF test (Gerreiro-Machado) becomes positive.
Recently a rapid slide flocculation test was compared with hemagglutination, immunofluorescence and CF tests and was found to be
useful for screening procedures in blood banks, and in field
conditions for the diagnosis of acute and chronic Chagas' disease.
Also studies done with the enzyme-linked immunosorbent assay
(ELISA) shows that this assay is a promising serologic test for
measuring antibodies to *T. cruzi* in individuals and populations.
Chronic Chagas' disease is diagnosed by CF, hemagglutination
inhibition, immunofluorescence antibodies and ELISA. X-rays
of chest, esophagus and colon will detect visceromegaly; functional tests when indicated will be helpful. Electrocardiographic
changes will indicate the existence of right bundle branch block
with left axis deviation and multifocal premature ventricular
contractions. About 20 percent of patients with chronic disease
will have a positive xenodiagnosis test.
    Differential diagnosis in the acute state will be the same
as Fever of Unknown Origin (FUO) with general adenopathy and
hepatosplenomegaly. Infectious mononucleosis, tuberculosis,
toxoplasmosis, salmonella infections, rheumatoid arthritis,
acute leukemia, lymphoma, and the collagen diseases have to
be ruled out.
    In congenital disease, syphilis, listeriosis, toxoplasmosis,
rubella and cytomegalovirus disease have to be considered in the
differential diagnosis. Rheumatic heart disease has to be considered, and hypertension, coronary artery disease and other

causes of cardiomegaly have to be excluded in the workup of chronic Chagas' disease. Carcinoma of the esophagus, idiopathic achalasia, toxic megacolon and ulcerative colitis must be considered in the evaluation of enteromegaly.

TREATMENT

In contrast with the relative success in the treatment of African trypanosomiasis, chemotherapy for Chagas' disease has been disappointing. Nitrofurans, pyrimethamine, primaquine, Bayer 2502 (Nifurtimox) and more recently metronidazole have been used with moderate success in removing parasites from the blood, in the acute phase. Table 1 summarizes data on some of the drugs used orally by Blandon and coworkers in Panamanian children. For the chronic state of the disease there are only general and symptomatic treatments. Congestive failure must be treated as well as cardiac arrhythmias. Digitalis must be used with great caution because of the extreme irritability of the myocardium, especially in the presence of hypokalemia. Symptomatic treatment is indicated for enteromegaly; dilatation of the esophagus and surgical resection are used in different stages of the disease; whereas resection of the colon or rectum are also used for treatment of volvulus of the colon.

Table 1. Drugs Used in Acute Chagas' Disease

Drug	Dosage	Duration
Primaquine	7.5-15.0 mg/kg/day	14-21 days
Bayer 2502 (Nifurtimox)	25 mg/kg/day (max 300-400 mg/day)	90 days
Levofuraltadone	25 mg/kd/day	40 days
Metronidazole	750-1000 mg/day (3-4 times a day)	180 days
Isopentaquine	5 mg/day	14 days

REMAINING PROBLEMS

Chagas' disease is primarily a socio-economic problem. Better housing is crucial, especially in rural areas. It is necessary to identify more precisely the transmission of the parasite to man and to improve ways and means of eradicating vectors. Blood transfusion transmitted infection is preventable and donors should be thoroughly screened in endemic areas. Money and human resources must be used for large clinical controlled trials in the search for chemotherapy of parasitemia and tissue forms.

REFERENCES

Bittencourt, A.L. (1976). Congenital Chagas disease. *Am. J. Dis. Chil. 130,* 97-103.
Blandón, R., Guevara, J.F., and Johnson, C.M. (1976). Enfermedad de Chagas aguda en niños, sintomatologia y tratamiento. *Rev. Med. Panamá 1(3),* 153-162.
Cerisola, J.A., Rabinovich, A., Alvarez, M., et al. (1972) Enfermedad de Chagas y la transfusión de sangre. *Bol. Ofic. Sanit. Panam. 73,* 203-221.
Chemotherapy of Chagas' disease. Chapter IX, 9.1-9.36. *In* The Chemotherapy of Protozoan Diseases (A. Steck). Walter Reed Army Institute.
Edgcomb, J.H., Johnson, C.M. (1976). American trypanosomiasis (Chagas' disease). *In* Pathology of Tropical and Extraordinary Diseases. H. Binford and H. Connor, Armed Forces Institute of Pathology, Washington, D.C.
Köberle, F. (1968). Chagas' disease and Chagas syndromes: The Pathology of American trypanosomiasis. *Advances Parasitol. Vol. 6,* 63-116.
Woody, N.C. and Woody, H.B. (1955). American trypanosomiasis (Chagas' disease). First indigenous case in the United States. *J. Amer. Med. Assoc. 159,* 476-477.

INFECTION AND DISEASE DUE TO <u>TOXOPLASMA GONDII</u>[1]

Jay P. Siegel[2]
Jack S. Remington

Division of Infectious Diseases
Department of Medicine
Stanford University School of Medicine
Stanford, California

Division of Immunology and Infectious Diseases
Research Institute, Palo Alto Medical Foundation
Palo Alto, California

INTRODUCTION

<u>Toxoplasma</u> <u>gondii</u> is one of the most common organisms which infects humans the world over. Despite this fact, physicians have only recently come to recognize the importance of this organism as a significant pathogen of humans. In its congenital form, toxoplasmosis may result in significant brain and eye damage. In older children and adults, toxoplasmosis may cause significant visual impairment; and in individuals with compromised immune defenses, the infection often causes life-threatening illness.

I. THE INFECTION AND THE DISEASE

A. *Epidemiology.*

T. <u>gondii</u> is an obligate intracellular protozoan which has as its definitive host members of the cat family. The oocyst form is excreted by cats in their feces and, after sporulation, is highly infectious for humans and other mammals. It can survive for months or years in warm, moist soil. Infection may be acquired through ingestion of undercooked meat containing tissue cysts or through ingestion of oocysts. During acute infection, the tachyzoites disseminate widely and ultimately they encyst in many organs but mainly in muscle and

[1] *This work was supported by Grant AI04717 from the National Institutes of Health.*

[2] *Recipient of a Leukemia Society of America, Inc. Fellowship and an Edith Milo Fellowship.*

brain.

When women acquire infection during pregancy, the fetus is at risk for congenital toxoplasmosis. The later in pregnancy that Toxoplasma infection is acquired, the more likely it is that placental transmission to the fetus will occur. The transmission rate is approximately 15% when infection is acquired in the first trimester, approximately 30% in the second trimester, and approximately 65% in the third trimester. Infected babies born of mothers who acquired their infection in the first trimester are generally severely abnormal; whereas those born of mothers who acquired their infection during the third trimester are almost always without signs of the infection. There is no concrete evidence that latent Toxoplasma infection acquired prior to pregnancy can be transmitted to the fetus; if this occurs, it must be exceedingly rare.

B.   *Clinical Features*

The vast majority of infections due to Toxoplasma in humans are asymptomatic. Although the term "toxoplasmosis" is often used improperly to include all infections due to Toxoplasma, it should be used only to refer to the disease which results when the infection becomes clinically apparent. Toxoplasmosis occurs as distinct entities: congenital toxoplasmosis, acquired toxoplasmosis, ocular toxoplasmosis, and acute toxoplasmosis in the immunocompromised patient.

1. Congenital Toxoplasmosis - Approximately 75% of newborns with congenital infection due to Toxoplasma are without signs of the infection at birth. Recent data suggest that more than 85% of these newborns will later manifest one or more sequelae of the infection including hearing loss, chorioretinitis, impaired vision, delayed psychomotor development, and mental retardation. Approximately 8% of newborns with congenital infection due to Toxoplasma have severe disease usually involving the eyes or the central nervous system or both. Neonates with clinically apparent disease may have any combination of the following: hydrocephalus, microcephaly, cerebral calcifications, seizure disorders, psychomotor retardation, microophthalmia, strabismus, cataracts, glaucoma, chorioretinitis, optic atrophy, deafness, lymphadenopathy, pneumonitis, jaundice, and rash.

2. Acquired Toxoplasmosis - In normal persons, acquired Toxoplasma infection most frequently is subclinical or presents with lymphadenopathy. The adenopathy is usually cervical and often only a single node is appreciably enlarged; however submental and pectoral adenopathy are not uncommon and the adenopathy may be in any location or may be generalized.

The nodes are discrete, nonsuppurative, and variable in tenderness and firmness. This lymphadenopathic form is self-limited and is most often asymptomatic; it may, however, be accompanied by fever, malaise, myalgia, sore throat, headache, rash, or hepatosplenomegaly. It rarely simulates infectious mononucleosis. Occasionally, in normal persons, acquired toxoplasmosis may cause serious infection manifested by myocarditis, pericarditis, hepatitis, polymyositis, pneumonitis, or encephalitis. Chorioretinitis occurs rarely.

3. Ocular Toxoplasmosis - Latent Toxoplasma infection is thought to account for approximately 35% of cases of chorioretinitis. The large majority of cases are congenital in origin; cases of Toxoplasma chorioretinitis in adolescents and adults usually represent reactivation of congenital infection. It has been estimated that chorioretinitis occurs in approximately 1% of patients with acute acquired infection. The acute lesions appear as yellow-white elevated patches with indistinct margins surrounded by hyperemia. Older lesions are gray-white plaques with distinct borders. Often multiple lesions of various ages are seen. Lesions are often perimacular.

4. Acute Toxoplasmosis in the Immunocompromised Patient - Immunocompromised patients (e.g. patients with hematologic malignancies, lymphomas, Hodgkin's disease, organ transplants, or patients receiving immunosuppressive therapy) may develop serious and often fatal disease due to reactivation of latent infection or, less often, as a result of the acute infection. In these patients clinical signs of the infection are most often referable to the central nervous system; encephalitis is the most common manifestation; myocarditis and pneumonitis are frequently seen; and a wide variety of organ systems may be involved. Cerebrospinal fluid studies, electroencephalogram and computer tomographic brain scan may present a picture consistent with encephalitis and/or brain abscess.

II. DIAGNOSIS

The various forms of toxoplasmosis may present with physical findings, abnormal complete blood count, abnormal cerebrospinal fluid, and abnormal radiologic studies; however, none of these need be present and none are diagnostic. The diagnosis may be definitively established by isolation of the organism, by demonstration of Toxoplasma in tissues, or by serological test results.

A. *Diagnostic Methods*

1. Isolation of T. gondii - This is accomplished by inoculation of body tissues or fluids from infected patients
into mice or tissue culture. Infected mice are identified by
seroconversion and by the presence of cysts in their brains.
In tissue culture, the organism may be seen intracellularly;
this method of diagnosis is not generally available or necessary but may be useful in select cases. Isolation of the organism from tissues may reflect latent infection with the
cyst form and does not necessarily prove the presence of
acute infection with tachyzoites; isolation from body fluids
however is strong evidence for active acute infection.

2. Histology - Demonstration of tachyzoites in tissue (e.g.
brain biopsy, bone marrow aspirate) or body fluids (e.g.
cerebrospinal fluid, amniotic fluid) is diagnostic of acute
toxoplasmosis. Immunospecific stains employing fluorescent
antibodies or peroxidase antiperoxidase reagents increase the
ability to identify tachyzoites which often stain poorly by
routine methods. The demonstration of the tissue cyst does
not distinguish between active and latent chronic infection.
A characteristic histological appearance has been described
which, when present, is diagnostic of Toxoplasma lymphadenitis.

3. Serology - Several useful serological tests are summarized in Table 1. In general, the Group 1 tests (DT, conventional IFA, CF, and IHA) become positive early in infection
and remain positive, often at high titers, for years. However,
IHA titers may not become positive until considerably later in
acute infection than the other titers; and therefore IHA should
not be used for diagnosis of infection with Toxoplasma in the neonate or in pregnant women. Group 2 tests (IgM-IFA and DS-IgM-
ELISA) become positive early and usually revert to negative or
low titers within several months.

A single high titer on a Group 2 test (IgM-IFA $\geq$ 1:64 or DS-
IgM-ELISA > 1:256) is diagnostic of infection acquired within
recent weeks or months. A single conventional IFA or DT titer
of 1:2000 or greater (or a very high CF titer) is strongly suggestive of infection acquired within recent months but occasionally may be seen years after infection. When sera obtained at
different times from a patient are run in parallel in any of these
tests, a serial two-tube rise in titer is diagnostic of recent
acute infection.

In some countries, it may be cost effective to screen
pregnant women serologically so that when acute infection acquired during pregnancy is demonstrated, early treatment of
the pregnant woman or abortion may be considered. Women who

TABLE 1. Guidelines for Interpretation of Results of Serological Tests for Antibodies against Toxoplasma[a]

	Positive titer	Titer in acute infection	Titer in chronic infection	Duration of elevation of titer
Group 1[b]				
Sabin-Feldman dye test (DT)[c]	1:4, undiluted[d]	$\geq$ 1:1000	1:4-1:2000	years
Indirect fluorescent antibody test (conventional IFA)	1:10	$\geq$ 1:1000	1:4-1:2000	years
Indirect hemagglutination test (IHA)[e]	1:16	$\geq$ 1:1000	1:16-1:256	years
Complement fixation test	1:4	Varies among laboratories	Negative to 1:8	years
Group 2				
IFA for IgM anti-Toxoplasma antibodies (IgM-IFA)[f]	1:2 infants 1:16 adults	$\geq$ 1:64	Negative to 1:20	weeks to months
Double sandwich ELISA for IgM (DS-IgM-ELISA)	1:64	$\geq$ 1:256	Negative to 1:64	months to years

[a] *Exceptions to those generalizations may occur. Also, values obtained in different laboratories may differ significantly.*

[b] *Measures mainly IgG antibodies.*

[c] *The World Health Organization has recommended that DT titers be expressed in international units per ml.*

[d] *In Toxoplasma chorioretinitis, the DT may be positive in undiluted serum only.*

[e] *The IHA may give false negative results early in infection. Therefore, IHA should not be used to detect congenital infection or infection during pregnancy.*

[f] *The IgM-IFA and the conventional IgM-ELISA (but not the DS-IgM-ELISA as described by Naot and Remington) may give false positive results in sera containing rheumatoid factor or antinuclear antibody.*

are seropositive in a Group 1 test before conception may be considered safe from transmission of Toxoplasma infection to the fetus. Women who are seronegative on an initial Group 1 test should take precautions to avoid infection during pregnancy. Where feasible, these women should have a Group 2 test performed at monthly intervals optimally or at the end of each trimester of pregnancy to detect newly acquired infection.

B. *Differential Diagnosis*

In the normal host, acute toxoplasmosis may be mistaken for lymphoma or for other conditions causing lymphadenopathy. Congenital toxoplasmosis most closely resembles congenital cytomegalovirus infection although occasionally it may mimic other congenital infections. In the immunocompromised patient where the manifestations of toxoplasmosis are legion but usually involve the central nervous system, the differential diagnosis includes infections caused by a wide range of opportunistic pathogens. In all immunocompromised patients with undiagnosed central nervous system disease, toxoplasmosis must be considered. Serological results may be misleading in these patients and a diagnosis by isolation or histology may be necessary.

III. PREVENTION AND THERAPY

A. *Prevention*

Pregnant women lacking serological evidence of prior infection with Toxoplasma can take a few simple precautions which will likely reduce the risk of infection during pregnancy: meat should be thoroughly cooked to 60°C or frozen at -20°C for 24 hours before ingestion (many freezers do not reach this temperature); hands should be washed carefully after handling raw meat or vegetables; raw fruits and vegetables should be washed to remove oocysts; contact with cat feces should be avoided; gloves should be worn when working in the garden. Dry heat to 66°C or boiling water will render oocysts noninfectious.

B. *Therapy*

1. When to Treat - Most immunologically normal patients with lymphadenopathic toxoplasmosis do not require treatment. When symptoms are severe or persistent or when vital organs are involved, specific therapy is indicated. Acute toxoplasmosis in immunocompromised patients should always be treated.

Data suggest that treatment of women infected during pregnancy reduces the risk of transmission to the fetus by approximately 50%. When considering the option of therapeutic abortion, the physician and patient should be aware of the risk of transmission to the fetus (see Section I. A), the expected severity of fetal involvement (see Section I. A), and the alternative of treatment of the pregnant woman. Congenital Toxoplasma infection in the neonate, whether overt or subclinical, should be treated.

2. Therapeutic Agents (see Table 2 for drugs and dosages) - Pyrimethamine is synergistic with either sulfadiazine or trisulfapyrimidines. Other sulfonamides may be less effective. Addition of folinic acid to this combination prevents the bone marrow toxicity of pyrimethamine. Because of its potential tetratogenic effect, pyrimethamine should not be used in the first trimester of pregnancy in which case sulfonamides alone may be used. Spiramycin is a macrolide antibiotic which has been used safely and apparently effectively during all trimesters of pregnancy. It is not presently available in the United States.

Clindamycin and the combination trimethoprim/sulfamethoxazole have activity against Toxoplasma but have not yet been shown to be equal or superior in efficacy to the drugs mentioned above and are not generally advised. Corticosteroids have been advised as an adjunct to specific therapy in cases of chorioretinitis when vision is threatened.

3. Duration of Therapy - Although optimal duration of therapy is unknown, the following practices have been advised. In immunologically normal patients who require such treatment, four to six weeks of therapy is advised and longer treatment may be necessary. In immunocompromised patients, it seems advisable to treat until at least four to six weeks beyond resolution of all signs and symptoms; we frequently treat for six months or longer. In France, Desmonts and Couvreur have treated pregnant women with three-week courses of spiramycin alternating with two-week intervals off therapy until term. Alternatively, in Germany, Kraubig has given pyrimethamine (except in the first trimester) plus sulfonamide for two or three, two-week courses alternating with three to four-week intervals.

In congenital toxoplasmosis, 21-day courses of pyrimethamine and sulfonamide should be alternated with 30 to 45 day courses of spiramycin (where available) for the entire first year of life. In healthy neonates whose mothers acquired the infection during pregnancy, Couvreur has recommended giving a single course of pyrimethamine and sulfonamide for 21 days followed by spiramycin for 30 to 45 days and to withhold further therapy until there is serological evidence of infection in the infant.

TABLE 2.   Specific Therapy for Toxoplasmosis

Drug	Oral Dosage	Major toxicity
Pyrimethamine	Loading. Adult: 100-200 mg/d in 2 divided doses Young children: 2 mg/kg/d for 2-3 d Infant: 1 mg/kg in 1 dose Maintenance. 1 mg/kg (max 25 mg) daily[a]	Bone marrow depression, possible teratogenicity
Sulfadiazine or trisulfapyrimidines	Loading. 50-75 mg/kg Infant: 50-100 mg/kg Maintenance. 75-100 mg/kg/d in 4 divided doses Infant: 50-150 mg/kg/d in 2 divided doses	Allergic reaction, cyrstalluria, hematuria
Folinic acid	5 to 10 mg/d Infant: 5 mg twice/week	None
Spiramycin	Adult: 2 to 4 g/d in 4 divided doses Infant: 50-100 mg/kg/d in 2-4 divided doses	Not fully known

[a] *For patients who are not very ill and who do not have active infection in the eye, it has been suggested that the maintenance dose of pyrimethamine be given at 2,3, or 4-day intervals.*

IV.   PERSPECTIVES ON FUTURE DEVELOPMENTS

The most promising immediate hope for decreasing the morbidity attributable to congenital toxoplasmosis lies in education of susceptible women on how to avoid infection during pregnancy. Development of a vaccine to prevent infection in susceptible women of childbearing age or in immunocompromised patients or to prevent oocyst development in cats could significantly decrease morbidity due to toxoplasmosis. Improved histological and serological methods of diagnosis are needed.

REFERENCES

Books

Frenkel, J.K.: Toxoplasmosis: parasite life cycle, pathology, and immunology. In Hammond DM, Long PL (eds): *The Coccidia: Eimeria, Isospora, Toxoplasma, and Related Genera*. Baltimore, University Park Press, 1973, pp 344-410.

Remington, J.S., Desmonts, G: Toxoplasmosis. In Remington, J.S., Klein, J.O. (eds): *Infectious Diseases of the Fetus and Newborn Infant*. First Edition. Philadelphia, W.B. Saunders, 1976, pp 191-332. (Second Edition, 1982, in press.)

Journals

Carey, R.M., Kimball, A.C., Armstrong, D., Lieberman, P.H.: Toxoplasmosis. Clinical experiences in a cancer hospital. *Am. J. Med. 54:*30-38, 1973.

Desmonts, G., Couvreur, J.: Congenital toxoplasmosis: a prospective study of 378 pregnancies. *N. Engl. J. Med. 290:* 1110-1116, 1974.

Feldman, H.A.: Toxoplasmosis. *N. Engl. J. Med. 279:*1370-1375, 1431-1437, 1968.

Naot, Y., Desmonts, G., Remington, J.S.: IgM enzyme-linked immunosorbent assay test for the diagnosis of congenital Toxoplasma infection. *J. Pediatr. 98:*32-36, 1981.

Naot, Y., Remington, J.S.: An enzyme-linked immunosorbent assay for detection of IgM antibodies to Toxoplasma gondii: use for diagnosis of acute acquired toxoplasmosis. *J. Infect. Dis. 142:*757-766, 1980.

Ruskin, J., Remington, J.S.: Toxoplasmosis in the compromised host. *Ann. Intern. Med. 84:*193-199, 1976.

Symposium on toxoplasmosis. *Bull. N.Y. Acad. Med. 50:*197-240, 1974.

Welch, P.C., Masur, H., Jones, T.C., Remington, J.S.: Serologic diagnosis of acute lymphadenopathic toxoplasmosis. *J. Infect. Dis. 142:*256-264, 1980.

Wilson, C.B., Remington, J.S.: What can be done to prevent congenital toxoplasmosis? *Am. J. Obstet. Gynecol. 138:* 357-363, 1980.

Wilson, C.B., Remington, J.S., Stagno, S., Reynolds, D.W.: Development of adverse sequelae in children born with subclinical congenital Toxoplasma infection. *Pediatrics 66:*767-774, 1980.

PART X
FUNGAL INFECTIONS OF SPECIAL IMPORTANCE

SYSTEMIC MYCOSES IN THE NORMAL HOST

John E. Bennett

Clinical Mycology Section
National Institute of Allergy
and Infectious Diseases
National Institutes of Health
Bethesda, Maryland

INTRODUCTION

The intent of this chapter is to provide an approach to the
diagnosis and treatment of systemic mycoses. Diagnosis is usually required prior to therapy because empiric treatment has
extremely limited use in the normal host. While the ultimate
diagnosis rests on identifying the fungus in culture, smear or
histopathologic section, clinical clues to the correct diagnosis
can be extremely helpful in deciding what approach to diagnosis
will be most productive and in deciding whether the laboratory
report is to be believed. Laboratory diagnosis is difficult
enough to permit mistakes in the best hands. When the clinical
picture is atypical, the clinician may wish to confirm the diagnosis by yet another approach or have a reference laboratory
confirm the result. Weighed against further diagnostic maneuvers
is the time, expense, disease progression and, occasionally,
antipathy by the laboratory whose diagnosis is being questioned.
Yet, incorrect diagnosis also has its penalties.

The discussion of diagnosis which follows will contain generalities which, like most generalities, contain exceptions.
Many of these exceptions are uncommon and will be ignored. Without taking a simplistic view, the physician may conclude that
clinical clues are useless: the infections are indistinguishable.
The situation is not at all so bleak.

EXPOSURE HISTORY

There are major endemic areas for some mycoses. Coccidioidomycosis is confined to certain arid areas of the Western Hemis-
phere. In the U.S.A., the major areas include Arizona, the
southern two-thirds of California, the western half of Texas and
New Mexico. Outside the U.S.A., there are endemic areas in
northern Mexico, South America and Central America. The endemic
areas of histoplasmosis and blastomycosis are broader and, in the
U.S.A., overlap each other. These mycoses are most common in the
central and southeastern states.

The patient's activity which preceded the illness may also
cast light on diagnostic possibilities. An acute pneumonia following by a week or two and exposure to bat droppings or to dust
from rich earth, particularly dirt containing bird droppings,
should suggest histoplasmosis. Exposure to arid dust in the endemic areas of coccidioidomycosis often precedes pulmonary infection with that fungus. On rare occasions, a young person shovel-
ing stored grain or hay will acquire an acute diffuse pneumonia
caused by Aspergillus. Gardeners, florists and horticulturists
may acquire cutaneous sporotrichosis from handling thorny or
prickly plants.

CLINICAL SYNDROMES

Several distinctive syndromes and their most frequent agents
are shown in Table I. Pathogens other than mycoses causing these
syndromes are omitted. Underlying conditions are generally omitted from the table because the patients referred to in this chapter are ostensibly normal. One exception seen in the table is a
history of cigarette smoking. This history is present in nearly
all patients with chronic progressive pulmonary histoplasmosis.
Underlying lung disease also precedes fungus ball of the lung.
Racial background is important in coccidioidomycosis. Disseminated infection is more common in blacks, filipinos and orientals.
Pregnancy also predisposes to dissemination in that mycosis.

DIAGNOSTIC TESTS

The most rapid approach to diagnosis of many syndromes is
visualizing the fungus in smear or biopsy. The appropriate test
varies with the specimen (Table II). At least 3-5 ml CSF should

TABLE I.   Clinical Syndromes in the Normal Host Which
Suggest a Mycosis

Syndrome	Most Likely Mycoses
Chronic meningitis	Ca, Cr, Co, H
Mediastinal fibrosis	H
Coin lesion of lung with calcification	H, Co
Thin-walled pulmonary cavity	Co, S
Chronic fibronodular apical pneumonia in a male smoker	H
Acute pneumonia	B, Co, H
Chronic pneumonia	B, Co, Cr, H, P, S
Fungus ball of the lung	A
Addison's disease	H, P
Chronic indurated ulcer of mouth, larynx, nose	H, B, P
Chronic arthritis	B, Ca, Co, S
Chronic skin lesions:	
Subcutaneous cold abscess	B, Co, Cr
Verrucoid plaque	B, Ch
Erythematous indurated area on hand with subsequent appearance of proximal nodules	S

A = aspergillosis, B = blastomycosis, Ca = candidiasis,
Ch = chromomycosis, Co = coccidioidomycosis, Cr = cryptococcosis,
H = histoplasmosis, P = paracoccidioidomycosis, S = sporotrichosis

TABLE II. Smears and Stains for Rapid Diagnosis

Test	Material
KOH smear	scrapings from skin, nails and mucosal lesions
Wet smear	pus, sputum, CSF
India ink	CSF
Giemsa or Wright's	bone marrow, oral ulcers
Gomorri methenamine silver	histopathologic section

be sent to laboratory in patients with chronic meningitis. A
syringe should be used to send pus to the laboratory, if at all
possible, not a dry swab or bandage. For sputums, first morning
specimens are preferred but, more importantly, a good deep cough
specimen is essential. Fungal serologic tests have some use
(Table III). Skin testing is nearly useless for diagnosis. A
positive histoplasmin skin test can create confusion by causing
an "m" band to appear on immunodiffusion testing of the patient's
serum. The complement fixation titer to histoplasmin may also
rise to 1:8 or 1:16.

Culture is slower but more accurate than histologic or serologic diagnosis. Blood should be cultured only in vented bottles.
Urine culture is helpful even when no urinary tract symptoms are
present. Cryptococcus neoformans may appear in sputum of patients with other lung disease.

TREATMENT

The two most useful recent regimens are flucytosine plus
amphotericin B (Table IV) and the new oral imidazole, ketoconazole (Table V). Intravenous miconazole is not listed because as
yet no situations have emerged where this preparation appears to
be indicated. The same can be said for rifampin plus amphotericin B. Details about administration of intravenous and intrathe-
cal amphotericin B are well reviewed in older publications.

TABLE III. Fungal Serologic Tests

Coccidioidomycosis

   Serum: Immunodiffusion tests useful for screening.

               Complement fixation titer over 1:16 suggests progressive infection.

               Falling complement fixation titer is good prognostic sign.

   CSF: Positive complement fixation titer indicates meningitis or, rarely, parameningeal focus.

Cryptococcosis

   Serum: Latex test positive in 2/3 meningitis, 1/3 pulmonary. Usually negative in bone or skin disease.

   CSF: Latex test positive in 90% of meningitis cases, titer falls with successful therapy. If control for rheumatoid factor positive at any dilution, latex test becomes uninterpretable.

Histoplasmosis

   Serum: Immunodiffusion good screening test. Complement fixation titer >1:16 should prompt search for histoplasmosis.

               Positive skin test boosts histoplasmin titer.

   CSF: Complement fixation test positive suggests diagnosis.

TABLE IV. Flucytosine Plus Amphotericin B

Dose: Flucytosine 37.5 mg/kg orally every 6 h
         Amphotericin B 0.3 mg/kg intravenously daily

Indications: Cryptococcal meningitis

               Systemic candidiasis

Pharmacology: Flucytosine rapidly, completely absorbed from G.I.
               tract and excreted unchanged in urine. Azotemia
               requires dose reduction in rough proportion to
               elevation of creatinine; viz., doubling of serum
               creatinine from 0.9 mg/dl to 1.8 mg/dl requires
               reducing flucytosine dose by half. Hemodialysis
               patients require about 37.5 mg/kg after each dial-
               ysis. Dose not altered in jaundiced patients.

               Amphotericin B clearance not altered by azotemia,
               jaundice or dialysis.

Side Effects: Flucytosine causes leukopenia or thrombocytopenia
               in some patients at blood levels over 100–125 µg/ml.
               Diarrhea, nausea and abdominal pain possibly are
               blood level related, but hepatic dysfunction ap-
               pears to be idiosyncratic and uncommon (4% or
               less). Rash is occasional.

               Amphotericin B usually causes nausea, anorexia,
               vomiting, chills, fever, azotemia, anemia, hypo-
               kalemia and phlebitis. Occasionally, mild leuko-
               penia occurs. Thrombocytopenia is rare and less
               clearly related to amphotericin B.

TABLE V.   Ketoconazole

Dose: 200-400 mg once daily by mouth

Indications: Chronic mucocutaneous candidiasis, griseofulvin
               resistant ringworm, chronic progressive coccidi-
               oidomycosis, chronic progressive histoplasmosis?
               blastomycosis?

Pharmacology: Gastric acid important for absorption. Dosage
               unchanged in azotemic and dialysed patients.
               Effect of jaundice unclear.

Side effects: Nausea, anorexia, pruritus, rash, and perhaps
               headache, nervousness and somnolence. Side ef-
               fects interfere with therapy in 10% of patients
               or less. A few patients have had hepatic dys-
               function clearly due to ketoconazole.

A PRACTICAL APPROACH TO INFECTIONS IN THE IMMUNOCOMPROMISED HOST[1]

William E. Hauser, Jr.[2]
Jack S. Remington

Division of Infectious Diseases
Department of Medicine
Stanford University School of Medicine
Stanford, California

Division of Immunology and Infectious Diseases
Research Institute, Palo Alto Medical Foundation
Palo Alto, California

INTRODUCTION

The clinical diagnostic and therapeutic approach to infections in immunocompromised patients is complicated by the fact that these patients are critically ill, immunosuppressed and have rapidly progressive clinical courses. The multiple physicians involved in their care are not always in communication, which unfortunately delays major decisions regarding management. For this reason we at Stanford University Hospital try to insure that one physician is ultimately responsible for, and coordinates the care of these critically ill patients. In addition, we consider the team approach to be optimal, but recognize that certain members of the team may not always be available. In this event, alternate physicians must be available. The necessity of having the appropriate technical and medical-surgical facilities has led a number of authors to recommend that these patients be cared for solely in major medical centers whenever possible. This necessity has unfortunately altered the quality of life for many patients in an untoward manner, especially where they have had to move themselves and their families to such centers.

The team may be rather extensive but most often consists of the patient's personal physician, housestaff, hematologist-oncologist, radiologist, infectious disease consultant, thoracic surgeon, laboratory microbiologist and pathologist. Coordination of such a team effort is not only a major responsibility but a necessity if these patients are to be cared for appropriately.

[1] *This work was supported by NIH grant AI04717.*

[2] *Recipient of an Edith Milo Fellowship.*

In the brief space afforded here, we will attempt to provide certain guidelines which we hope will be helpful for physicians caring for such patients. The necessity to be brief precludes the use of this chapter other than as a guide. For this reason the reader is referred to the bibliography for critical articles related to the subjects covered. What follows then will be a discussion, dealing with selected clinical, diagnostic and therapeutic considerations which the practicing physician may use in dealing with infections in high risk patients, primarily those with hematologic malignancy receiving high dose immunosuppressive drugs, including corticosteroids.

I.   CLINICAL AND DIAGNOSTIC APPROACHES

In the approach to the immunocompromised patient with suspected infection, it is helpful to have at least a superficial understanding of the immune defects associated with the patient's underlying disease and/or the drugs they are receiving since all of these factors may predispose to infection with a variety of bacteria, fungi, viruses, protozoa and helminths (Table I). The defects may be in humoral immunity, cell-mediated immunity (CMI) or both.

In normal individuals these two arms of the immune system may act alone or synergistically to both protect against and fight infection. It is important to recognize that these two arms of the immune system, often defend against different types of organisms. Differences between the two arms and the organisms against which they defend are shown in Tables II, III, and IV. Thus in the patient with multiple myeloma who presents with pneumonia, we suspect pneumococci as the primary etiology, since the immune defect is a deficiency in normal quantities of circulating immunoglobulins (antibodies). Such antibodies are necessary for opsonization of pneumococci for phagocytosis and killing. In contradistinction, when a patient with Hodgkin's disease or Hairy cell leukemia presents with pneumonia, the differential diagnosis includes certain of the facultative and obligate intracellular bacteria and fungi, defense against which is primarily cell-mediated. If these patients are also receiving cytotoxic agents and/or corticosteroids both humoral and cell-mediated immunity will be affected which thus will determine the etiology of the infection.

In dealing with infections in immunocompromised patients, clinicians must also be aware of the changing patterns and predominance of microbial isolates in their own hospitals. As outlined in Table V, certain epidemiologic factors may suggest the etiology of an infection in such patients. For instance, in certain institutions, such as Stanford University Hospital, the incidence of Aspergillus species as a cause of serious infections

Table I. Examples of Immune Defects and Common Pathogens in Patients with Malignancy

Neoplastic Disease	Immune Defect	Associated Pathogens	
Acute nonlymphocytic leukemia	Phagocyte (PMN)	Bacterial:	Staphylococcus aureus Gram-negative bacilli, especially Pseudomonas aeruginosa
		Fungal:	Candida spp., Aspergillus spp.
Hodgkin's disease Hairy cell leukemia	CMI	Bacterial:	Listeria monocytogenes Nocardia asteroides Pseudomonas aeruginosa Salmonella species Mycobacterium species
		Fungal:	Cryptococcus neoformans Candida species Coccidioides immitis Histoplasma capsulatum
		Protozoal:	Toxoplasma gondii Pneumocystis carinii Strongyloides stercoralis
		Viral:	Herpes simplex, Varicella-zoster, Cytomegalovirus
Chronic lymphocytic leukemia Multiple myeloma	HI	Bacterial:	Pneumococci Hemophilus influenzae Gram-negative enteric bacilli
		Protozoal:	Pneumocystis carinii

Adapted from Sotman et al. (2), Mackowiak et al. (3), Schimpff et al. (4), Ruckdeschel et al. (5), Schimpff et al. (6) and Notter et al. (7).

Table II. A Comparison of Certain Characteristics of the
Cellular and Humoral Immune Responses

Characteristics	Humoral Immunity	Cellular Immunity
Duration of time to maximal effect	Immediate to hours	Days
Mediator of effect	B-lymphocytes and plasma cells	T-lymphocytes
Effector	Antibody	Lymphocytes and macrophages
Effective against	Extracellular pathogens	Intracellular pathogens

Adapted from Wing, E.J. and Remington, J.S. (1)

in patients with acute nonlymphocytic leukemia is relatively
high, whereas in other institutions it is rarely seen. Another
example is the increasing number of nosocomial infections caused
by Legionella pneumophila, which in certain centers is nine times
more frequent in immunocompromised than in nonimmunocompromised
patients.

Some of the most common sources of nosocomial infections are
indwelling intravenous lines, urethral catheters and respiratory
care equipment. More recently transfusion as a source of life-
threatening infection other than hepatitis B and infection from
contaminated foodstuffs other has been emphasized. Cytomegalovirus
(CMV) infection acquired by transfusion or transplantation of a
previously infected kidney has predisposed to serious infection
and death in recipients. Colonization of the GI tract, the most
common origin of the etiologic agents which cause life-threatening
infection and death in patients with prolonged and severe granulocytopenia may occur when these patients are fed contaminated
foods such as salads, which are known to contain significant
numbers of Pseudomonas spp., Klebsiella spp., and E. coli.

In addition to the clinical history, the physical examination of these patients must be complete, including careful examination of the fundi (e.g. for the characteristic features of
Toxoplasmic, CMV or fungal retinitis) and skin (e.g. for the
characteristic or suggestive lesions of icthyma gangrenosa due to
Pseudomonas aeruginosa; Candida tropicalis; Candida albicans;
Herpes simplex and Herpes zoster) (Table VI). These two sites
which are so frequently missed, are excellent "windows" which afford us an insight into the diagnosis of the infection. Any new
skin lesions which cannot be easily explained to be due to drug
eruption or bleeding diatheses, should be biopsied or scraped and

Table III. Pathogens Against Which Cell-Mediated Immunity Appears to be Important in Host Defense

Bacteria	Viruses	Fungi	Protozoa	Helminths	Unclassified
Mycobacteria, including M. tuberculosis and M. leprae	Herpes simplex	Aspergillus species	Toxoplasma gondii	Schistosoma species	Pneumocystis carinii
Salmonella species	Herpes zoster	Candida species	Plasmodium species	Strongyloides stercoralis	
	Cytomegalovirus	Cryptococcus neoformans			
Listeria monocytogenes	Rubeola (measles)				
	Vaccinia	Phycomycetes species			
Francisella tularensis					
		Histoplasma capsulatum			
Brucella species					
Treponema pallidum		Coccidioides immitis			
Malleomyces pseudomallei (Meliodosis)					
Malleomyces mallei (Glanders)					

Adapted from Wing, E. J. and Remington, J. S. (1)

Table IV. Some Processes in Host Defense Against Infection in Which Antibody Has a Role

Process	Antibody Class(es) Participating	Pathogens Affected
Opsonization	IgG, IgM	Bacteria, especially encapsulated organisms: Pneumococci, Hemophilus influenzae type B, Meningococci, Group A streptococci, Pseudomonas species Fungi: Cryptococcus neoformans, Candida albicans Protozoa: Toxoplasma gondii Some viruses
Lysis	IgG, IgM	Gram-negative bacteria: Neisseria species, Hemophilus influenzae type B Some viruses and virus-infected host cells (Herpes simplex 1 and 2)
Toxin neutralization	IgG	Clostridium species, Corynebacterium diphtheriae ? Other bacteria, especially gram-negative bacilli
Inhibition of adherence	IgG	Gonococci, Streptococci ? Intestinal pathogens causing diarrhea
Virus inhibition (neutralization)	IgG, IgM, IgA	Varicella-zoster, Rubeola, Rubella Coxsackie virus Variola (smallpox) Enteroviruses

Table V. Nosocomial Pathogens in the Immunocompromised Host

Pathogens	Epidemiology		
	Endogenous	Exogenous	Device Associated
Bacterial			
S. aureus	++	+	+
S. epidermidis	+++	...	+
Corynebacterium species	+++	...	+
Gram-negative rods	++	+	+
Fungal			
Candida species	+++	...	+
Aspergillus species	...	+++	...
Viruses			
Herpes simplex	+++	...	...
Varicella-zoster	++	+	...
Cytomegalovirus	+	++	+ (blood or white cell transfusions)
Protozoa			
Pneumocystis carinii	++	+	...
Toxoplasma gondii	++	+	...

Adapted from Young, L. S. (9)

appropriately stained to assist in the definitive diagnosis.

The need for urgency in diagnosing infection in immunocompromised patients has been emphasized in clinical investigations of leukemic patients undergoing prolonged periods of granulocytopenia (< 1000 PMN/mm^3). In such patients, mortality approaches 40-50% and is significantly increased if the patient has bacteremia or pneumonia. A major predisposing factor to pneumonia in these patients is the fact that their oropharynx becomes colonized with enteric gram-negative bacteria. These bacteria are often nosocomial and therefore resistant to a variety of antimicrobial agents used in the hospital environment. Some general guidelines for the diagnostic approach to the febrile granulocytopenic patient are given in Table VII. These guidelines extend also to numerous other patient types in the growing legion of immunocompromised patients.

From the onset of fever to the time of death in the patients we are discussing here may be less than 24 hours. This is the reason for the organized and aggressive approach to the diagnosis.

Table VI.   Common Pathogens by Site of Infection
in Immunocompromised Patients

Site of Infection	Neoplastic Disease	Associated Pathogens
Oropharynx (including esophagus)	Acute nonlymphocytic leukemia	Bacteria: Streptococci Staphylococcus aureus Pseudomonas aeruginosa, Klebsiella pneumoniae, E. coli
		Fungi: Candida species Aspergillus species Mucor
		Viruses: Herpes simplex
Central nervous system	Acute nonlymphocytic leukemia	Bacteria: Gram-negative bacilli (Pseudomonas, Klebsiella, E. coli)
		Fungi: Aspergillus species Candida species Mucor
	Hodgkin's	Bacteria: Listeria monocytogenes
		Fungi: Cryptococcus neoformans Coccidioides immitis
		Protozoa: Toxoplasma gondii Strongyloides stercoralis
		Viruses: Varicella-zoster
Pulmonary	Acute nonlymphocytic leukemia	Bacteria: Staphylococcus aureus Gram-negative bacilli (Pseudomonas, Klebsiella, E. coli)
		Fungi: Aspergillus species Candida species Mucor
	Hodgkin's	Bacteria: Mycobacterium species Nocardia asteroides

(cont.)

Table VI (cont.)

Site of Infection	Neoplastic Disease	Associated Pathogens
Pulmonary	Hodgkin's	Bacteria: ? Legion- ella pneumophila
		Fungi: Cryptococcus neoformans Histoplasma capsu- latum Coccidioides immitis
		Protozoa: Pneumocystis carinii Strongyloides stercoralis
		Viruses: Herpes simplex Varicella-zoster Cytomegalovirus
		Other: Chlamydia trachomatis
	Chronic lymphocytic leukemia	Bacteria: Pneumococci Hemophilus influenzae
		Protozoa: Pneumocystis carinii
Cutaneous	Acute nonlymphocytic leukemia	Bacteria: Staphylo- coccus aureus Pseudomonas, Klebsi- ella, E. coli
		Fungi: Candida species Aspergillus species Mucor
		Viruses: Herpes simplex
	Hodgkin's	Bacteria: Mycobacterium species Nocardia asteroides
		Fungi: Cryptococcus neoformans Histoplasma capsu- latum Coccidioides immitis
		Viruses: Herpes simplex Varicella-zoster

Adapted from Armstrong, D. (12)

Even in the nonimmunosuppressed patient, approximately 50% of bacteremic patients who die, die within the first 24 hours. Following the obtaining of blood cultures, cultures of orifices and body fluids and appropriate staining of these materials, the physician may still be left without a diagnosis. This may occur in as many as 30-40% of patients. A special case in point is the patient with pulmonary infiltrates, for it is in these patients that we have observed the most costly waste of valuable time in making a decision as to the next diagnostic procedure. This decision must be made with intelligence and restraint, with a complete knowledge of the etiology of these pneumonias and the invasive procedures available for their diagnosis. This decision must also be based upon a careful consideration of the complications, potential risks and benefits of such procedures and upon the impact such a decision will have on the patient's quality of life.

Transtracheal aspiration (TTA) is a logical first alternative since there are few contraindications to its use and because it is a safe procedure if done by personnel familiar with the technique. If TTA cannot be done or is unsuccessful, more invasive procedures may be considered (Table VII). The type of procedure and the urgency with which it is done is dependent upon the clinical assessment of the patient's course, the type and location of the pulmonary infiltrate, the presence of bleeding diastheses and upon the expertise available at a given institution for performing such procedures. In addition, the physician's decision to obtain a diagnosis by one of these invasive techniques, must also be weighed against the possibility that the cause of the pulmonary infiltrate is noninfectious (Table VIII).

The handling of specimens obtained by any of the procedures should include immediate microscopic examination (including tissue silver stains for Pneumocystis carinii and fungi) and thorough culturing for routine and opportunistic pathogens (Table VII).

ANTIMICROBIAL THERAPY

It is beyond the scope of this paper to discuss specific antimicrobial therapy. The initial choice of antibiotics is often empiric and must be made without waiting for results of cultures. Here it should be evident that a clear knowledge of the types of organisms that infect these patients becomes critical in the proper choice of antibiotics. In all specialty centers in which such patients are cared for, combinations of antibiotics are employed to provide broad coverage and in an attempt to obtain synergy against the offending pathogen. This usually includes a cephalosporin, ticarcillin or carbenicillin and an aminoglycoside or either of the former three plus the latter.

Table VII. Some General Guidelines for the Diagnostic Approach
to the Febrile Granulocytopenic Patient

I. Initial Evaluation
   A. Thorough history and physical
      1. Possible etiologies suggested by physical findings
         or site of infection (Table VIII)
      2. Fundoscopic exam
         a) Endopthalmitis: Aspergillus species
                           Candida species
                           ? Bacteria
         b) Chorioretinitis: Toxoplasma gondii
                             Cytomegalovirus
   B. Laboratory and diagnostic tests (minimum)
      1. CBC with differential
      2. Chemistry panel with creatinine
      3. Urinalysis
      4. Blood culture(s)
      5. Chest x-ray (CXR)

II. Patient with Lung Infiltrate on CXR
   A. Productive or induced sputum
      1. Immediate examination of sputum by gram stain, acid-
         fast stain
   Culture for aerobes, fungi, mycobacteria
   B. Failure to expectorate or induce sputum or obtain useful
      information from (A)
      1. Consider invasive procedures in the following order:
         Transtracheal aspiration
         Flexible fiberoptic bronchoscopy with bronchial
           washings, brushings and biopsy
         Percutaneous needle aspiration and/or biopsy
         Open lung biopsy
   C. Handling of pulmonary specimens obtained by invasive
      procedures
      1. Immediate examination by:
         Gram stain, acid-fast stain and fungal wet mount
         (KOH)
         Gomori methenamine silver staining for pneumocystis
         Direct fluorescent antibody staining for Legionella
         or viruses if suspected
      2. Culture for aerobes and anaerobes, mycobacteria,
         fungi; Legionella and viruses if suspected clini-
         cally

III. Patient Without Lung Infiltrate on CXR
   A. No abnormal physical findings
      1. Initiate empiric antibiotic therapy after peripheral
         culturing complete

(cont.)

Table VII (cont.)

B. Skin or mucous membrane lesions
    1. Obtain material by scrapings, aspiration or biopsy
    2. Examination of material by gram stain, fungal wet
        mount, acid-fast stain, tissue stain for fungi,
        direct fluorescent antibody stain for herpes virus
        if suspected clinically
    3. Culture for aerobes and anaerobes, fungi, myco-
        bacteria, viruses if suspected
C. Central nervous system dysfunction
    1. No focal findings suggesting space occupying lesion
        Immediate lumbar puncture
        Direct CSF examination by gram stain, acid-fast
        stain, India ink
        CSF culture for aerobes and anaerobes, mycobacteria,
        fungi; viruses if suspected clinically
        CSF serology: complement fixation for Coccidioides
        immitis; antigen for Cryptococcus neoformans
    2. Focal findings suggesting space occupying lesions
        Immediate CT scan or radioisotope scan
        (I) If positive - proceed to immediate neurosurgical
        consultation with open biopsy if not contraindi-
        cated. Specimens should be handled as in II.C.
        above.
        (II) If negative - consider EEG to R/0 typical en-
        cephalographic changes of herpes encephalitis.
        Also consider detailed radiographic examination of
        entire neuraxis.

Table VIII. Noninfectious Causes of Pulmonary Infiltrates in
             Febrile, Immunosuppressed Patients

A. Recurrent tumor
B. Radiation pneumonitis and fibrosis
C. Drug-induced pneumonitis
    1. Bleomycin
    2. Cyclophosphamide
    3. Chloroambucil
    4. Busulfan
    5. Methotrexate
D. Miscellaneous
    1. Leukostasis
    2. Emboli
    3. Edema
    4. Hemorrhage

With the advent of the third generation cephalosporins our therapy may change, but not until results of carefully performed studies are available to offer the physician guidelines for their use. If staphylococcal infection is suspected, the above regimen may be modified to include an aminoglycoside plus an antistaphylococcal antibiotic. If an antifungal agent is to be included in the regimen, amphotericin B is the drug of choice. Except in rare instances, miconazole and ketoconazole should not be used until the data on these drugs for disseminated infection can be carefully and critically evaluated by authorities in the field. This has not yet been done, yet these drugs are being used inappropriately in these patients. Empiric therapy must also be based upon continuing review of a hospital's predominant microbial isolates and their antibiotic sensitivities. Consideration of these factors should allow antibiotic choices to be made rationally rather than in a "shot-gun" fashion.

Because these patients are at increased risk for the development of serious infections, empiric therapy should continue until granulocytopenia resolves, even if infection is not documented.

ANTIMICROBIAL PROPHYLAXIS

Since the risk of nosocomial infection is high in these patients, especially during prolonged periods of severe granulocytopenia, attempts have been made to suppress normal resident microbial flora (gram-negative enteric bacilli, S. aureus, C. albicans) which cause most of these infections.

Protective isolation is not available in most hospitals and will not be discussed here. Because of this unavailability, recent regimens have been directed against protection of patients on open wards and private rooms. These have included skin disinfection with povidone-iodine or chlorhexidine; nasopharyngeal sprays and mouth ointments containing either gentamicin, neomycin, polymyxin B or amphotericin B or combinations of these, and oral administration of either trimethoprim-sulfamethoxazole alone or in combination with nalidixic acid, polymyxin B or amphotericin B to reduce gut flora without affecting colonization resistance. These regimens have been remarkably effective in reducing the incidence of major infections in granulocytopenic patients and those undergoing induction chemotherapy. Further follow-up will be needed to determine the incidence of emergence of resistant organisms during and after such prophylactic measures.

In addition to its use to rid the gut of aerobes, oral trimethoprim-sulfamethoxazole combination when used prophylactically has been shown to significantly reduce the risk of infection by Pneumocystis carinii in a variety of immunosuppressed patients. For discussion of the patient population in whom this may be effective, the reader is referred to the article by Hughes.

A.   *Is There a Role for Granulocyte Transfusions in Prophylaxis and Treatment of Infections?*

This is perhaps the most controversial subject in relation to the management of the immunocompromised patient. To date it is generally agreed that prophylactic granulocyte transfusions should not be used, because they have not been demonstrated to significantly effect a reduction in the frequency of infections and in some instances have shown an increased risk of transfusion associated cytomegalovirus (CMV) infections. They also have caused sensitization of patients to platelets and leukocytes which have resulted in untoward reactions when patients have received platelet transfusions.

Results of investigations in which granulocytes have been given during periods of documented gram-negative bacterial or fungal infections together with antibiotics have not been consistent. Some studies have shown a beneficial effect but only in those patients with prolonged granulocytopenia and microbiologically documented infection. In those patients in whom marrow recovery occurred during granulocyte therapy, the administration of granulocytes did not enhance recovery from the infections over that obtained with antibiotics alone. It should be appreciated that the use of granulocyte transfusions is not without undue hazards to both donor and recipient. An example of this in the recipient is the recent report that severe, sometimes lethal, pulmonary reactions, notably intra-alveolar hemorrhage, have occurred in immunocompromised patients who were receiving amphotericin B concomitantly with granulocyte transfusions. The mechanisms are as yet unclear. If granulocyte transfusions are given to patients who also must receive amphotericin B, granulocytes should be administered slowly, at a different time than amphotericin B administration and in the setting of close pulmonary monitoring.

PROSPECTS FOR THE FUTURE: IMMUNOMODULATORS

The role of transfer factor (TF) in treatment of infections has never been satisfactorily defined. The first carefully performed study on its role as a preventive agent has recently been published: TF significantly reduced clinical chicken-pox during an outbreak of varicella in a cancer hospital. The effects of interferon (IF) have been notable in chronic hepatitis B infection, especially when given together with adenine arabinoside (Ara-A). The effect in other infections although present has not been remarkable, perhaps due to the lack of sufficient amounts of the agent, or purity, or both. This should be clarified with the purer preparations of IF now being produced. The role of other immunomodulators such as levamisole, thymosin, lithium, zinc and cimetidine has yet to be defined. Some of these agents look very promising.

REFERENCES

1. Wing, E. J., and J. S. Remington. 1977. Cell-mediated im-
    munity and its role in resistance to infection. West. J.
    Med. 126:14-31.
2. Sotman, S. B., S. C. Schimpff, and V. M. Young. 1980.
    Staphylococcus aureus bacteremia in patients with acute leu-
    kemia. Am. J. Med. 69:814-818.
3. Mackowiak, P. A., S. E. Demian, W. L. Sutker, et al. 1980.
    Infections in Hairy cell leukemia. Am. J. Med. 68:718-724.
4. Schimpff, S. C., M. J. O'Connell, W. H. Greene, and P. H.
    Wiernik. 1975. Infections in 92 splenectomized patients
    with Hodgkin's disease. Am. J. Med. 59:695-701.
5. Ruckdeschel, J. C., S. C. Schimpff, A. C. Smyth, and M. R.
    Mardiney, Jr. 1977. Herpes zoster and impaired cell-
    associated immunity to the Varicella-zoster virus in patients
    with Hodgkin's disease. Am. J. Med. 62:77-85.
6. Schimpff, S. C., W. H. Greene, V. M. Young, and P. H.
    Wiernik. 1974. Significance of Pseudomonas aeruginosa in
    the patient with leukemia or lymphoma. J. Infect. Dis. 130
    (Suppl.)S24-S31.
7. Notter, D. T., P. L. Grossman, S. A. Rosenberg, and J. S.
    Remington. 1980. Infections in patients with Hodgkin's
    disease: A clinical study of 300 consecutive adult patients.
    Rev. Infect. Dis. 2:761-800.
8. Schimpff, S. C., V. M. Young, W. H. Greene, et al. 1972.
    Origin of infection in acute nonlymphocytic leukemia: Sig-
    nificance of hospital acquisition of potential pathogens.
    Ann. Intern. Med. 77:707-714.
9. Young, L. S. 1981. Nosocomial infections in the immunocom-
    promised adult. Am. J. Med. 70:398-404.
10. Haley, C. E., M. L. Cohen, J. Halter and R. D. Meyer. 1979.
    Nosocomial Legionnaires' disease: A continuing common-source
    epidemic at Wadsworth Medical Center. Ann. Intern. Med. 90:
    583-586.
11. Remington, J. S., and S. C. Schimpff. 1981. Please don't
    eat the salads. N. Engl. J. Med. 304:433-435.
12. Armstrong, D. 1980. Infections in patients with neoplastic
    disease. In Infections in the Immunocompromised Host -
    Pathogenesis, Prevention and Therapy. J. Verhoef et al.
    editors. Elsevier/North-Holland Biomedical Press. pp. 129-
    158.
13. Bodey, G. P., V. Rodriguez, H. Chang, and G. Narboni. 1978.
    Fever and infection in leukemic patients: A study of 494
    consecutive patients. Cancer 41:1610-1622.

14. Singer, C., M. H. Kaplan and D. Armstrong. 1977. Bacter-
     emia and fungemia complicating neoplastic disease. Am. J.
     Med. 62:731-742.
15. Beam, T. R., Jr., and J. C. Allen. 1979. Patterns of in-
     fection in untreated acute leukemia: Impact of initial
     hospitalization. South. Med. J. 72:282-286.
16. Gurwith, M. J., J. L. Brunton, B. A. Lank, et al. 1978.
     Granulocytopenia in hospitalized patients: I. Prognostic
     factors and etiology of fever. Am. J. Med. 64: 121-126.
17. Johanson, W. G., A. K. Pierce, and J. P. Sanford. 1969.
     Changing pharyngeal bacterial flora of hospitalized patients:
     Emergence of gram-negative bacilli. N. Engl. J. Med. 281:
     1137-1140.
18. Kreger, B. E., D. E. Craven, and W. R. McCabe. 1980. Gram-
     negative bacteremia. IV. Re-evaluation of clinical features
     and treatment in 612 patients. Am. J. Med. 68:344-355.
19. Pennington, J. E., and N. T. Feldman. 1977. Pulmonary in-
     filtrates and fever in patients with hematologic malignancy:
     Assessment of transbronchial biopsy. Am. J. Med. 62:581-587.
20. Singer, C., D. Armstrong, P. P. Rosen, et al. 1979. Diffuse
     pulmonary infiltrates in immunosuppressed patients: Prospec-
     tive study of 80 cases. Am. J. Med. 66:110-120.
21. Phillips, M. J., R. K. Knight, and M. Green. 1980. Fibre-
     optic bronchoscopy and diagnosis of pulmonary lesions in
     lymphoma and leukaemia. Thorax 35:19-25.
22. Toledo-Pereyra, L. H., T. R. DeMeester, A. Kinealey, et al.
     1980. The benefits of open lung biopsy in patients with pre-
     vious non-diagnostic transbronchial lung biopsy. Chest 77:
     647-650.
23. Kilton, L. J., B. E. Fossieck, Jr., M. H. Cohen, and R. H.
     Parker. 1979. Bacteremia due to gram-positive cocci in pa-
     tients with neoplastic disease. Am. J. Med. 66:596-602.
24. Love, L. J., S. C. Schimpff, C. A. Schiffer, and P. H.
     Wiernik. 1980. Improved prognosis for granulocytopenic pa-
     tients with gram-negative bacteremia. Am. J. Med. 68:643-
     648.
25. Gurwith, M. J., J. L. Brunton, B. A. Lank, et al. 1979. A
     prospective controlled investigation of prophylactic tri-
     methoprim/sulfamethoxazole in hospitalized granulocytopenic
     patients. Am. J. Med. 66:248-256.
26. Bennett, J. E. and J. S. Remington. 1981. Miconazole in
     cryptococcosis and systemic candidiasis: A word of caution.
     Ann. Intern. Med. 94:708-709.
27. Pizzo, P. A., K. J. Robichaud, F. A. Gill, et al. 1979.
     Duration of empiric antibiotic therapy in granulocytopenic
     patients with cancer. Am. J. Med. 67:194-200.
28. Hahn, D. M., S. C. Schimpff, C. L. Fortner, et al. 1978.
     Infection in acute leukemia patients receiving oral nonab-
     sorbable antibiotics. Antimicrob. Ag. Chemother. 13:958-
     964.

29. Bodey, G. P., V. Rodriguez, F. Cabanillas, and E. J. Freireich. 1979. Protective environment-prophylactic antibiotic program for malignant lymphoma: Randomized trial during chemotherapy to induce remission. Am. J. Med. 66:74-81.

30. Bender, J. F., S. C. Schimpff, V. M. Young, et al. 1979. Role of Vancomycin as a component of oral nonabsorbable antibiotics for microbial suppression in leukemic patients. Antimicrob. Ag. Chemother. 15:455-460.

31. Schimpff, S. C., W. H. Greene, V. M. Young, et al. 1975. Infection prevention in acute nonlymphocytic leukemia. Ann. Intern. Med. 82:351-358.

32. Storring, R. A., T. J. McElwain, B. Jameson, et al. 1977. Oral non-absorbed antibiotics prevent infection in acute non-lymphoblastic leukaemia. Lancet ii:837-840.

33. Bender, J. F., S. C. Schimpff, V. M. Young, et al. 1979. A comparative trial of tobramycin vs. gentamicin in combination with vancomycin and nystatin for alimentary tract suppression in leukemic patients. Europ. J. Cancer 15:35-44.

34. Sleijfer, D. T., N. H. Mulder, H. G. de Vries-Hospers, et al. 1980. Infection prevention in granulocytopenic patients by selective decontamination of the digestive tract. Europ. J. Cancer 16:859-869.

35. Levine, A. S., S. E. Siegel, A. D. Schreiber, et al. 1973. Protected environments and prophylactic antibiotics: A prospective controlled study of their utility in the therapy of acute leukemia. N. Engl. J. Med. 288:477-483.

36. Yates, J. W., and J. F. Holland. 1973. A controlled study of isolation and endogenous microbial suppression in acute myelocytic leukemia patients. Cancer 32:1490-1498.

37. Guiot, H. F. L., J. W. M. van der Meer, and R. van Furth. 1981. Selective antimicrobial modulation of human microbial flora: Infection prevention in patients with decreased host defense mechanisms by selective elimination of potentially pathogenic bacteria. J. Infect. Dis. 143:644-654.

38. Hughes, W. A., S. Kuhn, S. Chaudhary, et al. 1977. Successful chemoprophylaxis for Pneumocystis carinii pneumonitis. N. Engl. J. Med. 297:1419-1426.

39. Alavi, J. B., R. K. Root, I. Djerassi, et al. 1977. A randomized clinical trial of granulocyte transfusions for infection in acute leukemia. N. Engl. J. Med. 296:706-711.

40. Strauss, R. G., J. E. Connett, R. P. Gale, et al. 1981. A controlled trial of prophylactic granulocyte transfusions during initial induction chemotherapy for acute myelogenous leukemia. N. Engl. J. Med. 305:597-603.

41. Winston, D. J., W. G. Ho, L. S. Young, and R. P. Gale. 1980. Prophylactic granulocyte transfusions during human bone marrow transplantation. Am. J. Med. 68:893-897.

42. Winston, D. J., W. G. Ho, and R. P. Gale. 1981. Prophylactic granulocyte transfusions during chemotherapy of acute nonlymphocytic leukemia. Ann. Intern. Med. 94:616-622.

43. Herzig, R. H., G. P. Herzig, R. G. Graw, Jr., et al. 1977.
    Successful granulocyte transfusion therapy for gram-negative
    septicemia: A prospectively randomized controlled study. N.
    Engl. J. Med. 296:701-705.
44. Vogler, W. R., and E. F. Winton. 1977. A controlled study
    of the efficacy of granulocyte transfusions in patients with
    neutropenia. Am. J. Med. 63:548-555.
45. Buchholz, D. H., N. Blumberg, J. R. Bove. 1979. Long-term
    granulocyte transfusion in patients with malignant neoplasms.
    Arch. Intern. Med. 139:317-320.
46. Wright, D. G., K. J. Robichaud, P. A. Pizzo, and A. B.
    Deisseroth. 1981. Lethal pulmonary reactions associated
    with the combined use of amphotericin B and leukocyte trans-
    fusions. N. Engl. J. Med. 304:1185-1189.
47. Steele, R. W., M. G. Myers, and M. M. Vincent. 1980. Trans-
    fer factor for the prevention of varicella-zoster infection
    in childhood leukemia. N. Engl. J. Med. 303:355-359.
48. Good, R. A., A. West, and G. Fernandes. 1980. Effects of
    nutritional factors on immunity. In Infections in the Im-
    munocompromised Host - Pathogenesis, Prevention and Therapy.
    J. Verhoef et al., editors. Elsevier/North-Holland Bio-
    medical Press. pp. 95-128.

DIAGNOSIS AND MANAGEMENT
OF IMMUNODEFICIENCY IN CHILDREN

Warren E. Regelmann
Paul G. Quie

Department of Pediatrics
Division of Infectious Diseases
University of Minnesota School of Medicine

I. INTRODUCTION

Early recognition of immunodeficiency in children is
necessary for appropriate treatment and may be critical for
the patient's survival. Clinical clues suggesting immunodeficiency include recurrent infections which do not respond appropriately to antibiotic therapy or serious lesions with
microbial species not usually considered to be pathogenic.
Persistence and severity of an infection also lead to suspicion of immunodeficiency and identify patients with abnormal
host defenses.

Persons with a normal immunological system, of course, may
have signs and symptoms that are progressive with exacerbations and remissions. Microbial species which produce chronic
relapsing symptoms in normal hosts include herpes viruses,
mycobacteria, fungi and protozoae.

Respiratory syncytial virus, adenovirus or cytomegalovirus
may result in damage to the upper respiratory tract in immunologically normal hosts which produces unusual susceptibility
to recurrent pneumonias with bacterial pathogens, i.e.,
Streptococcus pneumoniae or Staphylococcus aureus, Enterobac-
teriaecae, Pseudomonas and anaerobes. During the first year
of life Campylobacter and Salmonella species may also produce
recurrent symptoms and recurrent bouts of streptococcal pharyngitis and tonsillitis are frequent in older normal children.

Other epidemiologic factors should also be considered
before an extensive laboratory work-up of the immunological
system is begun. Younger children have a large number of infections. A study of childhood illness in a civilian population in Cleveland (1) showed that the median for children
age zero to one is 6-7 upper respiratory tract infections
(URI's) per year with a range of 0 - 15; median for age one to
three is 8 URI's per year; for age three to five, 6-7 URI's

359

per year; for ages six to nine, 5-6 per year and for ages ten to
sixteen, 4-5 per year. Thus, recurrent URI's alone do not define
a group at high risk for an underlying disorder. Late fall,
winter and spring are seasons which have the highest frequency of
viral and streptococcal upper respiratory tract infections.

Acute otitis media is a frequent complication. Approximately
two to 18 percent of children have one episode of otitis per year
and from 10 to 84 percent of children have had one episode of
acute otitis media by age five. Approximately 50% of children in
certain populations such as Eskimos have three or more episodes of
otitis per year. The average attack rate of acute otitis is from
.25 to 1.9 episodes per year up to age four in middle class populations in the United States (3,4). The higher rates of infection
are from studies in which prospective and systematic screening has
been done and otitis media is defined by the presence of middle
ear effusion. The incidence of recurrent otitis media is so high
in immunologically normal persons that its presence does not
suggest an underlying anatomic or immunologic abnormality.

II. CLINICAL MANIFESTATIONS OF POSSIBLE IMMUNODEFICIENCY

If a child is noted to have two to three times as many respiratory infections and losing two to three times as many days from
school as his siblings, immunologic screening tests are in order.
The pattern of symptoms is also of potential significance in
helping the clinician identify children with underlying defects in
host defense. Fevers above 101°F associated with cough, pharyngitis and other signs of respiratory infections are common in
normal children but recurrent or persistent fever greater than
100°F without pharyngitis in a child suggests a complication of a
viral respiratory illness or underlying defect.

A child who begins to have three to four episodes of acute
otitis media per year after age three may be demonstrating a progressively failing immune system. The recovery after tympanocentesis of unusual organisms such as Candida albicans should
motivate anatomic and immune evaluation. Recent evidence in our
laboratory has suggested that children with recurrent otitis media
may have dysfunction in neutrophil chemotaxis, oxidative metabolism and bactericidal capacity (5). These defects are transitory
but the patients may be susceptible to middle ear infection with
unusual bacterial pathogens.

Sinusitis may be a complication of viral URI's in normal
children, however, it is an unusual diagnosis before the age of
two years. Patients with sinusitis which does not respond to
antibiotics and systemic decongestant therapy should have their
sinuses aspirated and if unusual pathogens are recovered, the
patient may have a defect in immunologic defenses. Recurrent
symptomatic lower respiratory diseases, especially if severe
enough to require hospitalization, is a frequent presenting

illness in patients with immunodeficiency diseases (6,7). Pulmonary roentgenographic changes which are particularly significant
include lobar, segmental or diffuse infiltrates. When these
roentgenographic changes persist immunodeficiency should be considered. Similar x-ray findings, of course, are more frequently
observed in immunologically normal individuals and are associated
with reversible obstructive pulmonary disease, neonatal exposure
to high oxygen tensions, tracheoesophageal fistula, cystic fibrosis, Kartagener's syndrome, vascular anomalies, and tuberculosis.
The recovery of unusual organisms such as <u>Pneumocystis</u> <u>carinii</u> or
cytomegalovirus on sputum examination is highly indicative of an
underlying immune defect and/or malignant process. The sinopulmonary system is frequently the first to signal a child with a
detectable underlying defect.

Persistent diarrhea and gastroenteritis, especially in young
infants, is also a frequent signal of an underlying immune defect.
Diarrhea is extremely common in normals and indeed accounts for
about 15% of all illness in families with young children (1). From
ages one to ten years, two to three episodes of gastroenteritis
per year is the average. Like respiratory signs and symptoms,
gastroenteritis occurs more frequently in winter than summer but
has a midsummer increase in July and August. Gastroenteritis of
less than two weeks duration and manageable in the outpatient
setting, therefore, does not help to define a population at risk
for underlying illness. However, chronic diarrhea and malabsorption in infants less than two years of age may be associated with
defects in cell-mediated immunity, such as severe combined immune
deficiency, defects in phagocyte function, and defects in humoral
immunity. Bloody diarrhea associated with eczema and thrombocytopenia suggests Wiskott-Aldrich syndrome. Recovery of <u>Giardia</u>
<u>lamblia</u> from stools is often associated with defects in humoral
immunity.

Recurrent and severe stomatitis and gingivitis define a population at risk for underlying immune defects, especially neutropenia. Herpes simplex infections lead to recurrent oral ulceration in normal persons but unusual severity or persistence of herpetic infections are suggestive of an underlying host defense abnormality. Candidiasis of the mouth or "thrush" is not unusual
but recurrence of lesions in a child not receiving antibiotics or
resistance to topical anti-candidal therapy may be associated with
an underlying disorder of cell-mediated immunity.

Certain patterns of skin infections define populations at high
risk for underlying immunodeficiency (7). Recurrent abscesses,
especially if "cold" or associated with pneumonias and eczema
suggest the hyper IgE syndrome (Job's syndrome). Patients with
this syndrome have an intermittent defect in neutrophil chemotaxis. Recurrent skin abscesses associated with chronic lymphadenitis are highly indicative of defects in phagocyte bactericidal
mechanisms. This possibility is made more likely if <u>Serratia</u>
<u>marcescens</u> or other poorly virulent species are recovered from
aspirated abscess material.

Recurrence of meningitis that has been adequately treated or recovery of an unusual pathogen from the spinal fluid (the usual pathogens are E. coli and group B β hemolytic Streptococcus in the neonate and Hemophilus influenzae, Streptococcus pneumoniae and Neisseria meningitidis in the older child) is suggestive of an immunologic deficiency. An anatomic abnormality such as a cribriform plate defect must also be considered in these clinical circumstances.

TABLE I. Clinical Signs of Immunodeficiency

1. Recurrent signs and symptoms of infection with an infectious agent that does not typically cause relapsing or recurrent symptoms in normal children;

2. two to three times as many upper respiratory tract infections as his siblings or two to three times more than his age cohort at that particular season of the year;

3. acute otitis media occurring every two to three months or more, especially if the frequency increases with age or if it persists in the acute stage for more than four weeks and tympanocentesis reveals unusual pathogens or if associated with pneumonia, bronchitis or diarrhea;

4. sinusitis remaining symptomatic beyond two to four weeks or if it is recurrent by age two;

5. pneumonia with an infiltrate on chest roent- genogram that persists unchanged or worsens over two weeks of conventional therapy, or pneumonia that recurs after adequate treatment;

6. gastroenteritis of more than two weeks duration or more than six or seven episodes by age two; or a pattern of increasing frequency or severity with malabsorption and failure to thrive; or if bloody and associated with eczema and thrombocytopenia;

7. oral or perineal candidiasis that immediately relapses after appropriate topical therapy if the child is not receiving antibiotics;

TABLE I.   (continued)

8. recurrent skin abscesses associated with eczema and pneumonia;

9. recurrent non-mycobacterial lymphadenitis;

10. recurrent meningitis;

11. unusual organisms such as Pneumocystis carinii or cytomegalovirus from lung aspirates or Serratia marcescens from abscesses.

After clinical analysis, identification of infecting organisms and appropriate treatment, certain patients need to be screened for possible immune defects. Some of the more commonly available tests to screen these patients are listed in Tables II-IV.

Since infants born after 36 weeks or more of gestation have high levels of IgG placentally transferred from the mother, defects associated only with the production of endogenous immunoglobulin tend not to become apparent until after three months of age when the maternally derived IgG has decreased significantly. Signs and symptoms of IgA deficiency may be present earlier if the infant is not breast-fed.

Clinical clues are present at an early age in children with defects in thymic dependent lymphocyte function (cell-mediated immunity), phagocytic cell function and complement. These clinical signs are often related to response to infection and of course, some children may have less exposure to potential pathogens so that suspicion of immunodeficiency does not occur until later in childhood.

III. CELL-MEDIATED IMMUNITY

Cell-mediated immunity requires antigen processing by mononuclear phagocytes, antigen recognition by T (thymus dependent) lymphocytes, proliferation of this antigen specific clone of T cells, and secretion of biologically active mediators (lymphokines) which regulate mononuclear phagocytes and polymorphonuclear phagocytes. A normally functioning cell-mediated immune system in an infant who has been immunized to tetanus or had candidal diaper rash will result in 5 mm or more induration at 48 to 72 hours to intradermal tests with 1) tetanus toxoid adsorbed USP 1:10 dilution in a total dose of .1 ml or 2) Candida albicans extract (Greer) 5000 pnu/ml in a total dose of .1 ml. Other tests for cell-mediated immune function include phytohemagglutinin induced transformation of lymphocytes in tissue culture and skin tests

with other antigens such as SK-SD and mumps. Decreased T-lymphocyte or T-lymphocyte and B (bone marrow dependent) lymphocyte
numbers can often be observed in these immunodeficiencies. In
severe combined immunodeficiency there may be absolute lympho-
penia, however, a normal total lymphocyte count does not exclude
functional deficiencies of T-lymphocytes. Table II describes
available screening tests for evaluation of cell-mediated
immunity.

TABLE II. Immunologic tests for cell-mediated immunity

1. Delayed hypersensitivity skin tests

   a) tetanus toxoid - 1:10 dilution

   b) Candida albicans extract
      5000 pnu/ml

   c) PPd (intermediate)

   d) Streptokinase - Streptodornase

2. Quantitation of T-cells and B-cells

3. Phytohemagglutinin transformation of lymphocytes

4. T-cell response to specific antigens

5. Leukocyte enzymes, adenosine deaminase and
   nucleotide phosphorylase

Certain immune defects can be diagnosed without specific immunologic tests. Patients with chronic or recurrent pneumonitis,
with recovery of unusual organisms such as Pneumocystis carinii
from lung aspirate or biopsy or cryptococcus from spinal fluid
have immunodeficiency until proven otherwise. Abnormalities such
as small platelet size, purpura and thrombocytopenia suggest the
Wiskott-Aldrich syndrome and hypocalcemia due to parathyroid hypoplasia is present in the DiGeorge syndrome. Progressive ataxia
and mucosal telangiectasia are present in patients with ataxia
telangiectasia. In addition, 40 to 75 percent of these patients
have very low or absent serum IgA levels which do not increase
with age. Specific abnormalities in cell-mediated immunity to
Candida albicans are frequently demonstrable in patients with
mucocutaneous candidiasis and endocrine disorders are also
frequently associated with these disorders. An important disease
entity to consider in any child with recurrent pneumonia, diarrhea
and failure to thrive is cystic fibrosis. Clinical presentations
are similar in cell-mediated and antibody-mediated immunodeficiency diseases.

IV. PHAGOCYTE DISORDERS

Severe or persistent stomatitis can be an early sign of neutropenia from a variety of causes including congenital, immunologic
or therapeutic. Peripheral white blood cell count and differential is the simplest and most direct means of diagnosis. Cyclic
neutropenia can be documented by neutrophil counts weekly over the
period of six weeks. Recurrent pulmonary infections with organisms such as Staphylococcus aureus, Serratia marcescens, E. coli,
Klebsiella, Aspergillus, or Nocardia are frequently associated
with neutropenia. Lymph node, liver or bone abscesses, which
begin in early infancy, especially when any of the above organisms
are recovered, often are indicative of chronic granulomatous
disease of childhood. Confirmation of the diagnoses of chronic
granulomatous disease depends on the assessment of leukocyte metabolic response during phagocytosis and bactericidal capcity. A
good screening test for chronic granulomatous disease is to test
the ability of normal peripheral blood neutrophils to reduce the
dye nitroblue tetrazolium (NBT) during phagocytosis or when stimulated by soluble stimulators. Chronic granulomatous disease
neutrophils fail to reduce NBT when stimulated. Patients with defects in phagocytosis (engulfment) are rare but abnormal microbicidal function is also found in neutrophils with engulfment
defects.
Abnormalities of phagocytic cell locomotion are also associated
with recurrent and persistent infections. Patients with the
hyperimmunoglobulin E syndrome have eczema, recurrent skin lesions
with staphylococci and recurrent pneumonia or pulmonary abscesses
secondary to S. aureus. Extremely elevated levels of IgE are
present and there is a very high level of IgE antistaphyloccal
antibodies. An intermittent neutrophil chemotactic defect is also
characteristic of this syndrome (9,10). Methods for evaluating
phagocytic cell function are outlined in Table III.

TABLE III. Test for evaluating phagocytic cell function

   1. White blood cell count and differential

   2. Nitroblue tetrazolium (NBT) dye reduction
        during phagocytosis

   3. Assay of white cell chemiluminescence

   4. Chemotaxis
        Boyden chamber
        Under agarose

   5. Uptake of radiolabeled bacteria

   6. Adherence

   7. Microbicidal killing

V. COMPLEMENT DISORDERS

Recurrent severe pneumonias and meningitis in early infancy due to more common pathogens such as H. influenzae and S. pneumoniae are seen in deficiencies of complement, especially C3 or of C3b inactivator. Abnormally low values for C3 and total hemolytic complement activity are consistent with these deficiencies. A deficiency in factor B which is associated with the alternative complement pathway is also associated with severe recurrent pneumococcal and H. influenzae infections. In older children recurrent infections with Neisseria species may indicate deficiency of the "membrane attack units of complement" C6, 7, and 8 (11). Normal total hemolytic complement activity and C3 and 4 levels can be obtained in patients with abnormalities of the alternative pathway of complement activation and functional tests are necessary to determine if this system is intact. Total hemolytic complement activity is a good screen for evaluating the classical complement pathway.

VI. IMMUNOGLOBULIN DISORDERS

After four months of age, as maternally acquired IgG declines, clinical signs of deficiencies of immunoglobulin appear. Patients with immunoglobulin deficiencies have recurrent otitis media, pneumonitis and meningitis with H. influenzae and S. pneumoniae. Congenital X-linked (Bruton's) agammaglobulinemia occurs only in males but selective immunoglobulinemia deficiencies and the varied immunodeficiencies are found in both sexes and at all ages. Immunoglobulin synthesis and secretion is dependent on the ability of monocytes to process antigen, present it properly to the appropriate B-lymphocytes which then undergo proliferation and differentiation into B memory cells and into plasma cells which secrete antigen specific IgM and IgG or IgA antibodies. This process is initiated and/or modulated by T-lymphocytes acting as helper or suppressor cells.

The diagnosis of X-linked agammaglobulinemia is confirmed by very low or absent peripheral blood B-lymphocytes as determined by fluorescent anti-human immunoglobulin staining of the peripheral blood lymphocytes. Quantitative immunoglobulins may be obtained in most laboratories and normal values for IgG, IgM and IgA at different ages are given in Table IV.

TABLE IV. Pediatric Normal Immunoglobulin Ranges (mg/dl)

Age	IgA	IgG	IgM
cord blood	0	398-1248	0-29
1-3 mos.	0-23	96-502	11-116
4-6 mos.	3-42	52-393	29-107
7-12 mos.	8-54	179-705	32-155
13-24 mos.	14-85	82-773	29-221
25-36 mos.	16-75	309-936	60-225
3-5 yrs.	23-137	342-1112	42-212
6-8 yrs.	57-204	454-1180	44-242
9-11 yrs.	52-256	510-1261	36-240
12-16 yrs.	52-192	461-1220	39-330
Adult	40-468	372-1356	48-414

Selective immunoglobulin deficiencies are primarily made by
determining which immunoglobulin class or classes are absent or
abnormally low in serum (8). B-cell numbers may be normal or even
increased. Selective IgA deficiency is the most common of these
disorders and, although usually asymptomatic, patients may have
sinusitis, pneumonitis or reversible obstructive airway disease,
various allergic and autoimmune diseases or chronic diarrhea. If
IgG subclass deficiency is also present, the likelihood of recurrent infections in IgA deficiency may be greater (12). IgA
production with resolution of infections may occur as the patient
matures. Rarely, a specific lack of secretory IgA due to lack of
secretory piece may result in recurrent sinopulmonary infections
and/or diarrhea. Absent IgA in saliva or tears while present in
serum is consistent with this diagnosis. Methods for evaluating
immunoglobulins are listed in Table V.

TABLE V. Evaluation of Immunoglobulins

1. Quantitative analysis of IgG, IgM,
    IgA and IgE

2. Isohemagglutinins

3. Specific antibody response
    Pneumococcal polysacchride
    Tetanus
    Diphtheria

4. Number of B cells

Patients with recurrent sinopulmonary infections may have normal quantitative immunoglobulins but lack one of the four subclasses of IgG (Ig_1, IgGg, IgG_3 and IgG_4) (12). The availability of monoclonal antibodies to specific IgG subclass antibodies may make diagnosis of these disorders more available than presently. Antibody response to diphtheria, tetanus and pneumococcal capsular polysaccharide immunization provide presumptive evidence for normal antibody production.

Patients without spleens have impaired reticuloendothelial function which can result in recurrent bacteremia and overwhelming sepsis especially with S. pneumoniae and H. influenzae. Surgical splenectomy and certain hemoglobinopathies, such as sickle cell disease may result in increased susceptibility to infection. Osteomyelitis with S. pneumoniae and salmonella should prompt evaluation of splenic function.

VI. TREATMENT OF PATIENTS WITH IMMUNODEFICIENCIES

Successful treatment of immunodeficient patients depends on early diagnosis before recurrent infections and malnutrition result in irreversible tissue damage. The most successful treatment is replacement of immunoglobulin G in X-linked (Bruton's) hypogammaglobulinemia and in some of the common varied immunodeficiencies. Intravenous immunoglobulin preparations are now available and plasma therapy is used. Bone marrow transplantation has been successful in patients with severe combined immunodeficiency.

Thymic epithelium and thymic extracts are being used for treatment of disorders of maturation of T-lymphocytes. Early diagnosis of phagocytic defects permits earlier and more appropriate intervention with antimicrobial agents during episodes of infection. Granulocyte transfusions are effective therapy for life-threatening infections in patients with phagocytic cell disorders. The replacement of certain complement components by fresh frozen plasma can be used for patients with complement deficiencies during acute infections. A summary of current therapies for patients with immunodeficiencies is presented in Table VI.

TABLE VI. Specific therapy for patients with immunodeficiency

1. Aggressive appropriate antimicrobial therapy

2. Granulocyte transfusions

3. Immunoglobulin replacement
   Cohn FrII provides IgG
   Human breast milk provides IgA

4. Fresh plasma
   Provides complement components and
      immunoglobulins

5. Hyperimmune serum or IgG
   Provides specific antibodies

6. Thymic epithelium or extracts
   Restores T-lymphocyte function

7. Bone marrow transfusion
   Restores immunoglobulin producing stem cells

REFERENCES

1. Dingle, J.H., Badger, G.F., and Jordan, W.S., Jr., "Illness in the Home." (1964). Press of Case Western Reserve University, Cleveland, Ohio.
2. Giebink, G.S. and Quie, P.G. (1978). Ann. Review. Med. 29, 285.
3. Feigin, R.D. and Spector, G. (1981). In "Textbook of Infectious Diseases." (R.D. Feigin and J.D. Cherry, eds.) p. 122.
4. Perrin, J.M., et. al. (1974). N. Engl. J. Med. 291, 664.
5. Abramson, J.S., Giebink, G.S., and Quie, P.G. (1981). Pediatr. Res. 15(Part 2), 606.
6. Hill, H.R. (1980). Ped. Clin. North. Am. 27, 805.
7. Miller, M.E. (ed.) (1977). Ped. Clin. North. Am. 24, 277.
8. Report of a WHO Scientific Group. (1979). Clin. Immunol. and Immunopathol. 13, 296.
9. Schopfer, K., Baerlocher, K., Price, P., Krech, U., Quie, P.G., and Douglas, S.D. (1979). N. Engl. J. Med. 300, 835.
10. Abramson, J.S., Dahl, M.V., Walsh, G., Blumenthal, M.N., Douglas, S.D., and Quie, P.G. (1981). Submitted for publication.

11. Peterson, B.H., et. al.   (1979).   <u>Ann</u>. <u>Intern</u>. <u>Med</u>. 90, 917.
12. Oxelius, V.A., et. al.   (1981).   <u>N</u>. <u>Engl</u>. <u>J</u>. <u>Med</u>. 304, 1476.
13. Tiller, T.L., Jr., and Buckley, R.H.   (1978).   <u>J</u>. <u>Peds</u>. 92,
    347.

SYSTEMIC MYCOSES
IN THE IMMUNOCOMPROMISED HOST

John E. Bennett

Clinical Mycology Section
National Institute of Allergy
and Infectious Diseases
National Institutes of Health
Bethesda, Maryland

INTRODUCTION

It has become commonplace to note the rising incidence of systemic mycoses in immunosuppressed patients. This observation is usually followed by a note of despair about antemortem diagnosis and therapeutic response. Such nihilism has adequate support in experience with the severely compromised patient, such as a markedly neutropenic patient with systemic candidiasis, pulmonary aspergillosis or pulmonary mucormycosis. More success should be expected in less compromised patients and, for this reason, infections in these patients will be emphasized here.

This chapter will stress diagnosis. A summary of two newer treatment regimens is provided in another chapter. Although empiric antifungal therapy is now being evaluated in several cancer centers, indications for use of such regimens remains as yet undefined.

CLINICAL PRESENTATIONS

Pneumonia

Acute onset of one or more dense areas of pneumonia in a severely neutropenic patient raises the possibility of aspergillosis or mucormycosis. Progression despite broad spectrum

371

antibacterial therapy should enhance suspicion. Fever rarely
antedates the abnormal chest x-ray by more than two days. Survival beyond two weeks may be seen in patients with less severe
immunosuppression but true chronicity does not occur in pulmonary
mucormycosis. Chronic invasive pulmonary aspergillosis occurs in
chronic granulomatous disease but not in leukopenic patients.
Recovering patients with returning bone marrow function or with
decreasing doses of immunosuppressive drugs may excavate a necrotic area of lung and expectorate it partially. A movable
chunk can remain inside the cavity, resembling fungus ball of the
lung.

Pulmonary candidiasis is an acute, hematogenous infection.
The lung lesions cannot be seen on chest x-ray of most cases.
Occasionally, myriad abscesses are so numerous that a diffuse
interstitial infiltrate is seen.

Pulmonary cryptococcosis is of indolent onset and slow progression. A well defined margin and a dense infiltrate is most
suggestive but one or more patchy, poorly defined infiltrates
can also be found.

Disease of the Head and Neck

Craniofacial mucormycosis has such a distinctive progression
that diagnosis is usually made before death. As progression
makes the diagnosis easier, the patient's chance of avoiding
blindness, facial deformity and death become less likely. Aching
pain over a paranasal sinus of a diabetic should raise the question of mucormycosis. Fever is low-grade or absent early in the
disease. The patient is almost always hyperglycemic at onset
but is acidotic in only about a half the cases. The diabetes
mellitus in a patient with lymphoma or receiving adrenal corticosteroids may have been previously mild, not treated with
insulin. X-ray shows opacification of a paranasal sinus, usually
the maxillary sinus. A thin, serosanguinous nasal discharge may
be noted. As infection extends to the nasal turbinates, the mucosa becomes pale and boggy, then necrotic and purplish black.
The same color sequence can be seen in the hard palate, where the
lesion sharply respects the midline. Anterior extension to the
cheek causes erythema and induration early, rapidly followed by
purple necrosis. Often the first extension is to the orbit, with
double vision and pain. The globe becomes increasingly limited
in motion. Conjunctival edema appears. The patient's vision
becomes clouded as the fungus invades the globe or the ophthalmic
artery. Coma supervenes when the fungus reaches the brain by
direct extension to the frontal lobe or through the bloodstream,
by extension to the carotid artery in the siphon. Diagnosis can
rarely be made in any other way than by biopsy of infected tissue.

Biopsy of the sinus, nose, palate or cheek lesion should be
stained by Gomorri methenamine silver. The wide hyphae can also
be seen in wet smear of crushed tissue.

The clinical setting and fundoscopic picture of Candida
endophthalmitis is so characteristic that diagnosis can be
reasonably secure. The patient is rarely severely neutropenic
at time the lesion first occurs in the eye. Almost invariably,
the patient has had a plastic intravenous catheter in place.
Fever is usual at time of candidemia but may have disappeared
when the catheter was removed or replaced. Early symptoms may
have been missed because the patient was postoperative, had an
endotracheal tube in place, was comatose or otherwise unable to
communicate. When noted, early symptoms are a dull or sticking
eye pain, blurred vision or a scotoma. Ocular examination at
this time reveals one or more pale retinal lesions. These resemble diabetic exudates, cytoid bodies of systemic lupus erythematosus or leukemic exudates. Smaller lesions may look like
drüsen. Early lesions may resolve spontaneously over several
days. All too often, the infection spreads into the vitreous,
eventually destroying the eye. Lesions are unilateral in half
the cases. Progressive infection clouds the vitreous and extends
to the anterior chamber. Injection of deep scleral vessels
around the corneal limbus may be mistaken for conjunctivitis.
Vitreal extension makes prognosis for visual acuity more guarded
and requires more prolonged therapy with amphotericin B but also
makes possible confirmation of the diagnosis by pars plana vi-
trectomy. Some ophthalmologists feel that this procedure improves outcome as well as confirming the diagnosis.

Disease of the Gastrointestinal Tract and Liver

Endoscopy is being used increasingly to diagnose esophageal
and gastric lesions in the immunosuppressed host. Herpes simplex
and <u>Candida albicans</u> are both frequent causes of esophagitis in
this setting and respond well to specific therapy. Esophagram
may miss the lesions and does not reliably distinguish these two
from one another and from other causes, such as peptic esophagitis or aspergillosis. To complicate matters, Candida may invade
a herpetic lesion. Endoscopic biopsy and culture is optimal but
even a scraping and smear may show the pseudohyphae of Candida.
Once a diagnosis of candidiasis is established, the severely
neutropenic patient appears to warrant aggressive therapy in
order to prevent dissemination. While perforation of the esophagus or stomach is rare, the gastrointestinal tract is the most
frequent portal of systemic candidiasis in neutropenic patients.
Mucosal lesions due to Candida are usually asymptomatic below the
esophagus. While it has been difficult to prove that hematogenous dissemination can originate from the esophagus, treatment
can be justified also on the basis that asymptomatic lesions may

be present lower in the gastrointestinal tract. The most effective therapy is intravenous amphotericin B. Even doses of 10–15 mg/day can diminish symptoms in a few days. Radiologic healing may be seen after one to two weeks of this dose. Higher doses and more prolonged therapy may be required if the infection is already disseminated.

Patients with hematologic malignancies and gastrointestinal ulcerations due to Candida are prone to develop numerous small hepatic abscesses. Grossly, these are anywhere from barely visible to round white lesions a centimeter in diameter. Liver scan may show patchy uptake. Computer axial tomography and sonogram have not successfully visualized such small lesions. Liver function has been normal or shown small elevations of transaminase, but this patient group often has hepatic malfunction for other reasons. Diagnosis has required biopsy. Although this procedure may be risky in patients with hematologic malignancies, the presence of prolonged, unexplained fever in the proper setting may justify the procedure. Response to amphotericin B is very slow, in the author's experience, and relapse can be seen even after prolonged therapy.

Aspergillosis and mucormycosis sometimes enter the body through the gastrointestinal tract. These ulcerations have a strong propensity for perforation and may present as bacterial peritonitis. Bleeding diathesis due to underlying disease has made surgical diagnosis or treatment difficult.

DIAGNOSIS

Frequent reference has been made in the foregoing to diagnosis by biopsy. Despite great interest and numerous studies on serologic diagnosis, no one test has achieved any kind of a consensus that it is valuable. Detection of serum arabinitol in candidiasis and antigenemia in candidiasis and aspergillosis are attracting attention at present. It seems clear that some patients with the mycosis will be positive by these tests and that the problems are more likely to be false negatives than false positive tests, once account is taken of the effect of renal function on serum arabinitol. Widespread adoption, however, will require a better understanding of which patients have a positive test and just how common such patients are in a particular institution. With rapidly fatal mycoses, the test will have to be positive early in the infection and be simple enough to be done the day it is requested.

TREATMENT

The lack of new, helpful agents for treatment of systemic mycoses in immunosuppressed patients is probably excuse enough for adding very little to foregoing remarks about therapy. The encouraging new data about oral ketoconazole have been with mycoses other than systemic candidiasis and invasive aspergillosis. Discovery of aspergillosis and systemic candidiasis at autopsy of patients receiving ketoconazole prophylaxis has not raised expectations about successful therapy of established infections, though at present there are neither encouraging nor discouraging hard data on the subject. Studies in this area are difficult to do in a convincing way, a fact to which all the studies on miconazole stand in disarming witness. Hesitance of oncologists to use flucytosine-amphotericin B in neutropenic patients is probably appropriate, considering the difficulty with which it is to say whether flucytosine is adding to the patient's neutropenia or thrombocytopenia. Conceivably, frequent assessment of the blood flucytosine level could permit complete protection against flucytosine-induced bone marrow suppression. All current evidence indicates that this toxicity only occurs when the blood level exceeds 100–125 µg/ml. This extra trouble would be indicated were there good evidence that flucytosine-amphotericin B is superior to amphotericin B alone in candidiasis and aspergillosis. Without such evidence, amphotericin B remains the established drug for systemic mycoses in the immunosuppressed patient.

PART XII
SPECIAL DIAGNOSTIC CONSIDERATIONS

FEVERS THAT ARE DIFFICULT TO DIAGNOSE

Paul E. Hermans

Division of Infectious Diseases
Mayo Clinic and Mayo Foundation
Rochester, Minnesota

Most patients with fever of unknown origin (FUO)
challenge the clinical ability of the medical team; require
considerable time, effort, and testing; and thus incur
extremely high medical bills. Not all cases of fever in
which the cause is not rapidly established should be classified as FUO. The following criteria are helpful in
distinguishing patients who have FUO: (1) an illness of at
least 3 weeks' duration; (2) a temperature of at least 38.3°C
(101°F) rectally or 37.8°C (100°F) orally recorded several
times; and (3) an uncertain diagnosis after 1 week of systematic studies.

For the past 10 years, we kept records of Mayo Clinic
patients with fevers that were difficult to diagnose. Of the
256 patients, 202 fulfilled the aforementioned strict criteria
for FUO, and 54 did not but had conditions that were difficult
to diagnose. The diagnostic categories and the number of
patients in each category are listed in Table I for patients
with true FUO and in Table II for patients with fevers difficult to diagnose but not meeting the stringent criteria.

Obviously, despite intensive and prolonged efforts, no
diagnosis was made in about a fourth of the patients with FUO
and of those with fevers that were difficult to diagnose.
Other studies have shown that most patients in whom no diagnosis was made have a benign course and that the condition in
about two-thirds of these patients still remains undiagnosed
at subsequent follow-up examinations.

As shown in Table I, about 7% of patients with true FUO
had resolution of the fever during their hospitalization.
These patients were usually considered to have had an

infectious episode or hypersensitivity reaction that remained undiagnosed. Almost half of the patients with FUO were ultimately diagnosed as having an infection, a vasculitis-collagen type of illness, or a malignant lesion. These same diagnostic categories accounted for almost 60% of patients listed in Table II. Although this classification of patients with perplexing fevers is interesting, it is of little practical application in the diagnosis of any individual case.

Of some help is the information that an infection is much less likely to be present in patients who have had fever for more than 1 year than in those who have had fever for less than 1 year. Patients with perplexing fevers do not have unusual or esoteric illnesses. Most patients have relatively common illnesses that are manifested in an atypical manner or are in an early nondiagnosable phase of their disease.

The illnesses that were ultimately diagnosed in our patients with perplexing fevers are classified according to their cause in Table III. Clearly, in any specific patient with FUO, the diagnostic possibilities are numerous.

Fortunately, these possibilities can be limited by information obtained from the history (Table IV), the physical examination (Table V), the clinical course, and the results of routine and more specific testing (Tables VI through XII). As mentioned earlier, even extended efforts will not yield a diagnosis in about one in four patients. General rules for the approach to the problem of FUO are shown in Table XIII.

TABLE I.   Fever of Unknown Origin: Mayo Clinic Experience
           (202 Patients)

Diagnosis	Patients	
	No.	%
Infection	45	22.3
Hematologic malignant lesion	27	13.4
Vasculitis-collagen disease	13	6.4
Nonhematologic malignant lesion	12	5.9
Systemic arthritis	9	4.5
Idiopathic granulomatosis	8	4.0
Familial Mediterranean fever or periodic fever	8	4.0
Miscellaneous	15	7.4
Spontaneous resolution of fever	15	7.4
None	50	24.7

TABLE II. Difficult Fever: Mayo Clinic Experience (54 Patients)

Diagnosis	Patients	
	No.	%
Infection	18	33.3
Hematologic malignant lesion	3	5.6
Vasculitis-collagen disease or systemic arthritis	8	14.8
Nonhematologic malignant lesion	2	3.7
Idiopathic granulomatosis	0	0
Familial Mediterranean fever or periodic fever	0	0
Miscellaneous	6	11.1
Functional condition	3	5.6
None	14	25.9

TABLE III.   Fever of Unknown Origin: Etiologic Classification

---

Infections
  According to site: Heart (infective endocarditis), hepato-
  biliary region (liver abscess, cholangitis, cholecystitis),
  intra-abdominal extrahepatobiliary region (abscess,
  diverticulitis), upper urinary tract (pyelonephritis,
  xanthogranulomatous pyelonephritis), skeletal system
  (osteomyelitis, disk-space infection), head (paranasal
  sinusitis, mastoiditis), intestinal tract (infections from
  Clostridium difficile and *Campylobacter fetus jejuni*,
  Whipple's disease, others), reproductive system (prostatitis,
  pelvic inflammation, lymphogranuloma venereum)
  According to microorganisms:
  Bacteria: Tuberculosis, atypical mycobacteriosis, borreliosis
    (*Borrelia recurrentis* and others), bartonellosis, rat-bite
    fever (*Spirillum minus*), syphilis (*Treponema pallidum*),
    extragenital gonorrhea, meningococcemia
  Fungi: Histoplasmosis, blastomycosis, cryptococcosis,
    coccidioidomycosis, candidiasis, aspergillosis
  Plasmodia and parasitic: Malaria, toxoplasmosis,
    trypanosomiasis, leishmaniasis, trichinosis, amebiasis
  Chlamydiae: Psittacosis
  Rickettsiae: Q fever
  Viruses: Pleuropericarditis, hepatitis, encephalitis,
    cytomegalovirus, infectious mononucleosis, subacute
    thyroiditis, cat-scratch fever
Idiopathic granulomatosis
  Includes sarcoidosis, granulomatous hepatitis, and granuloma-
  tosis of unknown cause.   Tuberculosis, atypical mycobacterio-
  sis, fungal infections, cytomegalovirus, and infectious mono-
  nucleosis excluded.   Some investigators include temporal
  (cranial) arteritis, Wegener's granulomatosis, and regional
  enteritis
Vasculitis
  Temporal (cranial) arteritis, periarteritis nodosa, hypersensitivity vasculitis (Churg-Strauss syndrome), Takayasu's
  disease
Systemic arthritis
  Juvenile rheumatoid arthritis (Still's disease), adult
  Still's disease, atypical rheumatoid arthritis, rheumatic
  fever
Collagen (hypersensitivity) disorders
  Systemic lupus erythematosus, serum sickness, rheumatic
  fever, mixed connective tissue disease, erythema multiforme,
  idiopathic erythema nodosum
Hematologic malignant lesions
  Hodgkin's lymphoma, non-Hodgkin's lymphoma, acute myelomono-
  cytic leukemia, preleukemic leukemia, aleukemic leukemia,
  angio-immunoblastic lymphoma

Nonhematologic malignant lesions
  Hypernephroma, metastatic carcinomatosis, carcinoma of
  pancreas, hepatoma
Familial Mediterranean fever and periodic fever
  Usually, diagnoses made after exclusion of other causes;
  characterized by long duration, benign course, periodicity,
  and (occasionally) associated chest and abdominal distress
  without specific response but with response to colchicine or
  indomethacin. Mollaret's meningitis (recurrent, benign),
  cyclic neutropenia
Miscellaneous
  Physiologic hyperthermia (exaggerated circadian temperature
  variation), polymyalgia rheumatica, inflammatory bowel
  disease, interstitial pneumonitis (drug induced--cyclophos-
  phamide, others), chronic hepatitis, biliary cirrhosis,
  portal cirrhosis, thrombophlebitis, recurrent pulmonary
  emboli, pheochromocytoma, noninfectious postsurgical fever
  (halothane sensitization, postcardiotomy syndrome, aseptic
  meningitis after neurosurgical procedure or myelography),
  pheochromocytoma, hyperthyroidism, atrial myxoma, pancreatitis
Drug fever
  Antimicrobial agents: Any, but especially penicillins,
  isoniazid, nitrofurantoin
  Cardiovascular drugs: Hydralazine, methyldopa, procainamide,
  quinidine
  Miscellaneous: Antihistamines (over-the-counter preparations),
  barbiturates, phenytoin, iodides, mercaptopurine, salicylates
Factitious
  Two types of factitial fever: Manipulation of thermometer,
  factitial infection or inflammation (self-injection of
  microorganisms or irritants)

TABLE IV. The History

Detailed and repetitive
Interview of household family members and friends
Recent and past contacts (e.g., tuberculosis)
Detailed family history
Travel history (e.g., coccidioidomycosis, malaria)
Details of invasive procedures (e.g., common duct stone)
Use of medications and response
Pitfalls:
  True onset of illness
  Irritable bowel syndrome vs. inflammatory disease
  Nonacceptance of an unlikely detail
  Lack of specificity of questions
  The head (e.g., temporal or cranial arteritis)
  The abdomen (e.g., atypical cholecystitis, diverticulitis)
  The feet (e.g., mononeuritis multiplex due to periarteritis
  nodosa)

TABLE V. The Physical Examination

Documentation of fever
Pulse rate at time of fever (drug-induced fever, factitial fever)
A complete, thorough examination
Repeat examination a couple of times a week
Repeat examination before any invasive procedure
Pitfalls:
    Temporal regions (temporal arteritis)
    Mental status (subacute bacterial endocarditis, cryptococcal
     and tuberculous meningitis)
    Absence of neck stiffness (chronic meningitis)
    "Functional" or "hemic" heart murmur (in reality, subacute
     bacterial endocarditis)
    Small, firm lymph node (carcinoma, Hodgkin's disease)
    Evasive friction rub (idiopathic pericarditis)
    Briefly swollen joint (atypical rheumatoid arthritis)
    Percussible spleen (subacute bacterial endocarditis, lymphoma)
    Localized tenderness of the liver (abscess)
    Omitted rectal examination (diverticulitis)
    Presbyopic examiner (small petechiae, splinter lesions)
    Tender thyroid gland (subacute thyroiditis)

TABLE VI. The Routine Laboratory Tests

1. Hemoglobin level
    Red blood cells
    Indices
2. White blood cell count
    Differential count--the eosinophil
    Special hematology smear--the abnormal cell
3. Platelet count
4. Erythrocyte sedimentation rate
5. Urinalysis and repeat urinalysis
6. Blood chemistry
    Alkaline phosphatase
    Serum glutamic-oxalacetic transaminase
    Bilirubin--direct bilirubin
    Creatinine
    Uric acid
    Calcium
    Sodium, potassium, chloride
7. Automated reagin test
8. Chest roentgenography
9. Electrocardiography

TABLE VII. Cultures

Source	Routine	Acid-fast	Fungi	Brucella[a]
Blood	3x	...[b]	3x	3x
Urine	1x	3x	3x	2x
Sputum[c]	2x	3x	3x	...
Induced sputum with gastric washing	...	3x	3x	...
Biopsy material	Yes	Yes	Yes	Yes
Surgical tissue	Yes	Yes	Yes	Yes
Stool	Yes	...	...	...
Bone marrow	Yes	Yes	Yes	Yes
Cerebrospinal fluid	Yes	Yes	Yes	...

[a] Culture if indicated.
[b] Culture only if atypical mycobacteriosis is suspected.
[c] Culture also for *Nocardia* and *Actinomyces*.

TABLE VIII. Special Laboratory Tests[a]

1. Serum protein electrophoresis
2. Fungal serology
3. *Brucella* agglutination
4. Cytomegalovirus serology
5. Heterophil antibody test (infectious mononucleosis)
6. Antistreptolysin O titer
7. *Toxoplasma* serology
8. *Leptospira* serology
9. Hepatitis B surface antigen
10. Antinuclear antibody
11. Rheumatoid factor
12. Lupus erythematosus clot test
13. Stool for leukocytes
14. Stool for blood
15. Stool for parasites and ova
16. Malaria smear
17. Malaria serology
18. Center for Disease Control screening serology for parasites

[a] Tests 1, 2, 4, 5, 6, 10, 11, and 12 should be done in all patients. Need for other tests depends on circumstances.

TABLE IX.   Roentgenographic Studies

Plain film of abdomen
Excretory urography
Gallbladder
Intravenous cholangiography (past cholecystectomy)
Stomach
Small bowel
Colon
Paranasal sinuses
Mastoids
Skeletal survey for metastases

TABLE X.   Special Procedures[a]

Purified protein derivative (PPD) skin test[b]
Proctoscopic examination
Funduscopic examination

[a]These three procedures should be done in all patients.
[b]If result is negative and tuberculosis is still suspected, delayed-hypersensitivity skin tests should be done to determine whether the patient is capable of reacting.

TABLE XI.   Invasive Procedures[a]

Bone marrow aspiration and biopsy
Cerebrospinal fluid examination
Lymph node biopsy
Mediastinoscopy
Liver biopsy
Abdominal exploration
Lymphangiography
Muscle biopsy
Synovial biopsy
Pleural biopsy
Pericardial biopsy

[a]Invasive procedures should be done only when specifically indicated. Any tissue obtained by biopsy should be examined by a pathologist and should be cultured for "routine microorganisms," mycobacteria, fungi, and *Brucella*.

TABLE XII.   New Visualization Procedures

Lung perfusion-ventilation scan
Echocardiography (any patient with heart murmur)
Ultrasonography of abdomen
Liver-spleen scan
Gallium scan
Computed tomography scan of abdomen

TABLE XIII. General Rules for the Approach to the Problem of FUO

1. Realize the importance of the history and physical examination.
   The history and physical examination are always important.
   They should be especially detailed and complete in cases of FUO.
2. Establish the presence of a fever.
   Always establish that the patient indeed has a fever. Rule
   out habitual hyperthermia, preoccupation with temperature,
   variations with menstrual cycle, and factitial fever.
3. Rule out the possibility of a drug-induced fever.
   Early in the course of a workup, rule out a drug-related fever.
   This can be done by observing a pulse-rate deficit in relationship to the severity of the fever, by demonstrating eosinophilia, and by discontinuing the use of the most likely
   offending drugs. A meticulous history about recent drug
   intake should be elicited.
4. Realize that the episode may be self-limiting.
   One should remember that a considerable number of febrile
   episodes will be self-limiting and benign. Such episodes do
   not warrant the enormous expenses of an extensive workup.
5. Observe the course of the illness carefully.
   In the course of the workup of a patient with FUO, assess the
   patient's general condition from day to day. The workup
   should be expedited and intensified if the condition of the
   patient is deteriorating.
6. Determine why you order a test.
   If you order a test, you either want the test or you do not
   want it. If you do not want it, do not order it. If you
   want it, wait for the result.
7. Reexamine before performing an invasive procedure.
   Repeat a complete physical examination before carrying out an
   invasive procedure. A new physical finding may have developed
   since the last examination. Also reconsider all available
   data and the clinical course of the patient.
8. Order tests and procedures systematically.
   In the initial phase of the workup, use only those tests that
   are most likely to produce results based on information
   obtained from the history and physical examination. Also concentrate initially on potentially curable conditions--infec-
   tive endocarditis, acute cholecystitis, liver abscess, intra-
   abdominal abscess, urinary tract infection, fungal infections,
   tuberculosis, hypernephroma, xanthogranulomatous pyelonephritis, lymphoma, cranial arteritis.
9. Give precise instructions for processing tissue obtained by
   biopsy.
   It is critical to discuss in detail with the endoscopist, the
   surgeon, or the performer of a biopsy what should be done
   with the tissue that is obtained. The types of special stains
   and cultures must be reviewed. Occasionally, it is helpful to
   review the pathologic findings with the pathologist.

ACKNOWLEDGMENT

The patient data in Tables I and II are preliminary data that were derived from an ongoing collaborative study by the members of the Division of Infectious Diseases at the Mayo Clinic.

REFERENCES

Effersøe, P. (1968). *Dan. Med. Bull.* *15*, 240.
Petersdorf, R.G., and Beeson, P.B. (1961). *Medicine (Baltimore)* *40*, 1.
Sheon, R.P., and Van Ommen, R.A. (1963). *Am. J. Med.* *34*, 486.
Tumulty, P.A. (1967). *Johns Hopkins Med. J.* *120*, 95.

PREOPERATIVE AND POSTOPERATIVE FEVER

Robert E. Condon

Department of Surgery
The Medical College of Wisconsin
Milwaukee, Wisconsin

Not all fevers observed in association with an operation are due to infection. Indeed, the commonest cause of postoperative fever--atelectasis--clearly does not have an infectious basis. It behooves the physician encountering a patient with post-operative fever to keep the non-infectious as well as the infectious possibilities in mind. An expensive work-up for possible infection should not be undertaken before simpler causes of fever have been eliminated. The more common causes of fever occuring in association with an operation are listed below, more or less in the chronological order in which they might be encountered.

PRE-EXISTING SEPSIS

Ordinarily this situation does not cause any diagnostic con-fusion. The focus of infection will usually have been diagnosed and documented before the operation; in fact, the objective of the operation may have been to provide control of such infection. Pre-existing pneumonia will be worsened by a general anesthetic. Urinary tract infections which have been incompletely managed preoperatively result in a modest increase in fever postopera-tively, even though the urinary tract has not been manipulated. The presence of an uncontrolled septic focus at the time of operation provides a basis for bacteremia and preferential lodgement of bacteria in the operative wound.

MALIGNANT HYPERTHERMIA

This is a rare genetic syndrome, dominantly transmitted, triggered by administration of succinylcholine.
The onset is typically early during a general anesthetic and is characterized by tachycardia, an unstable blood pressure, a rapid rise in temperature to 105-107°F in less than 30 minutes, accompanied by muscle rigidity, hypoxia and eventual cardiac arrhythmias. The syndrome is thought to be due to uncoupling of oxidative phosphorylation leading to excess heat production.

OPERATIONS AROUND THE HYPOTHALMUS

Operations at the base of the brain may lead to temporary dysfunction of hypothalmic temperature regulation. Such patients may be poikilothermic, or nearly so. The more typical postoperative hypothalmic fever involves resetting of the thermostat approximately 2° above normal and persists for 3 to 7 days postoperatively.

THYROID STORM

Formerly a feared complication of operations on the thyroid, this syndrome is rarely seen today. The onset is in the immediate postoperative period, during and immediately after recovery from anesthesia. It is characterized by high fever, tachycardia, irritability, psychosis, vomiting, and high output cardiac failure.

INTRAOPERATIVE SEPTICEMIA

The operative maneuvers which necessarily manipulate a septic focus, such as drainage of an abscess or spillage of infected urine from an open bladder, contamination of the peritoneum or other serosal membranes and produce septicemia. Normal body responses--humoral, cellular and hypothalamic--are blunted while the patient is under anesthesia. As the anesthetic clears, fever, tachycardia and peripheral vasodilation may supervene in the recovery room.

TRANSFUSION REACTIONS

All varieties of transfusion reactions may be associated with fever. Reactions due to errors in cross-matching or bacterial contamination of banked blood are now very rare. The more common transfusion reactions are secondary to transfusion of antigens or pyrogens in plasma; administration of packed cells, and especially of washed packed red cells, markedly reduces the incidence of febrile transfusion reactions.

POST-TRAUMATIC HYPERMETABOLISM

Basal calorie comsumption is increased approximately three-fold (from 1500 calories to about 4500 calories per day in adults) after an operative procedure. The more extensive the operation, the greater the increase in basal metabolic rate, and the longer this alteration in metabolism will persist postoperatively. In typical cases, the hypermetabolic state reaches a peak on the operative day and thereafter declines, becoming nearly normal by the third or fourth postoperative day. Accompanying this hypermetabolism, a rise in basal body temperature of approximately 0.5 - 1°F is mediated by a resetting of the hypothalamic thermostat.

CLOSTRIDIAL MYONECROSIS

This complication typically accompanies operations on the colon, rectum, female pelvic organs, and the biliary tract. All these organs are sites in which endogenous clostridia are present. Shock accompanied by fever and severe toxemia appears in the first 24 hours postoperatively. There is crepitation and discoloration of skin surrounding the wound. When the wound is opened, there is a thin brownish malodorous discharge. This complication is lethal unless treated promptly.

ASPIRATION PNEUMONIA

Aspiration of gastric content while under anesthesia can lead to necrotizing pneumonia with its apparent onset at about the second postoperative day. Indeed, the regular occurrence of aspiration of small amounts of gastric contents in every patient undergoing a general anesthetic is the principle reason why modern anesthesiology techniques regularly involve the use of a cuffed endotracheal tube. Patients with impaired gastric acid barrier whose stomach lumen harbors an endogenous flora of mouth organisms and fecal aerobes are particularly liable to the development of this sort of postoperative pneumonia.

ATELECTASIS

This the the commonest cause of postoperative fever and occurs to some degree in every patient undergoing a general anesthetic. The degree of atelectasis is worse in patients afflicted with chronic bronchitis or emphysema, asthma, morbid obesity, and in quadraplegia and other neuromuscular disorders associated with weak respiratory effort. Fever typically begins 6-12 hours postoperatively; it may be as high as 102.5°F, and may persist for 3-4 days in nonsmokers, but for 5-8 days in smokers. Fever is accompanied by a modest increase in the respiratory rate and pulse; there are decreased breath sound at the lung bases with bronchial breath sounds noted, particularly posteriorly, accompaned by moist rales.

The clinical feature which distinguishes atelectasis from pneumonia is that the temperature can rapidly be reduced by coughing. Indeed, the temperature can be reduced from 102° to 100.5°F in less than 30 minutes by effective coughing or other measures which remove bronchial secretions. Although narcotics do depress the cough reflex, administration of adequate doses of narcotics is essential to reduce pain to permit effective voluntary coughing. In my experience, inadequate administration of narcotics is the prime reason for persistance of atelectasis in nonsmoking patients.

Since this is not an infectious process, antibiotic therapy is not indicated in the postoperative management of fever due to atelectasis.

EARLY WOUND CELLULITIS (Streptococcal, Clostridial)

This is an infectious process limited to the subcutaneous tissues and not involving muscle fascia. Symptoms typically appear about 72 hours postoperatively, with a spiking fever, increased pain and spreading erythema surrounding the wound. Clostridial cellulitis does not carry with it the marked systemic toxicity or grave prognosis which is associated with clostridial myonecrosis.

URINARY TRACT INFECTION

Postoperative urinary tract infection usually is limited to the bladder and urethra, almost always is secondary to catheterization, and can be delayed but not obviated by meticulous management of the catheter drainage system. Fever typically appears about the 5th postoperative day. Treatment of infected bladder urine while a catheter remains in place simply results in emergence of resistance.

POST SPLENECTOMY FEVER

This syndrome of low grade fever appearing early postoperatively and persisting for up to 2 weeks following splenectomy was thought in thepast to be related to a low grade pancreatitis involving only the tail of that gland, or to thrombosis of blood vessels in the hilum of the excised spleen. It is probable that most such febrile episodes are, in fact, related to low grade infection in a hematoma in the splenic bed.

POSTOPERATIVE PNEUMONIA

True pneumonia, that is invasion of pulmonary tissue by bacteria, usually has its onset 3-5 days postoperatively. Almost always there has been a preceding atelectasis which has been inadequately treated. Clinically persistant high fever accompanied by absent to bronchial breath sound and moist rales should lead one to suspect this diagnosis. Although fever is reduced somewhat with vigorous coughing, it usually stays above 101°F.

Confirmation of the diagnosis of pneumonia should be made by obtaining a transtracheal aspirate for culture. It is my view that transtracheal aspirates are essential to obtain reliable data for Gram stain and for both aerobic and anaerobic culture. The proximal airway is contaminated during the necessary peroral manipulations associated with conduct of anesthesia. This contamination persists for a relatively prolonged period postoperatively, so that sputum specimens, even deep-cough sputum specimens, are not reliable in identification of the involved pathogens.

THROMBOPHLEBITIS

Phlebitis related to an indwelling intravenous line inserted in the operating room typically begins about the third postoperative day. Much of this form of phlebitis can be obviated by removing all lines inserted in the operating room within the first 24 hours postoperatively.

Thrombophlebitis involving vessels in the calf typically has its onset 5-7 days postoperatively. Early clinical signs are some mild tenderness in the instep and assumption by the patients of unilateral or bilateral "frog leg" position in bed. Homans' sign (pain on stretching the gastrocnemius by sharp ankle dorsiflexion) is a late and unreliable sign of calf phlebitis.

Septic thrombophlebitis originating in pelvic vessels is a complication seen typically after operations on the female pelvic organs conducted in the face of established infection (septic abortion, tubo-ovarian abscess, etc.).

SUBCUTANEOUS WOUND INFECTION

This complication typically begins with an increase in wound pain noted beginning about the 3rd-4th day postoperatively. usually accompanied by some modest increase in periwound edema. More classic signs of erythema and heat may be minimal or absent. About the 5th postoperative day fever appears, and becomes spiking about the 7th postoperative day. It must be remembered that occasional wound infections may appear as late as three weeks postoperatively and follow a very indolent course. The risk of developing a subcutaneous wound infection is related to the relative blood supply in various body areas; less in incisions involving the scalp, head and neck, and perineum, and greater in operative wounds distally in the extremities or on the back, especially in older patients.

DEEP ABSCESS

This complication usually is heralded by spiking fever beginning 5-8 days postoperatively. The primary wound may heal without any evidence of infection, yet a deep abscess may be present. Anastomotic disruption is the commonest cause in elective bowel resection; exogenous or endogenous contamination is the commonest cause in emergency operations.

Intra-abdominal abscesses are most efficiently diagnosed by detection of appropriate physical signs, and by noting abnormalities on flat and upright plain films of the abdomen. Computerized tomography is very efficient in the diagnosis of intra-abdominal abscesses; the record of ultrasound is more variable in terms of diagnostic reliability in our experience. Contrast studies (UGI, Barium enema, arteriography) are much less useful. Gallium scans have not been helpful at all.

STARCH-TALC GRANULOMA

This is due to idiosyncratic reaction to the powder used on surgical gloves. Fever begins 1-3 weeks postoperatively, accompanied by ileus. The syndrome mimics a postoperative abscess or bowel obstruction.

DRUG FEVER

An uncommon cause of postoperative fever, but one that should be thought of whenever fever persists but the patient does not appear to be very ill. Antibiotics are notorious as a cause of drug fever. If antibiotics have been initiated on the basis of inadequate evidence because of fever early in the postoperative course, fever will persist as long as antibiotic administration is continued. The only way to sort out this problem is stop administering drugs.

FACTICIOUS FEVER

This problem rarely arises in a postoperative patient, factitious fever usually being induced by the patient much earlier in the course of hospitalization. But, whenever diagnostic efforts are of no avail, and the patient has persistant fever but does not otherwise appear ill, confirmation that fever is real can be obtained by measuring the temperature of freshly voided urine.

NON-INVASIVE DIAGNOSIS
OF OCCULT INTRA-ABDOMINAL INFECTION

Robert Fekety

Division of Infectious Diseases
Department of Internal Medicine
University of Michigan Medical School
and University Hospital
Ann Arbor, Michigan

INTRODUCTION

The presence of swelling, tenderness, erythema, or exudate
aids in the detection of most infections. Unfortunately, in
patients with intra-abdominal or other deep-seated infections,
these clues may not be present, and the patients present with
non-specific or vague complaints such as fever, night sweats,
malaise, fatigue, wasting, or pallor. Evaluation of these
patients has been greatly improved recently with the use of
various nuclear scans, ultrasonography, and computerized axial
tomography. These new techniques have presented their own
problems, primarily related to expense, reliability, and
interpretation, but they are drastically changing our attitudes
about the management of the FUO syndrome.

LOCALIZATION OF INFECTION IN PATIENTS
WITH FEVER OF UNKNOWN ORIGIN (FUO)

There are three criteria for the FUO syndrome: illness
lasting longer than three weeks, fever higher than 101°F rectally
on at least three occasions, and no diagnosis evident after
evaluation in the hospital for one week. Infections are the most
common cause of the FUO syndrome. They accounted for 36 percent
of patients in one series (1), where eleven patients had tuberculosis, seven had liver or biliary tract infections, five had
bacterial endocarditis, four had intra-abdominal abscesses, and
three had pyelonephritis. Five infections were not detected

ante-mortem, and three of these unfortunate individuals had treatable pyogenic intra-abdominal infections. Nine additional infections were diagnosed at exploratory laparotomy, and three patients with disseminated tuberculosis were diagnosed by percutaneous liver biopsy. In all, 15 (42%) of the 36 infections were intra-abdominal and required invasive procedures for diagnosis. Until recently, abdominal exploration often has been performed in patients with the FUO syndrome when all other studies have been non-diagnostic. Some diagnosis is obtained at laparotomy in the majority of properly selected patients with FUO, especially when there are clues pointing to an abdominal process. A complete exploration of the abdomen along with indicated biopsies is associated with a morbidity rate of up to 15 percent, but operative deaths are unusual except in patients with disseminated incurable diseases.

It is now evident that many occult intra-abdominal infections can be located (but not necessarily specifically diagnosed or treated) using newer non-invasive methods. Thus, the concept of a "medical laporatomy" has become popular, and exploration often is required only for obtaining a tissue diagnosis or for definitive treatment. Some experts believe exploration should be resorted to only when patients are elderly, have clues pointing to the abdomen, or multiple bouts of fever, or fail to improve with conservative or medical therapy.

Occult abscesses are important causes of the FUO syndrome, not only because they are treatable, but also because they account for about 10 percent of the diagnoses made at laparotomy. Early diagnosis, definition of microbial etiology, and precise localization are the keys to improving therapeutic results. The diagnosis is sometimes based upon conventional x-rays demonstrating an immobile, high diaphragm, or gas outside the alimentary tract (2). More often, however, these findings are absent and the diagnosis is suggested by scanning techniques.

Liver-Spleen Scans

All liver-imaging nuclide preparations of clinical importance utilize the principle of RES trapping. Technetium (Tc 99m) sulfur colloid is most popular. The whole body dose of 0.05 rads with a Tc99M liver scan is low. About 95 percent of administered TC 99m goes to Kupffer cells in liver, and 5 percent to spleen (3). Imaging is done 10 minutes after injection; anterior, posterior, and right lateral views (LAO for spleen) should be obtained.

The main use of technetium liver scans is in diagnosis of primary or metastatic tumors, and pyogenic or parasitic abscess. Abscesses are characterized by areas of decreased uptake. This finding is non-specific, and abscesses are indistinguishable from neoplasms and cysts. Granulomatous and parenchymal diseases such as cirrhosis and hepatitis can produce similar results

("pseudotumors"), and even normal variants can be troublesome.
Lesions no larger than 2-3 cm can be detected on technetium scan,
but lesions as large as 6 cm can be missed, especially if deep,
and the significance of a positive scan is much greater than that
of a negative scan.

Liver-Lung Scans

Combined liver-lung scans using Tc 99m-macroaggregated
albumin (for lung) and Tc 99m-sulfur colloid or diphosphonate (for
liver) have been used successfully in detecting subphrenic
abscesses, especially on the right (4). Conditions other than
abscesses (such as hematomas) can cause similar defects, so that
follow-up of abnormal liver-lung scans with other studies is often
desirable. Left subphrenic abscesses are more difficult to
diagnose than those on the right. It should be emphasized that a
negative study does not rule out subphrenic abscess.

Gallium Scans

While radio-gallium scans were first used to detect primary or
metastatic cancers, early users noted that abscesses also took up
the isotope (5). Gallium scans are now an important part of the
FUO work-up. Gallium accumulates in the reticuloendothelial cells
of liver and spleen, in certain tumors, and at sites of inflammation. No adverse reactions have been reported. A dose of 1 to
2.5 millicuries is used, and the total body dose is only about
1 rad. The half-life of radio-gallium is 78 hours following oral
administration, and 5 hours following IV administration. Scans
are usually performed routinely 6, 24 and 48 hours after dosing.
There is still controversy concerning the mechanisms of accumulation of gallium at infected sites. It is notable that
inflammatory sites may be visualized even in patients with
granulocytopenia.

Radioactive gallium accumulates normally in the liver, spleen,
bone marrow, nasopharyngeal region, breasts, sternum, and media-
stinum. Normal lymph nodes do not take up appreciable amounts of
gallium. The usefulness of gallium scans in detecting infections
in the abdomen is less than at other sites because gallium 67 is
excreted into the gastrointestinal tract, and the background
radioactivity detected may obscure disease process. Gallium scans
are of little value in patients with pelvic inflammatory disease
(6). This problem can be minimized by preparing patients carefully with a liquid diet, enemas, laxatives, and by use of serial
scans. In particular, scans should be done 6 hours after giving
the isotope in patients with FUO, since uptake in abscesses is
usually good by then, but background radioactivity is minimal.

Littenberg and colleagues (7) published one of the first
reports on the use of gallium scans for detecting deep infection.
Of their 12 patients with suspect infection, the probable focus
was detected in 10. This report was soon followed by many others
confirming the value of gallium in detecting occult infections
(8,9,10). Intra-abdominal abscesses, empyema of the gallbladder,
and liver abscesses are readily detected (5,9,11). Gallium is also
useful in detecting brain abscesses and osteomyelitis (6). Silva
and Harvey (11) reported a series of 28 patients in 21 of whom
inflammatory foci were correctly localized using total body
gallium scans 48 to 72 hours after dosing. Infections of aortic
prostheses can be detected with gallium. Liver abscesses smaller
than 1.5 cm in diameter usually do not visualize with gallium,
probably because the background radioactivity of the liver obscures
detection of small lesions. It must be emphasized that large
abscesses in the lesser sac and spleen can be missed with gallium.
    As mentioned above, early (6 hour) scans are being done more
and more routinely in patients with FUO, and may provide information that is helpful in deciding whether surgical intervention for
drainage of abscesses is indicated in critically ill patients. In
a recent report of 62 patients scanned both at 6 hours and at 24
to 48 hours, 31 of 33 abscesses were detected on the early scan.
There were only two false-positives in the 62 scans (3 percent);
in retrospect, both represented errors in interpretation due to
colonic uptake of the isotope (12).
    One serious limitation of gallium in looking for deep
infections in post-operative patients is that infected, and sometimes noninfected, surgical incisions may be visualized for long
periods following surgery. The outside limits are not well-
defined. Accordingly, physicians reading gallium scans should be
familiar with the patient and be aware of incisions, colostomies,
wound infections, and other factors that may lead to artefacts.
    Various investigators have attempted to improve the
sensitivities and specificity of gallium scans by injecting
patients with autologous peripheral blood leukocytes labeled
in vitro with Ga^{67} citrate. Indium (^{111}In) labeled leukocytes
also have been used recently in attempts to localize abscesses.
This promising innovation has the advantage of minimal background
activity due to intestinal uptake but is still investigational.
    The subphrenic area is an especially difficult one for
detection of infection with gallium because of the normal accumulation of gallium and other isotopes in the liver. Liver-lung
scans and gallium-technetium subtraction scans have been studied
in an attempt to improve the accuracy of diagnosis of right
subphrenic abscess (13). The latter technique takes advantage of
the fact that a liver abscess is "cold" with Tc, and "hot" with
Ga^{67}. Technical advances permitting electronic subtraction of the
hepatic technetium signal from the display of the gallium scan
largely eliminates the problem of hepatic background, thus aiding
in detection of small abscesses in or adjacent to the liver.

Among the recent reports confirming the utility of gallium scans in managing patients with infectious diseases, the report by Teates (10) was of special interest. Seventeen (40 percent) of 42 patients they studied with fever had positive gallium scans, and in 9 of the 17 (or 21 percent of patients scanned), new information of importance in managing the patient was obtained.

Diagnostic Ultrasound

Ultrasonography is a conceptually simple and yet amazingly powerful diagnostic tool. Sonograms are rapid and safe, and able to localize or suggest many lesions not detectable by other methods.

Ultrasonic scanning (or echography) utilizes reflected high-frequency sound waves (1-15,000,000 cpsec) to distinguish between fluid-filled and solid structures, which have different acoustical impedances. Density variations of as little as 1 percent can be revealed. A crystalline transducer placed on the skin intermittently emits pulsed sound waves and also receives the reflected signals of echoes. The echoes are transformed into a visible image on an oscilloscope, either one-dimensionally in a distance oriented way, or two-dimensionally (B mode) so as to yield a cross-sectional picture in which organ outlines are displayed (14). Echoes originate both from organ borders and from internal structures such as septae and vessels. Solid organs present inner echoes and appear dense, while hematomas, cysts and abscesses appear as echo-free areas or holes. With appropriate equipment, it is possible to generate and display hundreds of scan images per second and thus to scan objects in motion, such as the heart (TM mode). Echography plays an important role in study of intra-abdominal and cardiac diseases. Unfortunately, bony structures and organs filled with air or barium cannot be studied, and echography is of little value in patients with marked abdominal distension due to gas-filled intestines or postoperatively.

Ultrasonography is a safe, rapid, and effective means of detecting and characterizing deep abscesses (14). The amount of energy used in diagnostic ultrasound is small, and no harmful effects have been seen. Even seriously ill patients may be examined. Lesions as small as 1-2 cm may be located. Cysts and abscesses in the pancreas or kidneys can be distinguished. Ultrasound cannot distinguish abscesses from cysts or hematomas with certainty, but abscesses are often more irregular than cysts. Since serial examinations are feasible, the effects of antibiotic treatment can be followed. In patients with renal transplants and unexplained fever (15), ultrasound may help distinguish between rejection and perirenal infection. The development of so-called "gray scale" or "density-slicing" ultrasound equipment has greatly increased resolution of liver lesions, and has even permitted "color conversion", or artificial display in color of the internal structure of large organs. The resolution obtainable in the liver in now approaching two millimeters. This allows for evaluation of the liver for metastatic disease, abscess, and dilated intrahepatic biliary ducts.

Jensen and Pedersen (16) reported their results with ultrasonic examination of 34 patients with suspected abdominal abscess or hematoma. Their diagnosis was confirmed in 31 (91%). Twelve (75%) of 16 patients with negative scans were subsequently shown not to have abscesses. Thus, 31 (89%) of 35 abscesses (or hematomas) were detected. Lesions were detected all over the abdomen, and 25 percent were smaller than 6 cm. Results like theirs have been found by many others, and it is not surprising that ultrasound has become a routine diagnostic modality in a variety of abdominal conditions.

An important innovation in ultrasonographic techniques concerns a central-channeled aspirating transducer, which may be used to biopsy lesions or to aspirate abscesses with a fine gauge needle under accurate ultrasonic guidance. Smear and culture of aspirated material can be performed immediately upon detection of a lesion, and the diagnosis may be definitely established in a matter of minutes (17).

Angiography

Angiography is sometimes invaluable in defining occult abscesses. However, it is an invasive procedure and not as safe as ultrasound or nuclear scans, and thus it is usually reserved for special situations in which non-invasive techniques have not been helpful.

Lymphangiography

The lymphangiogram is most useful in diagnosing and managing patients with lymphomas and other malignant diseases. Carcinomatous deposits must be at least 5 to 10 mm in size before they can be identified. While lymphangiograms are useful in evaluation of fever of unknown origin, they are of limited value in identifying infectious causes of the syndrome. They are being performed less and less often, and are usually considered only when other scans are negative.

Computerized Axial Tomography

Computerized tomography is undoubtedly the most sophisticated, sensitive, and helpful technique for identifying intra-abdominal septic foci. It is also the most expensive; especially when the newer sophisticated and rapid equipment is used. Therefore, in most situations, abdominal CT is not used as a screening technique, but for evaluation of suspicious areas located by other scans, or when other scans are negative. Used in this way, it may be cost-effective.

CT utilizes minute x-ray beams emitted and collected by a rotating device that enables examination of each of a series of anatomical cross-sections hundreds of times. With the aid of a computer, the hundreds of thousands of signals received are collected, analyzed and mapped. An image can then be generated on a cathode ray tube in which brightness is proportional to density of tissue. Hematomas and abscesses can be distinguished from edema, tumors, cysts, and other lesions. An enhancement or augmentation study can be performed while the patient is receiving an intravenous radio-opaque dye, which can demonstrate a vascular capsule, and increase the likelihood of detecting an abscess.

One of the first reports of use of CT in abdominal abscess indicated a higher diagnostic yield with it than with gallium, technetium, or ultrasonic scans (18). A later report (19) showed CT (96%), ultrasound (90%), and nuclear scans (92%) were highly but equally useful, and that many patients needed more than one of these studies to define their disease. Our experience suggests that if there are no palpable abdominal masses or other localizing findings, a nuclear scan should be done before CT scans to pinpoint a lesion for study with it or other techniques when patients are not critically ill. CT is especially useful diagnostically in post-operative patients. CT can even be used to guide aspiration and non-surgical drainage by means of a catheter. Using improved equipment, 93 of 94 intra-abdominal abscesses were detected with CT, with only two confirmed false-positives (19,20).

CONCLUSION

It is apparent that occult septic processes now can be located more safely and quickly than ever before, but also at greater immediate cost. Many believe that these newer scanning techniques will ultimately lower the cost of evaluation and treatment of these patients, because they will result in shorter hospitalization, and aid in avoidance of unnecessary surgery. In addition, they may return patients to an active healthy life earlier and more often. These beliefs are not overly optimistic, but careful application and evaluation of the role of these newer procedures will be required for realization of their extraordinary promise.

REFERENCES

1. Petersdorf, R.G., and Beeson, P.B.   (1961)   Fever of
    unexplained origin: report of 100 cases.   Medicine 40, 1.
2. Rice, R.P., and Masters, S.J.   (1973) Intra-abdominal
    abscess.   Seminars in Roentgenology 8, 365.
3. Braunstein, P., and Song, C.S.   (1975) The uses and limitations
    of radioisotopes in the investigation of gastrointestinal
    diseases.   Digestive Diseases 20, 53.
4. Gold, R.P., and Johnson, P.M.   (1975) Efficacy of combined
    liver-lung scintillation imaging.   Radiology 117, 105.
5. Lomas, F., and Wagner, H.N.   (1972) Accumulation of ionic
    ^{67}Ga in empyema of the gallbladder.   Radiology 105, 689.
6. Deysine, M., Rafkin, H., Teicher, I., et al.   (1975) Diagnosis
    of chronic and postoperative osteomyelitis with gallium 67
    citrate scans.   Amer. J. Surg 129, 632.
7. Littenberg, R.L., Taketa, R.M., Alazraki, N., et al.   (1973)
    Gallium-67 for localization of septic lesions.   Ann. Int.
    Med. 79, 403.
8. Blair, D.C., Carroll, M., Silva, J., et al.   (1974)
    Localization of infectious processes with gallium
    citrate Ga67.   J. Amer. Med. Assoc. 230, 82.
9. Habibian, M.R., Staab, E.V., and Matthews, H.A.   (1975)
    Gallium citrate Ga^{67} scans in febrile patients.   J. Amer.
    Med. Assoc. 233, 1073.
10. Teates, C.D., and Hunter, J.G.   (1975) Gallium scanning as a
    screening test for inflammatory lesions.   Radiology 116,
    383.
11. Silva, J., and Harvey, W.C. (1974) Detection of infections
    with Gallium-67 and scintigraphic imaging.   J. Infect.
    Dis. 130, 125.
12. Hopkins, G.B., Kan, M., and Mende, C.W.   (1975) Early ^{67}Ga
    scintigraphy for the localization of abdominal abscesses.
    J. Nucl. Med. 16, 990.
13. Damron, J.R., Beihn, R.M., Selby, J.B., et al.   (1974)
    Gallium-technetium subtraction scanning for the
    localization of subphrenic abscess.   Radiology 113, 117.
14. Friday, R.O., Barriga, P., and Crummy, A.B.   (1975)
    Detection and localization of intra-abdominal abscesses
    by diagnostic ultrasound.   Arch. Surg. 110, 335.
15. Winterberger, A.R., Palma, L.D., and Murphy, G.P.   (1972)
    Ultrasonic testing in human renal allografts.   J. Amer.
    Med. Assoc. 219, 475.
16. Jensen, F., and Pedersen, J.F.   (1974) The value of ultrasonic
    scanning in the diagnosis of intra-abdominal abscesses and
    hematomas.   Surg. Gynec. and Obstet. 139, 326.
17. Smith, E.H., and Bartrum, R.J.   (1974) Ultrasonically guided
    percutaneous aspiration of abscesses.   Amer. J. Roentgen.
    122, 308.

18. Haaga, J.R., et al.   (1977) CT detection and aspiration of
        abdominal abscesses.   Am. J. Roentgenol. 128, 465.
19. Knochel, J.Q., et al.   (1980) Diagnosis of abdominal
        abscesses with computed tomography, ultrasound, and [111]In
        leukocyte scans.   Radiology 137, 425.
20. Koehler, R.P., et al.   (1980) Diagnosis of intra-abdominal
        and pelvic abscesses by computerized tomography.   JAMA
        244, 49

PART XIII
SPECIAL THERAPEUTIC CONSIDERATIONS

CLINICAL CONCEPTS IN ANTIBIOTIC SELECTION

William A. Craig

Department of Medicine
University of Wisconsin
Madison, Wisconsin

I. ESTABLISHING THE ETIOLOGIC DIAGNOSIS

The rational selection of antimicrobial agents for the
therapy of infectious diseases is a multistep process that is
always dependent on the clinical setting with each individual
patient. The first step in the process is to establish the
etiologic diagnosis. Cultures of blood and other body fluids
and tissues are necessary to identify the specific causative
pathogen. Since therapy is often required before the precise
etiologic diagnosis can be established, the physician must be
able to formulate the most likely causative organisms for the
infection. The likely pathogens are dependent on a variety of
factors listed below in Table I.

The site of infection is a major determinant in establishing
the likely pathogens. Organisms vary in their ability to

TABLE I. Factors to be Considered in Establishing
the Likely Etiologies of Infection

Site of Infection
Age of patient
Predisposing host factors
Predisposing mechanical factors
Epidemiologic considerations

---

colonize and infect different tissues. For example, Staphylococcus aureus is a common cause of osteomyelitis but an uncommon
etiology of urinary tract infections. Infections near mucosal
surfaces should suggest the possibility of anaerobic infection.
At many infection sites, the age of the patient markedly modifies
the list of likely pathogens. For instance, in meningitis the
predominant organisms are the Group B streptococcus and Gram-
negative bacilli in newborns, H. influenzae and the meningococcus in young children, the meningococcus in young adults, and
the pneumococcus and Gram-negative bacilli in older adults.

   There are a variety of predisposing host factors that
increase the likelihood of infection with specific organisms.
These are summarized in Table II. Thus, a patient with sepsis
in the presence of leukopenia has a greater risk of infection
with Pseudomonas aeruginosa, and antimicrobial therapy should be
tailored appropriately. Similarly, the postsplenectomy patient
with sepsis has an increased chance of infection with the
pneumococcus, and coverage of this organism with initial antimicrobial therapy is necessary.

   A list of the many predisposing mechanical factors are
listed in Table III. In most situations, mechanical factors
provide access of the patient's endogenous normal flora
to deeper tissues. Thus, abdominal trauma, especially

TABLE II. Predisposing Host Factors

Predisposing factor	Organism
Diabetes	Staphylococci
Rheumatoid arthritis	Staphylococci
Splenectomy	Pneumococci
Ascites	Pneumococci
Hemoglobinopathy	Salmonella
COPD	Pneumococci + Haemophilus
Chronic alcoholism	GNB (Klebsiella)
CNS disorders	Aspiration (anaerobes)
IV drug addicts	Staphylococci, GNB (Pseudomonas), + Fungi
Burns	Staphylococci + Pseudomonas
Leukopenia	GNB (Pseudomonas) + Fungi
Malignancy	Opportunistic organisms
Immunosuppressive therapy	Opportunistic organisms
Valvular heart disease	Streptococci
Prosthetic heart valves	Staphylococci, GNB + Candida

GNB = Gram negative bacilli

TABLE III. Predisposing Mechanical Factors

Predisposing factor	Organism
IV catheter	Staphylococci
IV fluid	Klebsiella-Enterobacter
Hyperalimentation	Candida
Arterial catheter-pressure monitoring catheters	Unusual GNB
Urinary catheters	GNB
Hemodialysis	Staphylococci + GNB
Intracerebral pressure monitors	Staphylococci
Mechanical ventilation	GNB
Abdominal trauma	Anaerobes + GNB
Recent surgery:	
abdominal	Anaerobes + GNB
gynecological	Anaerobes + GNB
orthopedic	Staphylococci + GNB

penetrating wounds, allow the intestinal flora to contaminate the peritoneal cavity. Antimicrobial therapy should, therefore, be based on covering the primary organisms in the intestinal flora (anaerobes and gram-negative bacilli). In other situations, the mechanical device becomes colonized with organisms that can survive in it. For example, yeasts such as Candida albicans can survive in hyperalimentation fluids, and these organisms account for the majority of infections associated with total parenteral nutrition.

The patient's occupational and travel history and history of animal exposure can often provide important clues as to the likely etiologies. Whether the infection was community or hospital acquired can greatly alter the likely pathogens. A list of some of the epidemiologic factors that should generate suspicion of specific organisms is provided in Table IV.

II. IDENTIFICATION OF INFECTING ORGANISM

Although cultures are the major method for definitive identification of pathogenic organisms, there are a number of methods for the rapid identification of microorganisms. The Gram stain of body fluids is the simplest and cheapest of these tests. It can be used to identify the presence and morphology of microorganisms that should enable the physician to narrow the etiologic possibilities in a specific patient. For certain body

TABLE IV.   Epidemiologic Considerations

Epidemiologic clue	Organism or disease
Global travel	Malaria and parasites
US travel	Deep mycoses
Military recruit	Meningococcus
Abatoir worker	Brucellosis
Rancher or farmer	Q-fever, brucellosis
Small animal hunter	Tularemia
Bird fancier	Psittacosis
Tick bite	Tularemia, rickettsial disease, Lyme disease
Cat bite	Pasteurella multocida
Ingestion of raw pork	Trichinosis
Hospital acquired	GNB, staphylococci

fluids the Gram stain can also determine the adequacy of the specimen for culture. For example, a Gram stain of sputum in a patient with pneumonia that reveals many squamous epithelial cells suggests that the specimen is primarily saliva and a poor specimen to culture. On the other hand, a sputum Gram stain that reveals very few epithelial cells and/or numerous polymorphonuclear leukocytes is representative of an appropriate specimen for culture.

Other tests such as counterimmunoelectrophoresis (CIE), immunofluorescent staining, and special stains of biopsy material can also aid in the rapid identification of the infecting pathogens. As with many tests, a positive result is very helpful in establishing the etiology, but a negative result does not eliminate the organisms from consideration.

III. SELECTION OF THE ANTIMICROBIAL

Once the likely pathogens have been ascertained by clinical and laboratory features, the physician must next decide on the appropriate antimicrobial. One needs, therefore, a working knowledge of the activity of different antimicrobials against the commonly encountered pathogens. Such lists are found in most textbooks. Data of this type are also published periodically in publications such as the Medical Letter on Drugs and Therapeutics. However, it is important to remember that there are significant geographic differences in antimicrobial susceptibility than can alter antimicrobial selection. For example, in areas with a high incidence of methicillin-resistant

staphylococci, vancomycin would be a more appropriate choice for
empiric therapy of staphylococcal sepsis than a penicillinase-
resistant penicillin or cephalosporin. Thus, the physician
should have knowledge of the local resistance patterns for the
various antimicrobials.

Even then, there are a variety of drug factors besides
in vitro sensitivity that must be considered to ensure optimal
chemotherapy of the infection. Should the drug be bactericidal
or is bacteriostatic activity alone sufficient? Generally
speaking, bactericidal drugs are preferred. However, with most
infections in patients with relatively normal host defenses,
bacteriostatic and bactericidal antimicrobials are equally
effective. Notable exceptions would be endocarditis and meningitis. In addition, patients with significant leukopenia should
receive bactericidal drugs as the white cell is an important host
defense for bacterial and even many fungal infections.

Should a single drug or a combination of antimicrobials be
used? There are several reasons for using a combination of
drugs. Combinations of antimicrobials are used in tuberculosis
to delay the emergence of resistant organisms. Treatment of
mixed bacterial infections often requires antibiotic combinations.
For example, treatment of abdominal sepsis with clindamycin and
an aminoglycoside is necessary to provide effective therapy for
both anaerobes and enteric gram-negative bacilli. However, it
should be emphasized that most infections involving the lung,
kidney, meninges, heart, bone and joints are single pathogen
infections. Combinations of antimicrobials may also give an
enhanced efficacy in the treatment of an infection. The combination of penicillin G with an aminoglycoside such as streptomycin
or gentamicin for the treatment of enterococcal endocarditis is
a classic example. Similarly, the combination of an antipseudomonal penicillin with an antipseudomonal aminoglycoside
improves the results of treatment of pseudomonas infections in
leukopenic patients. The most common reason by far for combinations of antimicrobials is to broaden the coverage of likely
pathogens until culture results return. This use of antimicrobial combinations may decrease in the future as the pharmaceutical industry develops new drugs with much wider antimicrobial
spectrums.

Of primary importance in antimicrobial selection is whether
the drug can penetrate to the site of infection. This is not a
major problem with most infectious sites as the capillaries
supplying tissues have pores that readily allow for passage of
drug into the area of infection. Providing adequate concentrations in serum usually ensures that adequate levels are reached
at the site of infection. There are, however, some sites in the
body such as the central nervous systems and the eye that are
supplied by capillaries that lack the usual pores. In order for
an antimicrobial to penetrate well into these sites, it needs
to be lipid soluble enough to pass across the capillary membranes.

Antimicrobials that penetrate poorly into CSF even in the presence of inflammation include the aminoglycosides, cephalosporins and clindamycin.

Disease states can also affect the ability of a drug to reach the site of infection. For example, renal impairment may limit some drugs from reaching adequate concentrations in the urine for treatment of urinary tract infections. In severe renal impairment urinary concentrations of nitrofurantoin, doxycycline and minocycline are below the MIC for common urinary tract pathogens. In contrast, the aminopenicillins, cephalosporins, and trimethoprim-sulfamethoxazole provide therapeutic levels in the urine of uremic patients.

The last major drug factor to consider is the potential of the drug to produce toxicity. The incidence of adverse reactions is dependent on many host factors such as age, genetic predisposition, previous drug allergy, underlying disease states and concomitant drug therapy (drug interactions). Several examples for each modifying host factor are summarized in Table V. Interactions of antimicrobials with other drugs is of sufficient magnitude to deserve separate presentation (Table VI).

The ability of the liver to conjugate chloramphenicol is dependent on age. In newborns, this mechanism of chloramphenicol inactivation is inadequately developed and administration of high doses of the drug can produce vascular collapse (Gray syndrome). The incidence of isoniazid hepatitis is age-related with the highest rate in elderly adults. Genetic factors may also make some patients more susceptible to toxicity. For example, the red blood cells of patients with glucose-6-phosphate dehydrogenase deficiency are more susceptible to hemolysis by antimicrobials such as nitrofurantoin and sulfonamides that act as oxidants. Previous drug allergy may also alter antibiotic selection. Although the frequency of cross-reactivity between cephalosporins and penicillins is relatively low, any patient who has had an anaphylactic reaction to penicillin should be given a cephalosporin with great caution, if at all.

There are a variety of disease states that can enhance the risk of toxicity. The diseases of major importance are those that affect the elimination of antimicrobials such as renal impairment and hepatic dysfunction. Renal impairment would primarily affect those drugs which are eliminated primarily by the kidney. This would include the aminoglycosides, several cephalosporins, carbenicillin, ticarcillin, vancomycin and flucytosine. These drugs can still be used when appropriate but the dosage needs to be modified for the degree of renal impairment. There are some drugs that should be avoided in the presence of renal disease because of increased toxicity. For example, the tetracyclines (except doxycycline) produce an antianabolic effect in patients with renal impairment resulting in further azotemia. For that reason, doxycycline is the tetracycline of choice in patients with renal impairment. Other drugs that should be avoided in the presence of significant renal impairment are listed in Table V. There are several antimicrobials that have increased hepatotoxicity in patients with underlying hepatic dysfunction. This includes tetracycline, erythromycin, isoniazid and rifampin. Tetracycline can usually be avoided, but the other drugs are often needed for specific infections such as Legionnaire's disease and tuberculosis. The dose of these drugs along with clindamycin and chloramphenicol should be moderately reduced in patients with hepatic impairment as these drugs are primarily excreted or detoxified in the liver. Tetracycline, sulfonamides and metronidazole should be avoided during pregnancy. Large doses of tetracycline during pregnancy can produce hepatotoxicity as well as stain and enamel hypoplasia of teeth in the fetus. Sulfonamides are safe until just prior to delivery. If administered then it can displace

TABLE V. Host Factors Potentiating Toxicity

Host factor	Antimicrobial	Result
Age	Chloramphenicol	Gray syndrome in newborns
	Tetracycline	Teeth staining in children
	Isoniazid	Hepatitis in adults
Genetic predisposition	Sulfonamides + nitrofurantoin	Hemolysis in patients with G6PD deficiency
Previous drug allergy	Penicillins and cephalosporins	Cross-reactivity
Renal disease	Tetracycline	Azotemia and hepatotoxicity
	Nitrofurantoin	Neuropathy
	Cephaloridine	Renal impairment
	Nalidixic acid	Metabolic acidosis
Hepatic disease	Tetracycline	Hepatotoxicity
	Erythromycin	Hepatotoxicity
	Isoniazid	Hepatotoxicity
	Rifampin	Hepatotoxicity
Pregnancy	Tetracycline	Hepatotoxicity + teeth staining
	Sulfonamides	Kernicterus
	Metronidazole	Mutagenic

TABLE VI. Drug Interactions Resulting in Toxicity

Drug	Antimicrobial	Result
Methotrexate	Sulfonamides	Bone marrow depression
Phenytoin	Sulfonamides Chloramphenicol Isoniazid	Phenytoin toxicity
Tolbutamide	Sulfonamides Chloramphenicol	Hypoglycemia
	Rifampin	Hyperglycemia
Warfarin	Sulfonamides Chloramphenicol Nalidixic acid Metronidazole	Bleeding
	Rifampin	Poor anticoagulation
Barbiturates	Sulfonamides Chloramphenicol	Sedation
Methadone	Rifampin	Withdrawal
Cortisone	Rifampin	Addison's disease
Oral contraceptives	Rifampin	Pregnancy
Cyclophosphamide	Chloramphenicol	Decreased activity
Gentamicin and tobramycin	β-lactams	Inactivation of aminoglycoside
Digoxin	Intestinal antibiotics	Digoxin toxicity

bilirubin from binding sites resulting in hyperbilirubinemia and kernicterus. Metronidazole is mutagenic and may be teratogenic as well.

Two different types of drug interactions involving antimicrobials can lead to drug toxicity. In the first type the antimicrobial either displaces the drug from binding sites or inhibits its metabolism so that an enhanced activity of the drug is observed. The drug interactions with chloramphenicol and the sulfonamides are major examples. In the second type of interaction the antimicrobial either increases the metabolism of the drug or inactivates it resulting in a decrease in the pharmacologic effect of the drug. Rifampin is an inducer of liver microsomal enzymes and can enhance the metabolism of several drugs. The resulting effect of rifampin-stimulated enzyme induction with the oral contraceptives is pregnancy. The classic example for direct interaction is the inactivation of tobramycin and gentamicin by β-lactam antibiotics such as carbenicillin and ticarcillin. In vivo inactivation is insignificant if renal function is normal or moderately impaired. However, in patients

with significant renal dysfunction carbenicillin or ticarcillin
will shorten the elimination half-life of these two aminoglycosides necessitating more frequent dosing of the drug. Amikacin
is not inactivated by these β-lactam antibiotics and may be the
preferred drug when aminoglycosides plus carbenicillin or
ticarcillin are needed in the patient with renal impairment.

IV. SUMMARY

This brief review has outlined in tabular form the variety
of host, drug and laboratory factors that can interact and
affect antimicrobial selection. A better appreciation and
understanding of these factors should enable the physician to
establish the likely etiology of the infection and select the
appropriate antimicrobials that will be most effective and
associated with the least toxicity.

ANTIBIOTIC PROPHYLAXIS IN SURGICAL PATIENTS

Robert E. Condon

Department of Surgery
The Medical College of Wisconsin
Milwaukee, Wisconsin

Between 24% and 75% of all antibiotic prescriptions, depending on the class of drugs being examined, are written for surgical prophylaxis. Although surgical antibiotic prophylaxis practices used to be characterized as unwarranted, useless, and even harmful, numerous controlled trials published over the past two decades have firmly established that antibiotic prophylaxis, under appropriate circumstances and constraints, reduces the risk of wound infection and other septic complications associated with operations.

INDICATIONS

1. Clean-contaminated Operations. For short-hand purposes, these can be thought of as any operation which opens into one of the hollow visceral systems of the body which harbors an endogenous flora. In addition, operations for trauma in which gross spillage from a hollow viscus is absent also are viewed as clean-contaminated cases. In this type of operation, the bacterial density in the wound exceeds 10^6 organisms/gram tissue, but rarely is much higher than 10^8 or 10^9 organisms/gram tissue. Thus, tissue contamination is sufficiently heavy that an increased risk of septic complications is present, but the contamination is not so dense as to make suppuration inevitable.

2. Clean Operations involving Insertion of a Prosthesis or other Foreign Body. The presence of the prosthesis disables wound healing and other local defense mechanisms, resulting in a doubling of the underlying wound infection risk. This moves the risk from clean to the "clean-contaminated" class. Effective antibiotic prophylaxis will reduce the infection risk to that obtaining with an otherwise identical strictly clean operation not involving insertion of a prosthesis.

3. <u>Clean Operation in a Patient with Impaired Host Defenses</u>.
4. <u>Clean Operation in which any Infection Constitutes a</u>
<u>Disaster</u>. Many operations in the field of neurosurgery, cardiac surgery, and ophthalmology fall into this class. Of all of the indications for surgical prophylaxis, this group remains most controversial.

SELECTION OF ANTIBIOTIC

Choice of antibiotic depends on a thorough knowledge of the bacteria which constitute the endogenous flora at various body sites, as well as knowledge of the pathogenic organisms which are predominantly associated with septic complications following the various classes of operations. Further, up-to-date knowledge concerning the antimicrobial sensitivity of the various pathogens is essential.

TABLE I.   Typical Pathogens of the Endogenous Flora

MOUTH-PHARYNX
     Strep. viridans
     Staph. epidermidis

     Candida sp.
     Actinomyces sp.

     Peptostreptococci
     Peptococci
     Bacteroides sp. (PCN sens)
     Veillonella sp.
     Fusobacterium sp.

BILIARY TRACT
     E. coli
     Klebsiella sp.
     Enterococcus
     Proteus sp.

     Clostridium sp.

     Peptostreptococci
     Bacteroides sp.

COLON
     (including appendix, distal small bowel, female genital
     tract)
     E. coli
     Proteus sp.
     Pseudomonas sp.
     Klebsiella sp.
     Enterococcus
     Streptococcus sp.
     Enterobacter sp.
     Staph aureus
     Candida sp.

     Bacteroides fragilis sp.
     Bacteroides melaninogenicus
     other Bacteroides sp.
     Peptostreptococci
     Peptococci
     Clostridium sp.
     Eubacterium sp.
     Fusobacterium sp.

The bacterial flora are relatively predictable and are summarized in Table 1. Antibiotic sensitivity patterns change with time, so that information concerning this aspect of antibiotic selection needs to be updated constantly by each practitioner.

TIMING AND DURATION OF ANTIBIOTIC PROPHYLAXIS

The classic work of Miles and Burke[1] established that prophylactic antibiotics needed to be present in tissue at the time contamination occurred. In his classic experiments, Burke showed experimentally that administration of antibiotics before or at the time of tissue contamination was associated with a negligibly increased infection risk; as antibiotic administration was delayed, infection risk increased; antibiotics administered more than four hours after tissue contamination had no effect. Burke's observations were of Staphylococcus aureus and have long been believed to be applicable to all aerobic organisms. More recently, the fact that this principle also applies to prophylaxis against anaerobic organisms was established by the work of Shapiro and colleagues[2] studying a similar model in which the pathogen inoculated was <u>Bacteroides fragilis</u>.

Numerous clinical studies have confirmed the experimental observations. For example, Stone's study[3] recorded a decrease in wound infection rate from 14% in controls to 3.5% in patients receiving antibiotic prophylaxis in association with a variety of abdominal operations.

The duration of antibiotic prophylaxis is a much less settled matter because data concerning many classes of operations is lacking. But, whenever this issue has been examined critically, short-term prophylaxis has been shown to be as effective as long term prophylaxis. Several studies have established the efficacy of short-term prophylaxis in orthopaedic surgery, as well as in gynecologic operations[4] and in cardiac surgery[5]. Recently, the report of Strachan and colleagues[6] has demonstrated that short-term prophylaxis is as effective as longer term therapy in patients undergoing cholecystectomy. Dellinger and associates[7] have shown that 12 hours of doxycycline and penicillin prophylaxis was as effective in patients with penetrating abdominal trauma as five days of this antibiotic therapy.

ESOPHAGUS

The esophagus lacks a serosa and has a poor blood supply so that leaks of esophageal anastomoses are relatively frequent. Cyclic negative intra-thoracic pressure exerted on the postoperative esophagus also doesn't help much. Careful studies demonstrate that about 40% of all esophageal anastomoses and closures of esophageal wounds develop at least a minor leak; up to 10% have a major leak with some degree of mediastinitis. Therefore, the potential for mediastinal contamination following operations on the open esophagus is great.

The esophagus does not have a resident flora, but is regularly contaminated by swallowed microorganisms. Effective peristalsis sweeps most of these organisms into the stomach. Postoperatively, however, the degree of oral contamination is increased and the effectiveness of esophageal swallowing-sweeping is reduced, thereby enhancing the infection risk. The swallowed bacteria are predominantly mouth and pharyngeal organisms, usually with the addition of moderate numbers of E. coli. If the patient has been receiving antibiotics for more than 4 or 5 days, the numbers of swallowed Candida also markedly increase. In the presence of esophageal obstruction--either mechanical or functional--the esophagus acquires a resident flora composed of a mixture of fecal aerobes plus oral aerobes and anaerobes.

STOMACH

The normal stomach is an effective sterilizer of swallowed bacteria. Indeed, 30 minutes of contact with normal gastric acid juice serves to kill even relatively protected encapsulated organisms, such as M. tuberculosis. The transit time across the normal fasting stomach is 30 minutes. Thus, essentially no microorganisms are passed into the duodenum or upper small bowel in the fasting state in a patient whose gastric acid barrier is intact, and no resident flora occupies the lumen of the normal stomach.

Diseases involving the gastric mucus membrane--chronic gastritis, gastric ulcer, gastric carcinoma--all are associated with diminished to absent secretion of hydrochloric acid and consequent impairment of the gastric barrier. In patients with these gastric mucosal diseases, viable bacteria are transmitted across the stomach and contaminate the duodenum and upper small bowel in the fasting state, and resident flora comes to occupy the lumen of the stomach. Other patients have acute disorders which also interfere with the acid gastric barrier. Patients with bleeding duodenal ulcer and those with gastric outlet obstruction (abnormal motility) may be capable of normal acid secretion, but nonetheless have an ineffective gastric barrier due to dilution or buffering.

Clinically, all patients with gastric mucosal disease, hemorrhage as an indication for operation, or gastric outlet obstruction, are at risk to acquire a resident flora in the lumen of the stomach. The organism involved in the "failed barrier" patient are both aerobic and anaerobic oral bacteria together with moderate numbers of fecal aerobes, especially E. coli.

SMALL BOWEL

Because of the effective gastric acid barrier in normal individuals, the upper small bowel in the fasting state possesses no resident flora. The upper small bowel is transiently contaminated with swallowed microorganisms during and for 1-2 hours after ingestion of a meal, but then the normal state of near sterility is restored.

Beginning in the mid-ileum, the distal small bowel acquires a resident flora due to backwash from the cecum through the ileocecal valve. In the distal two feet of ileum, a fecal aerobic-anaerobic microflora is always resident.

Obstructed small bowel rapidly acquires a large volume of contaminated fluid which, essentially, can be viewed as fluid feces. The source of microorganisms in small bowel obstruction is not precisely known, but most of the organisms probably are derived from distal small bowel and contaminate proximal small bowel retrogradely just prior to complete bowel obstruction. Every effort should be made intraoperatively in the management of small bowel obstruction not to open the bowel. Bowel decompression by open suction, or any enterotomy, is associated with a six-fold increase in the risk of septic complications. As an alternative, a long tube can be passed through the nose preoperatively. Or, a tube such as the Nelson-Baker tube can be passed through a gastrostomy. On occasion, entry into obstructed small bowel or resection of obstructed segments is necessary; in such cases, the operation should be viewed as contaminated.

APPENDIX

The appendix contains a rich and varied fecal flora, identical to that of the rest of the colon and rectum. A variety of antibiotics have been prescribed for prophylaxis in association with appendectomy; nearly all of them seem to have a positive effect, whether administered topically or systemically!

COLON

The colon contains a rich and varied aerobic-anaerobic microflora. Operations on the colon without the benefits of prophylactic antibiotic cover are associated with a 40% risk of wound infection or other major septic complication. Reduction in the risk of infectious complications involves thorough mechanical cleansing of gross feces from the colon lumen, followed by administration of antibiotics. Both mechanical cleansing and antibiotic administration are essential; either alone is much less effective. Indeed, mechanical preparation alone without antibiotics is almost as risky as no preparation at all.

Our preference, supported by our own clinical trials as well as the experience of others, is for oral antibiotic preparation in elective cases. Combination chemotherapy with an amino-glycoside (neomycin or kanamycin) together with a drug effective against anaerobes (erythromycin base, metronidazole, tetracycline) is consistently effective. Systemic administration of antibiotics has a more mixed record. We do not use systemic antibiotics in patients who can be successfully prepared with oral antibiotics for elective operations, reserving systemic administration of antibiotics for patients who have high grade colon obstruction or who are undergoing an emergency operation which obviates oral bowel preparation.

BILIARY TRACT

The flora of importance in the biliary tract varies with the state of disease. Although a variety of fecal organisms can be recovered from gallbladder mucosa or from fluid gallbladder bile, E. coli is the organism which causes nearly all infectious complications associated with cholecystectomy. The risk of infection in cholecystectomy also depends on whether or not acute cholecystitis is present or has recently subsided; the risk is high in all such cases. Further, in chronic cholecystitis, the risk of infection is dependent on the patient's age, and also on whether or not the gallbladder is removed intact. Several studies have shown that the risks of infection correlate with the presence of bactibilia, which progressively increases from 10-20% below age 60 to 100% at and above age 80.

In patients with common duct obstruction, particularly those in whom the obstruction is due to stone or stricture disease, the flora of concern is more varied; in addition to E. coli, Klebsiella, Enterococcus, Proteus and Clostridium species are regularly associated with septic complications.

In cholangitis (temperature +101°F, bilirubin +3.0 mg/%, chills) bile should be viewed as dilute fluid feces. Although aerobes are still the predominant organism, anaerobes are more numerous in this clinical situation than in other forms of biliary tract disease; the anaerobic microflora includes not only clostridia, but relatively high numbers of peptostreptococci and, occasionally, Bacteroides fragilis.

PANCREAS

The normal pancreas is sterile. Edematous (acute or relapsing) pancreatitis is not usually a septic disease. Hemorrhagic, necrotic pancreatitis, on the other hand, is associated with a high incidence of pancreatic abscess; indeed, one-fourth of deaths associated with this serious form of pancreatitis are due to septic complications.

Controlled clinical trials which have looked at the issue of antibiotic prophylaxis have all been trials of chronic relapsing edematous alcohol-related pancreatitis, in which infection is rarely a consideration. Not surprisingly, these trials have indicated that antibiotics are unwarranted in the management of this form of pancreatitis. Unfortunately, principally because the number of cases is relatively small, the issue of whether or not to prescribe antibiotics in patients with more serious necrotic forms of pancreatitis remains unsettled. My personal practice is to administer antibiotics if patients are hemodynamically unstable, require blood transfusion or albumin transfusion as part of resuscitation, or require peritoneal lavage as part of their therapy.

As well as the specific clinical circumstances involving gastrointestinal surgery briefly outlined above, information concerning antibiotic prophylaxis in gynecologic surgery, vascular surgery, orthopedics, etc. is very extensive. A review of all of these considerations is beyond the scope of this presentation, but entree to the literature is provided by recent reviews(8,9).

REFERENCES

1. Miles, A.A., Miles, E.M., Burke, J. (1957). Brit. J. Exp. Path. 38:79.
2. Shapiro, J. et al. (1980). J. Inf. Dis. 141:532.
3. Stone, H.H. et al. (1976). Ann. Surg. 184:443.
4. Mendelson J. et al (1979). Obst. Gynecol. 53:31.
5. Conte, J.E., Jr. et al (1972). Ann. Int. Med. 76:943.
6. Strachan, C.J.L. et al (1977). Brit. J. Med. 1:1254.

7. Oreskovich, C. et al (1981). Presented to Surgical Infection Society, Chicago, April 25.
8. DiPrio, J.T. et al (1981). Amer. J. Hosp. Pharm. 38:320.
9. Berger, S.A. et al (1978). SGO 146:469.

WHEN AND HOW TO USE CEPHALOSPORINS AND AMINOGLYCOSIDES

Paul E. Hermans
Randall Edson

Division of Infectious Diseases
Mayo Clinic and Mayo Foundation
Rochester, Minnesota

A discussion of the relative merits of the cephalosporin-like antibiotics and the aminoglycosides is timely. New cephalosporins are being investigated and are being or will be marketed because of their extended spectrum of activity. Some of the so-called third-generation cephalosporins have antimicrobial activity that is comparable to that of aminoglycosides such as gentamicin, tobramycin, and amikacin. Nevertheless, existing differences must be realized in order to prescribe these new agents correctly. Table I lists the most important agents of both classes.

The terms "cephalosporin-like antibiotics" and "cephalosporins" are used interchangeably. These antibiotics include actual cephalosporins, cephamycins such as cefoxitin, and oxa-beta-lactams such as moxalactam.

In this review, cefazolin is used as a prototype for all first-generation cephalosporins, which are interchangeable as far as antimicrobial activity is concerned. The cephalosporins of the second and third generation have distinguishing individual antimicrobial properties and are therefore not interchangeable.

With regard to the aminoglycosides, the emphasis will be on gentamicin, tobramycin, and amikacin. Compared with the older aminoglycosides, these three agents have a wider spectrum of activity, which includes almost all strains of *Pseudomonas aeruginosa* and *Serratia marcescens*. Several investigational aminoglycosides and cephalosporins have been included in Table I for the sake of completeness.

TABLE I. Aminoglycosides and Cephalosporins

Aminoglycosides
1. Streptomycin (streptomycin sulfate, USP)
2. Neomycin (Mycifradin, neomycin sulfate)
3. Kanamycin (Kantrex)
4. Gentamicin (Garamycin)
5. Tobramycin (Nebcin)
6. Amikacin (Amikin)
7. Netilmicin[a]
8. Sisomicin[a]

Cephalosporin-like antibiotics

First generation	Second generation	Third generation
1. Cephalothin (Keflin)	1. Cefamandole (Mandol)	1. Cefotaxime (Claforan)
2. Cephapirin (Cefadyl)	2. Cefoxitin (Mefoxin)	2. Cefoperazone[a]
3. Cefazolin (Ancef, Kefzol)		3. Ceftizoxime[a]
4. Cephaloridine (Loridine)		4. Cefsulodin[a]
5. Cephradine (Velosef)		5. Ceftriaxone[a]
6. Cefaclor (Ceclor)		6. Ceforanide[a]
7. Cephalexin (Keflex)		7. Moxalactam[a]
Parenteral 1-5	1,2	1-6
Oral 5,6,7	...	?

[a]Experimental agents.

ANTIMICROBIAL ACTIVITY OF AMINOGLYCOSIDES AND CEPHALOSPORINS

Table II gives the percentage of relatively common isolates susceptible to the listed antibiotics at the minimal inhibitory concentration (MIC). These MIC breakpoints represent concentrations that can be exceeded twofold to fourfold with standard therapeutic doses of the antimicrobial agents listed. Table III allows comparison of the susceptibility of relatively uncommon isolates for the three aminoglycosides and the three cephalosporins listed in Table II.

ANTIMICROBIAL ACTIVITY OF AMPICILLIN, CARBENICILLIN, CHLORAMPHENICOL, AND TETRACYCLINE

As background information for comparison, the susceptibility of relatively common and uncommon isolates is listed for the older agents ampicillin, carbenicillin, chloramphenicol, and tetracycline in Tables IV and V.

GRAM-POSITIVE COCCI AND *BACTEROIDES FRAGILIS*

Tables II through V do not include information about susceptibility against aerobic gram-positive cocci and anaerobic microorganisms. The emphasis is on comparison of susceptibility patterns of aerobic gram-negative bacilli. All cephalosporins have antistaphylococcal activity. The second- and third-generation cephalosporins, however, have been introduced because of their expanded gram-negative spectrum. The cephalosporins are not active against *Streptococcus faecalis*, but their antibacterial spectrum includes other streptococci. The aminoglycosides gentamicin, tobramycin, and amikacin also have substantial antistaphylococcal activity but are too toxic for primary use as antistaphylococcal agents. Combinations of vancomycin or nafcillin and gentamicin have synergistic activity against some strains of *Staphylococcus aureus* and *S. epidermidis*. An interesting and important expansion of antimicrobial activity is the susceptibility of *Bacteroides fragilis* to some of the new cephalosporins, specifically cefoxitin and moxalactam.

A comparison of the most important differences in activity among the various generations of cephalosporins is given in Table VI.

TABLE II. Percentage of Relatively Common Isolates Susceptible to Listed Antibiotics[a]

Species	Aminoglycosides			Cephalosporins		
	Amikacin ($\leq$8)	Gentamicin ($\leq$2)	Tobramycin ($\leq$2)	Cefamandole ($\leq$8)	Cefazolin ($\leq$8)	Cefoxitin ($\leq$8)
Enterobacter aerogenes	100	93	95	73	11	4
Escherichia coli	98	97	94	94	90	90
Klebsiella pneumoniae	100	96	96	95	94	95
Morganella morganii	100	100	100	68	3	39
Proteus mirabilis	99	98	98	98	96	97
Proteus vulgaris	100	99	96	5	2	95
Providencia rettgeri	93	97	87	93	36	78
Pseudomonas aeruginosa	96	86	96	0	0	0
Serratia marcescens	96	95	76	15	0	44

[a]Numbers in parentheses denote minimal inhibitory concentration (μg/ml).

TABLE III. Percentage of Relatively Uncommon Isolates Susceptible to Listed Antibiotics[a]

Species	Aminoglycosides			Cephalosporins		
	Amikacin (≤8)	Gentamicin (≤2)	Tobramycin (≤2)	Cefamandole (≤8)	Cefazolin (≤8)	Cefoxitin (≤8)
Acinetobacter calcoaceticus	94	94	90	28	11	29
Aeromonas spp.	100	94	85	91	45	67
Alcaligenes spp.	96	93	86	93	54	75
Citrobacter diversus	100	100	100	95	94	97
Citrobacter freundii	97	93	95	77	24	19
Enterobacter agglomerans	100	100	100	95	71	86
Enterobacter cloacae	99	96	97	80	10	8
Klebsiella oxytoca	100	100	99	98	75	97
Pseudomonas alcaligenes	65	55	45	40	20	50
Pseudomonas fluorescens	100	98	100	0	5	0
Pseudomonas maltophilia	21	15	16	3	0	2
Pseudomonas stutzeri	98	98	98	60	44	54
Salmonella enteritidis	100	86	86	95	100	100
Serratia liquefaciens	100	100	100	100	0	92

[a] Numbers in parentheses denote minimal inhibitory concentration (μg/ml).

TABLE IV. Percentage of Relatively Common Isolates Susceptible to Listed Antibiotics[a]

Species	Ampicillin (≤8)	Carbenicillin (≤64)	Chloramphenicol (≤8)	Tetracycline (≤4)
Enterobacter aerogenes	7	87	84	89
Escherichia coli	74	81	92	74
Klebsiella pneumoniae	5	18	90	88
Morganella morganii	2	96	70	72
Proteus mirabilis	99	99	87	76
Proteus vulgaris	4	92	71	84
Providencia rettgeri	28	87	23	21
Pseudomonas aeruginosa	0	84	0	0
Serratia marcescens	6	84	26	19

[a]Numbers in parentheses denote minimal inhibitory concentration (μg/ml).

TABLE V. Percentage of Relatively Uncommon Isolates Susceptible to Listed Antibiotics[a]

Species	Ampicillin (<8)	Carbenicillin (<64)	Chloramphenicol (<8)	Tetracycline (<4)
Acinetobacter calcoaceticus	46	99	30	95
Aeromonas spp.	12	21	97	97
Alcaligenes spp.	86	96	41	68
Citrobacter diversus	3	21	98	91
Citrobacter freundii	37	86	85	82
Enterobacter agglomerans	62	74	99	100
Enterobacter cloacae	19	90	92	92
Klebsiella oxytoca	4	19	99	95
Pseudomonas alcaligenes	40	85	55	90
Pseudomonas fluorescens	5	12	12	82
Pseudomonas maltophilia	2	55	57	25
Pseudomonas stutzeri	38	77	69	74
Salmonella enteritidis	82	82	93	75
Serratia liquefaciens	67	100	100	92

[a]Numbers in parentheses denote minimal inhibitory concentration ($\mu g/ml$).

TABLE VI.   Spectrum of Activity of the Cephalosporins

First-generation cephalosporins
  E. coli, *K. pneumoniae*, *P. mirabilis*, *C. diversus*, *Salmonella*
  species, gram-positive cocci
Second-generation cephalosporins
  Above species, including some strains resistant to first-
  generation cephalosporins. Variable activity against indole-
  positive *Proteus* species, *S. marcescens*, and *Enterobacter*.
  Not active against *P. aeruginosa*. Cefoxitin: *B. fragilis*
Third-generation cephalosporins
  Not interchangeable. Some (moxalactam) active against *P.*
  aeruginosa, *B. fragilis*, indole-positive *Proteus* species,
  Haemophilus, and *Neisseria gonorrhoeae*. Cefotaxime not active
  against *P. aeruginosa* and minimally active against *B. fragilis*
The following species are "holdouts" against all cephalosporins:
A. calcoaceticus and *S. faecalis*. As the spectrum includes more
gram-negative bacillary species, activity against *S. aureus*
strains is diminished

BACTERIOSTATIC AND BACTERICIDAL PROPERTIES

In severe infections, especially in immunocompromised patients
and in endocarditis, bactericidal therapy is usually necessitated.
Table VII gives the range of MICs and minimal bactericidal concentrations (MBCs) for moxalactam against strains of several
bacteria. It is apparent that, especially for most strains of *S.*
marcescens and *P. aeruginosa*, the MBCs are unattainable in the
serum in vivo with use of standard dosages.
    This potential therapeutic problem is further illustrated in
Table VIII. The bacteriostatic and bactericidal concentrations
of three new cephalosporins and of gentamicin were compared for
strains of *P. aeruginosa*. Gentamicin was superior as a bactericidal agent in these in vitro studies.

SPECIAL THERAPEUTIC INDICATIONS FOR AMINOGLYCOSIDES

Table IX lists many special therapeutic applications of older
and newer aminoglycosides.

TABLE VII. Minimal Inhibitory Concentration (MIC) and Minimal
            Bactericidal Concentration (MBC) of Moxalactam for
            Various Blood Isolates

Species	No. of strains	Range (μg/ml) MIC	MBC
S. aureus	4	4–8	8–32
K. pneumoniae	3	0.13–1	0.5–16
E. aerogenes	1	1	1
S. marcescens	4	0.25–16	1->128
E. coli	7	0.13–2	0.13–4
P. aeruginosa	5	4–32	8->128[a]

[a]MBC = 8 in one of five strains and >128 in four of five strains.

TABLE VIII. Minimal Inhibitory Concentration (MIC) and Minimal
             Bactericidal Concentration (MBC) of Three Third-
             Generation Cephalosporins and Gentamicin for 12
             Strains of *Pseudomonas aeruginosa*

Drug	Range (μg/ml) MIC	MBC	No. of strains with MBC >128
Moxalactam	8–64	32->128	7 of 12
Cefoperazone	4–8	8->128	11 of 12
Cefotaxime	16–128	32->128	11 of 12
Gentamicin[a]	0.5–1[b]	1–4[b]	MBC <2 in 8 of 12, 4 in 2 of 12, and >128 in 2 of 12

[a]The MBC was tested for 12 strains, including 2 strains with high-level gentamicin resistance.
[b]Applies to the 10 gentamicin-susceptible strains.

TOXIC SIDE EFFECTS OF AMINOGLYCOSIDES

The toxicity of aminoglycosides is summarized in Table X.
Although any of the aminoglycosides can cause cochlear or
vestibular damage (or both), the predominant type of toxicity is
as listed. For the average patient, adjusting to vestibular
damage is easier than adjusting to cochlear damage. In our
opinion, the theory that tobramycin is less nephrotoxic than
gentamicin has not been clearly demonstrated.

CONSIDERATIONS FOR CHOOSING BETWEEN AMINOGLYCOSIDES AND CEPHALOSPORINS

Table XI provides an overview of the advantages and disadvantages of the aminoglycosides and the cephalosporins. On the basis of these considerations, it is our practice to use gentamicin, tobramycin, or amikacin in the initial phase of treatment when an aerobic gram-negative bacillus is suspected as the causative microorganism. The initial phase of treatment corresponds to the time between making the clinical diagnosis and obtaining the microbiologic information. If the microorganism is shown to be susceptible to ampicillin, a cephalosporin, or tetracycline, we replace the aminoglycoside with the most appropriate of these three less toxic agents.

TABLE IX. Special Therapeutic Applications of Aminoglycosides

---

Streptomycin
  Tuberculosis (combined with one or two other antituberculous agents), brucellosis (combined with tetracycline), tularemia, plague, endocarditis due to *S. faecalis* (combined with penicillin or ampicillin when the *Streptococcus* is relatively susceptible to streptomycin), short-course (2-week) therapy for endocarditis due to viridans streptococci (combined with penicillin G)
Neomycin
  Topical application, irrigation of wounds, urinary bladder and "bowel prep," reduction of bowel flora in severe liver disease
Kanamycin
  Rarely used. *P. aeruginosa* not susceptible
Gentamicin
  Serious aerobic gram-negative bacillary infections, including those caused by *P. aeruginosa* (the latter in combination with carbenicillin or ticarcillin). Endocarditis due to *S. faecalis* (combined with penicillin or ampicillin when the *Streptococcus* is not sensitive to streptomycin)
Tobramycin
  Same as for gentamicin; use when microorganism is resistant to gentamicin but susceptible to tobramycin
Amikacin
  Same as for gentamicin and tobramycin; use when microorganism is not susceptible to another aminoglycoside and in certain atypical mycobacterioses

TABLE X. Toxicity of Aminoglycosides

Cochlear[a]	Vestibular[b]	Renal[c]
Tinnitus	Dizziness	Proteinuria
"Fullness" of ears	Nystagmus	Urinary casts
Hearing loss	Vomiting	Increased serum creatinine

[a]Kanamycin, amikacin.
[b]Streptomycin, gentamicin, tobramycin.
[c]Kanamycin, gentamicin, tobramycin, amikacin.

TABLE XI. Comparison of Advantages and Disadvantages of Aminoglycosides and Cephalosporins

Factor	Aminoglycosides	Cephalosporins
Spectrum of activity	Wider, more consistent; includes most strains of *P. aeruginosa*; not active against anaerobes	Variable activity of newer cephalosporins against *P. aeruginosa* and *B. fragilis*
Bacteriostatic versus bactericidal activity	Usually bactericidal	Bactericidal against most strains of some species (*E. coli*); usually only bacteriostatic against certain strains of some species (*P. aeruginosa, S. marcescens*)
Toxicity	Relatively high—ototoxicity, nephrotoxicity	Very low—mainly allergic reactions
Margin between therapeutic and toxic level	Narrow	Wide
Dosage requirements	Close attention required; serum levels must be measured	Not strict, as long as therapeutic levels are achieved
Costs	Relatively low	High, especially for third-generation drugs

If the microorganism is not sensitive to an alternative non-aminoglycoside agent or if the microorganism is *P. aeruginosa* or *S. marcescens*, we prefer to continue treatment with an appropriate aminoglycoside. In cases of severe infections caused by *P. aeruginosa*, we add either carbenicillin or ticarcillin because of frequent synergism against *P. aeruginosa*.

In our hospital setting, almost all common gram-negative aerobic bacillary isolates are susceptible to gentamicin. In a recent review at our institution, 191 of 210 strains of *P. aeruginosa* were susceptible to all three aminoglycosides. Of the 19 gentamicin-resistant strains, 5 were susceptible to tobramycin and amikacin, 7 were susceptible to amikacin only, and 7 were also resistant to tobramycin and amikacin. Our concern is that extensive use of tobramycin and amikacin may lead to an increase in the number of strains resistant to either or both agents.

Obviously, if an upsurge of infections occurs in a nosocomial setting because of a gentamicin-resistant strain, tobramycin or amikacin, depending on susceptibility patterns, will be the agent of first choice.

DOSAGE OF CEPHALOSPORINS

Because of the low toxicity of the cephalosporins, determining the dosage of these agents is not difficult. In the presence of renal failure, high levels may be found in the blood and various tissues, but this rarely leads to adverse effects. Although it has often been stated that the dosage of cephalosporins needs little adjustment when renal failure is present, this practice leads to unnecessarily high levels and thus antibiotic waste and unwarranted expense to the patient. See the formula to estimate dosage, based on age and renal function, in the next section ("Dosage of Aminoglycosides").

DOSAGE OF AMINOGLYCOSIDES

Ascertaining the appropriate dosage of aminoglycosides is complicated because one must aim to achieve levels that are therapeutic and attempt to avoid toxicity. The following factors should be considered in determination of the appropriate dosage of aminoglycosides.

1. The relatively common practice of administering gentamicin or tobramycin in a dosage of 80 mg intramuscularly or intravenously three times a day to adult patients often leads to suboptimal serum and tissue levels and thus less than optimal therapy.

2. The dosage of aminoglycosides should be calculated on the basis of the patient's weight, as shown in Table XII.

3. The dosage of aminoglycosides should be reduced in older patients and in those with decreased renal function. The following formula allows an estimate of a patient's creatinine clearance, based on age and serum creatinine concentrations. (For women this is multiplied by 0.9.)

$$\frac{140 - \text{age (yr)}}{\text{serum creatinine concentration (mg/dl)}}$$

4. Serum peak levels and trough levels should be measured after administration of a few doses because no formula or nomogram can guarantee reliable dosage. The following serum peak levels are considered safe and effective in most instances: gentamicin and tobramycin, 5 to 6 μg/ml; amikacin, 15 to 20 μg/ml.

Trough levels of 2 μg/ml or more for gentamicin and tobramycin and of 5 μg/ml or more for amikacin strongly suggest decreased renal clearance. This may be due to preexisting decreased renal clearance or may be caused by the aminoglycoside itself (or a combination of both factors). When the trough level is increased, the next peak level will also be increased because of a cumulative effect. Consistency between trough level and the next peak level (provided the drug is administered intravenously) permits quality control of the laboratory procedure.

5. For obtaining reproducible and more reliable serum levels, the aminoglycosides should be administered rapidly intravenously (read package insert for details).

6. At any age and regardless of the clearance capability of the kidneys, the first dose is not reduced but subsequent doses are adjusted downward.

7. It is better not to exceed a dose of 130 mg every 8 hours in obese patients. Higher doses may be given if measurement of serum levels indicates suboptimal dosage.

8. If an infection is not under control after 10 days of treatment with an aminoglycoside, one should reevaluate the clinical situation and the need for further aminoglycoside therapy. Table XIII shows an example of calculation of a dosage schedule for gentamicin.

TABLE XII.   Calculation of the Dosage of Aminoglycosides on the Basis of the Patient's Weight

Antibiotic	Dose (mg/kg) per 24 hours
Streptomycin	15 (one-half every 12 hours)
Kanamycin	15 (one-half every 12 hours)
Gentamicin	5 (one-third every 8 hours)
Tobramycin	5 (one-third every 8 hours)
Amikacin	15 (one-half every 12 hours)

TABLE XIII.   Examples of Calculation of a Dosage Schedule for
Gentamicin

A woman, age 70 years, has a serum creatinine level of 1.0 mg/dl
and weighs 60 kg
Estimate of creatinine clearance:

$$\frac{140 - age\ (yr)}{serum\ creatinine\ (mg/dl)} \times 0.9 = \frac{140 - 70}{1.0} \times 0.9 = 63\%$$

Daily dose 60 x 5 = 300 mg or 100 mg every 8 hours (based on
weight only)
Because of reduced creatinine clearance, the dosage should be:
First dose--100 mg
Thereafter--60 mg every 8 hours, intravenously
If the same patient's serum creatinine would be 3 mg/dl, her
estimated creatinine clearance would be:

$$\frac{140 - 70}{3} \times 0.9 = 21\%$$

First dose--100 mg (same as above)
Thereafter--20 mg every 8 hours, intravenously

ACKNOWLEDGMENTS

    The microbiologic data in Tables II through V were obtained
from the Section of Clinical Microbiology and modified from an
information booklet provided to residents of Mayo Foundation
(John P. Anhalt, Ph.D., M.D., John A. Washington II, M.D., and
Paul E. Hermans, M.D.). Data in Table VII are the result of a
collaborative clinical and laboratory study of moxalactam in
patients with bacteremia conducted by all members of the Division
of Infectious Diseases (Walter R. Wilson, M.D., and Thomas F.
Keys, M.D., principal investigators). Data in Table VIII
summarize the results of studies by Randall S. Edson, M.D.,
trainee, Division of Infectious Diseases, done in the Clinical
Microbiology Laboratory (head, John A. Washington II, M.D.).

REFERENCES

Cephalosporins

Bodey, G.P., Fainstein, V., and Hinkle, A. M. (1981). *Antimicrob.*
    Agents Chemother. 20, 226.
Edson, R., Washington, J.A. II, and Hermans, P.E. (In press).
    Antimicrob. Agents Chemother.
Kurtz, T.O., Winston, D.J., Hindler, J.A., Young, L.S., Hewitt,
    W.L., and Martin, W.J. (1980). *Antimicrob. Agents Chemother.*
    18, 645.
Thompson, R.L. (1977). *Mayo Clin. Proc. 52*, 625.

Aminoglycosides

Brewer, N.S. (1977). *Mayo Clin. Proc. 52*, 675.
Feld, R., Valdivieso, M., Bodey, G.P., and Rodriguez, V. (1977).
    J. Infect. Dis. 135, 61.
Jackson, G.G. (1977). *Clin. Ther. 1*, 200.
Keys, T.F., Kurtz, S.B., Jones, J.D., and Muller, S.M. (1981).
    Mayo Clin. Proc. 56, 556.
Kurtz, T.O., Winston, D.J., Hindler, J.A., Young, L.S., Hewitt,
    W.L., and Martin, W.J. (1980). *Antimicrob. Agents Chemother.*
    18, 645.
Smith, C.R., Baughman, K.L., Edwards, C.Q., Rogers, J.F., and
    Lietman, P.S. (1977). *N. Engl. J. Med. 296*, 349.

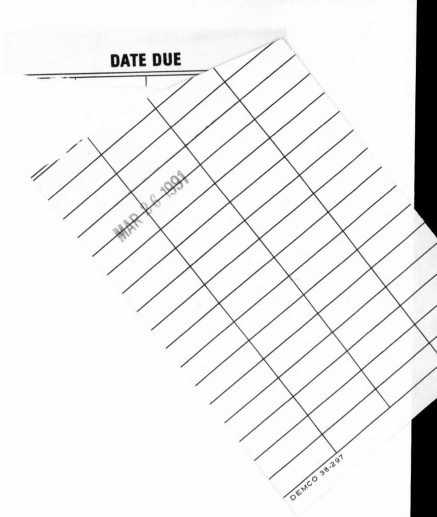